HANDBOOK OF COMMONLY PRESCRIBED DRUGS

Fifteenth Edition

G. John DiGregorio, M.D., Ph.D.
National Medical Services
Willow Grove, Pennsylvania
and
Professor of Pharmacology and Medicine
MCP Hahnemann University
Philadelphia, Pennsylvania

Edward J. Barbieri, Ph.D.
National Medical Services
Willow Grove, Pennsylvania
and
Adjunct Associate Professor of Pharmacology
MCP Hahnemann University
Philadelphia, Pennsylvania

2000

HANDBOOK OF COMMONLY PRESCRIBED DRUGS

Fifteenth Edition

ISBN 0-942447-35-2

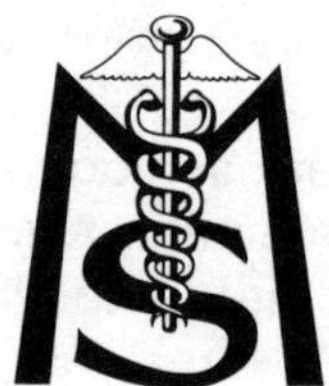

*The **HANDBOOK OF COMMONLY PRESCRIBED DRUGS, Fifteenth Edition,** attempts to present the most common trade names and adult doses, and should be used only as a guideline to these; it should not be considered as an official therapeutic document. If there is a discrepancy in therapeutic category, preparations, and dosages, the reader is advised to obtain official and more complete information from the pharmaceutical manufacturer.*

The Authors or Publisher are not responsible for typographical errors within the contents of this booklet.

PREFACE

The **Fifteenth Edition** of the **HANDBOOK OF COMMONLY PRESCRIBED DRUGS** includes a several new therapeutic agents and new dosage forms. Listed below are some of the new individual therapeutic agents that have been added to this edition:

Alitretinoin (PANRETIN) – a new topical antineoplastic for cutaneous lesions associated with AIDS-related Kaposi's sarcoma

Amprenavir (AGENERASE) – a new oral HIV protease inhibitor

Entacapone (COMTAN) – a new oral antiparkinson drug used as an adjunct to levodopa/carbidopa therapy

Eprosartan Mesylate (TEVETEN) – a new angiotensin II receptor antagonist for the treatment of hypertension

Estradiol Hemihydrate (VAGIFEM) – new oral estradiol derivative for the treatment of atrophic vaginitis

Exemestane (AROMASIN) – a new oral antineoplastic agent for the treatment of breast cancer

Gatifloxacin Sesquihydrate (TEQUIN) and Moxifloxacin Hydrochloride (AVELOX) – two new fluoroquinolone antibacterial drugs

Interferon Alfa-n1 Lymphoblastoid (WELLFERON) – a new interferon for the treatment of chronic hepatitis C virus infection

Ketotifen Fumarate (ZADITOR) – a new ophthalmic drug for the treatment of allergic conjunctivitis

Leflunomide (ARAVA) – a new oral therapy for rheumatoid arthritis

Levalbuterol Hydrochloride (XOPENEX) – a bronchodilator for treating bronchospasm

Levetiracetam (KEPPRA) – a new oral antiepileptic drug for treatment of partial onset seizures

Orlistat (XENICAL) – a novel lipase inhibitor for the management of obesity

Oseltamivir Phosphate (TAMIFLU) – a oral therapy for treating patients with influenza virus infection

Pioglitazone Hydrochloride (ACTOS) and Rosiglitazone Maleate (AVANDIA) – two new insulin resistance reducers for diabetic patients

Polyethylene Glycol 3350 (MIRALAX) – a new laxative

Rabeprazole Sodium (ACIPHEX) – a new proton-pump inhibitor for the treatment of ulcers

Rofecoxib (VIOXX) – a new cyclooxygenase-2 (COX-2) inhibitor for the treatment of acute pain, primary dysmenorrhea, and osteoarthritis

Zaleplon (SONATA) – a new oral hypnotic agent

Zinamivir (RELENZA) – an inhalation therapy for treating patients with influenza virus infection

---

Some of the new combination products that have been added include:

AGGRENOX — a platelet aggregation inhibitor containing aspirin and dipyridamole
AVALIDE 150/12.5 and AVALIDE 300/12.5 — two fixed-dose strengths of the antihypertensive combination preparation of irbesartan and hydrochlorothiazide
CLARITIN-D 24-HOUR — a longer-acting preparation of the popular CLARITIN-D
COSOPT — a topical ophthalmic combination solution of dorzolamide hydrochloride and timolol maleate for the treatment of glaucoma
ORTHO-PREFEST — an estrogen-progestin combination for treating women with symptoms associated with menopause
RYNATAN Tablets — reformulated to now contain pseudoephedrine sulfate and azatadine maleate
SYNERCID — a combination of two new antibacterial compounds, quinupristin and dalfopristin for treating vancomycin-resistant *E. faecium* bacteremia and complicated skin and skin-structure infections

---

During the past year, some drugs have received approval for new indications and a few examples of these products which are now included in the text, are:

Allopurinol Sodium (ALOPRIM) — approved for use as an antineoplastic adjunct (cytoprotective agent)
Cefepime HCl (MAXIPIME) — approved for use as an empiric therapy for febrile neutropenic patients
Dalteparin Sodium (FRAGMIN) — approved for use in hip replacement surgery and for systemic anticoagulation
Levonorgestrel (PLAN B) — approved for use as an emergency contraceptive
Paroxetine (PAXIL) — approved for use in the treatment of panic disorder and social anxiety disorder

---

Examples of a few new dosage forms of existing drugs that were marketed in the United States and have been added to this edition include:

Betamethasone Valerate (LUXIQ) — available as a foam for application to the scalp
Itraconazole (SPORANOX) — now available in an injectable form
Ketoconazole (NIZORAL A-D) — now available as an antidandruff shampoo
Nedocromil Sodium (ALOCRIL) — an ophthalmic solution used as an antiallergic
Paroxetine (PAXIL CR) — now available in controlled-release tablets

This booklet is intended to provide medical personnel with a concise reference source for drug names, the preparations available, and common dosages in adults in a tabular format. The pocket size of the handbook has been exceptionally popular (with over 1,000,000 copies in circulation of over the 15 years of publication). In each new edition new drugs, new dosage forms, and new indications that become available each year will be added. We are committed to publishing this booklet in the pocket-size design so that it can be placed in a jacket or laboratory coat pocket and carried throughout the hospital or used in the office, emergency room, and classroom. We hope that you will use this handbook in this way.

We attempt to present the most common trade names and adult dosages, and this handbook should be used only as a guideline to these; it should not be considered as an official therapeutic document. If there is a discrepancy in therapeutic category, preparations, and dosages, the reader is advised to obtain official and more complete information from the pharmaceutical manufacturer.

As always, we are most grateful for your continued interest and support.

G. John DiGregorio, M.D., Ph.D.
Edward J. Barbieri, Ph.D.

TABLE OF CONTENTS

THERAPEUTIC CATEGORY LISTING[a]

[a] This section lists, by Therapeutic Category, drugs found in the **SELECTED INDIVIDUAL DRUG PREPARATIONS** (pp. 27 to 208) and the **SELECTED COMBINATION DRUG PREPARATIONS** (pp. 209 to 252) sections only. Refer to the **INDEX** for a more complete listing of drugs.

Drug names in UPPER CASE represent TRADE NAMES; the TRADE NAMES without generic names preceeding them are COMBINATION PRODUCTS.

ANALGESICS, OPIOID

ANTIDIARRHEALS

ANTIEMETICS

ANTI-ENURETIC AGENTS

ANTIEPILEPTICS and ANTICONVULSANTS

CYTOPROTECTIVE AGENTS see **ANTINEOPLASTIC ADJUNCTS**

DECONGESTANTS, NASAL

DECONGESTANTS, OCULAR

SELECTED INDIVIDUAL DRUG PREPARATIONS

GENERIC NAME	COMMON TRADE NAMES	THERAPEUTIC CATEGORY	PREPARATIONS	COMMON ADULT DOSAGE
Abacavir Sulfate	ZIAGEN	Antiviral	**Oral Solution**: 20 mg/mL **Tab**: 300 mg	300 mg bid po in combination with other antiretroviral agents.
Acarbose	PRECOSE	Hypoglycemic Agent	**Tab**: 50, 100 mg	**Initial**: 25 mg tid po at the start (with the first bite) of each main meal. **Maintenance**: Adjust the dosage at 4 - 8 week intervals. The dosage may be increased to 50 mg tid po; in some the dosage may be raised to 100 mg tid po. Maximums: 50 mg tid for patients ≤ 60 kg; 100 mg tid for patients > 60 kg.
Acebutolol Hydrochloride	SECTRAL	Antihypertensive, Antiarrhythmic	**Cpsl**: 200, 400 mg	**Hypertension**: Initially, 400 mg once daily po. An optimal response is usually achieved with 400 - 800 mg daily. **Ventricular Arrhythmias**: Initially, 200 mg bid po; increase dosage gradually until an optimal clinical response is obtained, generally at 600 - 1200 mg daily.
Acetaminophen	ANACIN, ASPIRIN FREE	Non-Opioid Analgesic, Antipyretic	**Cplt, Tab & Gelcap**: 500 mg	1000 mg tid or qid po.
	PANADOL, MAXIMUM STRENGTH		**Cplt & Tab**: 500 mg	1000 mg q 4 h po.
	TYLENOL, REGULAR STRENGTH		**Cplt & Tab**: 325 mg	325 - 650 mg tid or qid po.
	TYLENOL, EXTRA-STRENGTH		**Cplt, Tab, Gelcap & Geltab**: 500 mg	1000 mg tid or qid po.
			Liquid: 500 mg/15 mL (7% alcohol)	30 mL (1000 mg) q 4 - 6 h po.
	TYLENOL ARTHRITIS EXTENDED RELIEF		**Extended-Rel. Cplt**: 650 mg	1300 mg q 8 h po.
	FEVERALL, JUNIOR STRENGTH		**Rectal Suppos**: 325 mg	Insert 2 rectally q 4 - 6 h.

	ACETAMINOPHEN UNISERTS		**Rectal Suppos**: 650 mg	Insert 1 rectally q 4 - 6 h.
Acetazolamide	DIAMOX	Diuretic, Antiepileptic, Anti-Glaucoma Agent	**Tab**: 125, 250 mg **Inj**: 500 mg	**Diuresis in CHF**: 250 - 375 mg once daily in the morning po or IV. Best results occur when given on alternate days, or for 2 days alternating with a day of rest. **Drug-induced Edema**: 250 - 375 mg once daily po or IV for 1 or 2 days. **Epilepsy**: 8 - 30 mg/kg/day in divided doses po (optimum range: 375 to 1000 mg daily). **Glaucoma**: 250 - 1000 mg per day usually in divided doses po.
	DIAMOX SEQUELS	Anti-Glaucoma Agent	**Sustained-Rel. Cpsl**: 500 mg	**Glaucoma**: 500 mg bid po.
Acetic Acid	VOSOL	Antibacterial, Antifungal	**Otic Solution**: 2%	Carefully remove all cerumen and debris. Insert a wick saturated with the solution into the ear canal. Keep in for at least 24 h and keep moist by adding 3 - 5 drops of solution q 4 - 6 h.
Acetohexamide	DYMELOR	Hypoglycemic Agent	**Tab**: 250, 500 mg	250 - 1500 mg once daily po.
Acetylcysteine Sodium	MUCOMYST, MUCOSIL	Mucolytic	**Solution**: 10, 20%	**Nebulization (tracheostomy, mask or mouth piece)**: 3 - 5 mL (of 20% solution) or 6 - 10 mL (of 10% solution) tid to qid. **Direct Instillation**: 1 - 2 mL (of 10 or 20% solution) q 1 - 4 h.
Acetylsalicylic Acid [see Aspirin]				
Acitretin	SORIATANE	Anti-Psoriasis Agent	**Cpsl**: 10, 25 mg	25 - 50 mg once daily po with main meal. May cease when psoriatic lesions resolve.

GENERIC NAME	COMMON TRADE NAMES	THERAPEUTIC CATEGORY	PREPARATIONS	COMMON ADULT DOSAGE
Acyclovir	ZOVIRAX	Antiviral	**Cpsl**: 200 mg **Susp**: 200 mg/5 mL **Tab**: 400, 800 mg	***Herpes simplex***: **Initial Genital Herpes**: 200 mg q 4 h (5 times daily) po for 10 days. **Chronic Suppressive Therapy for Recurrent Disease**: 400 mg bid po for up to 1 year. **Intermittent Therapy**: 200 mg q 4 h (5 times daily for 5 days. ***Herpes zoster*, Acute Treatment**: 800 mg q 4 h (5 times daily) po for 7 to 10 days. **Chickenpox**: 20 mg/kg (not to exceed 800 mg) qid po for 5 days.
			Oint: 5%	Apply sufficient quantity to adequately cover all lesions q 3 h, 6 times daily for 7 days.
Acyclovir Sodium	ZOVIRAX	Antiviral	**Powd for Inj**: 500, 1000 mg	**Mucosal and Cutaneous *Herpes simplex* Infections in Immunocompromised Patients**: 5 mg/kg infused IV at a constant rate over 1 h, q 8 h (15 mg/kg/day) for 7 days. ***Herpes simplex* Encephalitis**: 10 mg/kg infused IV at a constant rate over at least 1 h, q 8 h for 10 days. ***Varicella zoster* in Immunocompromised Patients**: 10 mg/kg infused IV at a constant rate over at 1 h, q 8 h for 7 days.
Adapalene	DIFFERIN	Anti-Acne Agent	**Gel**: 0.1%	After washing, apply a thin film once daily to the affected areas in the evening before bed.
Adenosine	ADENOCARD	Antiarrhythmic	**Inj**: 3 mg/mL	Initial dose is 6 mg (rapid IV bolus given over a 1 - 2 second period). If the first dose does not stop the arrhythmia within 1 - 2 minutes, 12 mg should be given (by rapid IV bolus). The 12 mg dose may be repeated a second time if required.

Alatrofloxacin Mesylate [see Trovafloxacin Mesylate (TROVAN)]

Albendazole	ALBENZA	Anthelmintic	**Tab**: 200 mg	**Hydatid Disease**: Administer in a 28-day cycle followed by a 14-day albendazole-free interval, for a total of 3 cycles. < **60 kg**: 15 mg/kg/day po in divided doses (bid) with meals (Maximum: 800 mg/day). ≥ **60 kg**: 400 mg bid po with meals. **Neurocysticercosis**: Administer for 8 - 30 days. < **60 kg**: 15 mg/kg/day po in divided doses (bid) with meals (Maximum: 800 mg/day). ≥ **60 kg**: 400 mg bid po with meals.
Albuterol	PROVENTIL, VENTOLIN	Bronchodilator	**Aerosol**: 90 μg/spray	**Bronchospasm**: 2 inhalations q 4 - 6 h. **Prevention of Exercise-Induced Bronchospasm**: 2 inhalations 15 minutes prior to exercise.
Albuterol Sulfate	PROVENTIL, VENTOLIN NEBULES	Bronchodilator	**Solution for Inhalation**: 0.083% (1 mg/mL, equal to 0.83 mg/mL of albuterol base)	2.5 mg tid - qid by nebulization. This solution requires no dilution prior to administration.
	PROVENTIL, VENTOLIN		**Solution for Inhalation**: 0.5% (6 mg/mL, equal to 5 mg/mL of albuterol base)	2.5 mg tid - qid by nebulization. Dilute 0.5 mL of the 0.5% solution with 2.5 mL of sterile normal saline before administration.
			Syrup: 2 mg (of albuterol base)/5 mL **Tab**: 2, 4 mg (of albuterol base)	2 - 4 mg tid or qid po. For those who do not respond to 2 mg qid, the dose may be cautiously increased stepwise, but not to exceed 8 mg qid as tolerated.
	VENTOLIN ROTACAPS		**Cpsl for Inhalation**: 200 μg	200 μg inhaled q 4 - 6 h using a Rotahaler inhalation device. In some, 400 μg inhaled q 4 - 6 h may be required.
	PROVENTIL REPETABS		**Extended-Rel. Tab**: 4 mg	4 - 8 mg q 12 h po.
	VOLMAX		**Extended-Rel. Tab**: 4, 8 mg	8 mg q 12 h po.

GENERIC NAME	COMMON TRADE NAMES	THERAPEUTIC CATEGORY	PREPARATIONS	COMMON ADULT DOSAGE
Alclometasone Dipropionate	ACLOVATE	Corticosteroid	**Cream & Oint**: 0.05%	Apply a thin film to affected skin areas bid to tid; massage gently until the medication disappears.
Alendronate Sodium	FOSAMAX	Bone Stabilizer	**Tab**: 5, 10, 40 mg	Take at least 30 min. before the first food, beverage, or medication of the day. **Osteoporosis in Postmenopausal Women**: **Treatment**: 10 mg once daily po. **Prevention**: 5 mg once daily po. **Paget's Disease**: 40 mg once daily po for 6 months.
Alfentanil Hydrochloride (C-II)	ALFENTA	Opioid Analgesic	**Inj**: 500 μg/mL	**Duration of Anesthesia**: **Under 30 min**: 8 - 20 μg/kg IV, followed by increments of 3 - 5 μg/kg IV q 5 - 20 minutes or 0.5 - 1 μg/kg\min IV. **30 - 60 min**: 20 - 50 μg/kg IV, followed by increments of 5 - 15 μg/kg IV q 5 - 20 minutes.
Alitretinoin	PANRETIN	Antineoplastic	**Gel**: 0.1%	Initially, apply bid to Kaposi's Sarcoma cutaneous lesions. Application frequency can be gradually increased to tid or qid. Apply sufficient gel to cover lesion; allow the gel to dry for 3 - 5 min. before covering with clothing.
Allopurinol	ZYLOPRIM	Antigout Agent	**Tab**: 100, 300 mg	**Mild Gout**: 200 - 300 mg daily po. **Moderately Severe Gout**: 400 - 600 mg daily po.
Allopurinol Sodium	ALOPRIM	Antineoplastic Adjunct (Cytoprotective Agent)	**Powd for Inj**: 500 mg	200 - 400 mg/m^2/day by IV infusion. Can be given as a single injection or in equally divided infusions at 6-, 8-, or 12-h intervals. Maximum: 600 mg/day.
Alprazolam (C-IV)	XANAX	Antianxiety Agent	**Tab**: 0.25, 0.5, 1, 2 mg	0.25 - 0.5 mg tid po.

Alteplase, Recombinant	ACTIVASE	Thrombolytic	**Powd for Inj**: 50, 100 mg	**Acute Myocardial Infarction**: **3-Hour Infusion**: 100 mg IV given as: 60 mg in the first hour (of which 6 - 10 mg is given as an IV bolus over the first 1 - 2 min), 20 mg over the second hour and 20 mg over the third hour. **Accelerated Infusion**: > **67 kg**: 100 mg as a 15 mg IV bolus, followed by 50 mg infused over the next 30 min and then 35 mg infused over the next 60 min. ≤ **67 kg**: 15 mg IV bolus, followed by 0.75 mg/kg infused over the next 30 min not to exceed 50 mg and then 0.5 mg/kg over the next 60 min not to exceed 35 mg. **Acute Ischemic Stroke**: 0.9 mg/kg (maximum: 90 mg) IV (infused over 60 min) with 10% of the total dose administered as an IV bolus (over 1 min). **Pulmonary Embolism**: 100 mg by IV infusion over 2 hours.
Altretamine	HEXALEN	Antineoplastic	**Cpsl**: 50 mg	260 mg/m^2/day po in 4 divided doses after meals and hs. Administer either for 14 or 21 consecutive days in a 28 day cycle.
Aluminum Hydroxide Gel	ALTERNAGEL	Antacid	**Liquid**: 600 mg/5 mL	5 - 10 mL po, prn, between meals & hs.
	ALU-CAP		**Cpsl**: 475 mg	3 capsules tid po.
	ALU-TAB		**Tab**: 600 mg	3 tablets tid po.
	AMPHOJEL		**Susp**: 320 mg/5 mL	10 mL (640 mg) 5 or 6 times daily po, between meals & hs.
			Tab: 300, 600 mg	600 mg 5 or 6 times daily po, between meals & hs.
Amantadine Hydrochloride	SYMMETREL	Antiparkinsonian, Antiviral	**Tab**: 100 mg **Syrup**: 50 mg/5 mL	**Parkinsonism**: 100 mg bid po. **Influenza Virus**: 200 mg once daily po or 100 mg bid po.

GENERIC NAME	COMMON TRADE NAMES	THERAPEUTIC CATEGORY	PREPARATIONS	COMMON ADULT DOSAGE
Ambenonium Chloride	MYTELASE	Cholinomimetic	**Tab**: 10 mg	5 - 25 mg tid to qid po. Start with 5 mg and gradually increase dosage.
Amcinonide	CYCLOCORT	Corticosteroid	**Cream & Oint**: 0.1% **Lotion**: 0.1%	Apply to affected areas bid to tid. Rub into affected areas bid.
Amikacin Sulfate	AMIKIN	Antibacterial	**Inj (per mL)**: 50, 250 mg	**Usual Dosage**: 15 mg/kg/day IM or by IV infusion (over 30 - 60 min) divided in 2 or 3 equal doses at equal intervals. **Uncomplicated UTI**: 250 mg bid IM or by IV infusion (over 30 - 60 min).
Amiloride Hydrochloride	MIDAMOR	Diuretic	**Tab**: 5 mg	5 mg once daily po with food. The dosage may be increased to 10 mg daily if needed.
Aminocaproic Acid	AMICAR	Systemic Hemostatic	**Syrup**: 250 mg/mL **Tab**: 500 mg	5 g po during the first hour, followed by 1 to 1.25 g po per hour for about 8 h or until bleeding has been controlled.
			Inj: 250 mg/mL	4 - 5 g by IV infusion during the first hour, followed by a continuing infusion at the rate of 1 g/h in 50 mL of diluent for about 8 h or until bleeding has been controlled.
Aminophylline		Bronchodilator	**Liquid**: 105 mg/5 mL	See Oral Aminophylline Doses Table, p. 261.
			Tab: 100, 200 mg	See Oral Aminophylline Doses Table, p. 261.
			Inj: 250 mg/10 mL	See IV Aminophylline Doses Table, p. 262.
			Rectal Suppos: 250, 500 mg	500 mg daily or bid rectally.
Amiodarone Hydrochloride	CORDARONE	Antiarrhythmic	**Tab**: 200 mg	**Loading Doses**: 800 - 1600 mg/day po for 1 to 3 weeks (sometimes longer) until therapeutic response occurs. Administer in divided doses with meals if daily dose ≥ 1000 mg, or when gastrointestinal upset occurs. For life-threatening arrhythmias, administer loading doses in a hospital.

				Dosage Adjustment and Daily Maintenance Dose: For approximately 1 month, 600 - 800 mg po; then 400 mg daily po.
	CORDARONE INTRAVENOUS		**Inj**: 50 mg/mL	**First 24 Hours:** **Loading Infusions**: 150 mg IV over the FIRST 10 minutes (15 mg/min) (concentration = 1.5 mg/mL), followed by 360 mg IV over the NEXT 6 hours (1 mg/min) (concentration = 1.8 mg/mL). **Maintenance Infusion**: 540 mg IV over the REMAINING 18 hours (0.5 mg/min). **After the First 24 Hours**: The maintenance infusion rate of 0.5 mg/min (720 mg/24 h) should be continued at a concentration of 1 - 6 mg/mL.
Amitriptyline Hydrochloride	ELAVIL	Antidepressant	**Tab**: 10, 25, 50, 75, 100, 150 mg	**Outpatients**: Initially, 75 mg daily po in divided doses; may be increased to 150 mg daily po in divided doses if needed; increases are preferably made in the late afternoon or hs. Alternatively, begin with 50 to 100 mg po hs; may increase by 25 or 50 mg prn hs to a total dose of 150 mg per day. The usual maintenance dose is 50 - 100 mg daily po. **Hospitalized Patients**: Initially, these patients may require up to 100 mg daily po; may be raised to 200 mg daily if necessary. Usual maintenance dose is 50 - 100 mg daily po. **Adolescent Patients**: 10 mg tid po, with 20 mg hs, may be satisfactory.
	ELAVIL		**Inj**: 10 mg/mL	Initially, 20 - 30 mg qid IM. Amitriptyline tablets should replace the injection as soon as possible.
Amlexanox	APHTHASOL	Antinflammatory (Topical)	**Oral Paste**: 5%	**Aphthous Ulcers (Canker Sores)**: Apply 1/4 inch to each ulcer qid (preferably following oral hygeine after breakfast, lunch, dinner, and at bedtime). Continue until ulcer heals.

GENERIC NAME	COMMON TRADE NAMES	THERAPEUTIC CATEGORY	PREPARATIONS	COMMON ADULT DOSAGE
Amlodipine Besylate	NORVASC	Antihypertensive, Antianginal	**Tab**: 2.5, 5, 10 mg	**Hypertension**: 2.5 - 5 mg once daily po. **Angina**: 5 - 10 mg once daily po.
Amoxapine	ASENDIN	Antidepressant	**Tab**: 25, 50, 100, 150 mg	Initially, 50 mg bid or tid po. Depending upon tolerance, dosage may be increased to 100 mg bid or tid po by the end of the first week. When an effective dosage is established, the drug may be given in a single dose (not to exceed 300 mg) hs.
Amoxicillin	AMOXIL	Antibacterial	**Cpsl**: 250, 500 mg **Tab**: 500, 875 mg **Chewable Tab**: 125, 250 mg **Powd for Susp (per 5 mL)**: 125, 250 mg	**Infections of the Lower Respiratory Tract**: 500 mg q 8 h po or 875 mg q 12 h po. **Gonorrheal Infections, Acute Uncomplicated**: 3 grams (plus 1 g of probenecid) as a single po dose. **Other Susceptible Infections**: **Mild to Moderate**: 250 mg q 8 h po or 500 mg q 12 h po. **Severe**: 500 mg q 8 h po or 875 mg q 12 h po.
	WYMOX		**Cpsl**: 250, 500 mg **Powd for Susp (per 5 mL)**: 125, 250 mg	Same dosages as for AMOXIL above.
Amphetamine Sulfate (C-II)		CNS Stimulant, Anorexiant	**Tab**: 5, 10 mg	**Narcolepsy**: Start with 10 mg daily po; raise dosage in increments of 10 mg daily at weekly intervals. **Exogenous Obesity**: 5 - 10 mg once daily to tid 30 - 60 minutes ac po.
Amphotericin B	FUNGIZONE	Antifungal	**Cream, Lotion & Oint**: 3%	Apply topically bid - qid.
	FUNGIZONE ORAL SUSPENSION		**Susp**: 100 mg/mL	1 mL qid po. If possible, administer between meals.

Amphotericin B Cholesteryl	AMPHOTEC	Antifungal	**Powd for Inj**: 50, 100 mg	Initially, 3 - 4 mg/kg/day by slow IV infusion (rate 1 mg/kg/h) diluted in 5% Dextrose for Injection. A test dose immediately before the first dose is advisable when beginning all new courses of treatment.
Amphotericin B Deoxycholate	FUNGIZONE INTRAVENOUS	Antifungal	**Powd for Inj**: 50 mg	Initially, 0.25 mg/kg/day by slow IV infusion (given over 6 h); dose may be increased gradually as tolerance permits. A 1 mg test dose (by slow IV infusion) is advisable to determine patient tolerance.
Amphotericin B Lipid Complex	ABELCET	Antifungal	**Powd for Inj**: 100 mg	**Aspergillosis**: 5 mg/kg daily as a single IV infusion at 2.5 mg/kg/h.
Amphotericin B Liposomal	AMBISOME	Antifungal	**Powd for Inj**: 50 mg	**Empirical Therapy**: Initially, 3.0 mg/kg/day by slow IV infusion (given over 2 h); the dose should be individualized as tolerance permits. **Systemic Fungal Infections**: Initially, 3.0 - 5.0 mg/kg/day by slow IV infusion (given over 2 h); the dose should be individualized as tolerance permits.
Ampicillin Anhydrous	OMNIPEN	Antibacterial	**Cpsl**: 250, 500 mg **Powd for Susp (per 5 mL)**: 125, 250 mg	**Respiratory Tract and Soft Tissue Infections**: 250 mg q 6 h po. **Genitourinary or Gastrointestinal Tract Infect. other than Gonorrhea**: 500 mg q 6 h po. **Gonorrhea**: 3.5 g (plus 1.0 g of probenecid) as as a single po dose.
Ampicillin Sodium	OMNIPEN-N	Antibacterial	**Powd for Inj**: 125, 250, 500 mg; 1, 2 g	**Respiratory Tract and Soft Tissue Infections**: **Under 40 kg**: 25 - 50 mg/kg/day in equally divided doses at 6 - 8 h intervals IM or IV. **Over 40 kg**: 250 - 500 mg q 6 h IM or IV. **Genitourinary or Gastrointestinal Tract Infections including Gonorrhea in Females**: **Under 40 kg**: 50 mg/kg/day in equally divided doses at 6 - 8 h intervals IM or IV. **Over 40 kg**: 500 mg q 6 h IM or IV.

[Continued on the next page]

GENERIC NAME	COMMON TRADE NAMES	THERAPEUTIC CATEGORY	PREPARATIONS	COMMON ADULT DOSAGE
Ampicillin Sodium [Continued]	OMNIPEN-N			**Urethritis in Males due to *N. gonorrhoeae***: Two doses of 500 mg each IM or IV at an interval of 8 - 12 h. Repeat if necessary. **Bacterial Meningitis**: 150 - 200 mg/kg/day in equally divided doses q 3 - 4 h. Treatment may be initiated with IV drip and continued with IM injections. **Septicemia**: 150 - 200 mg/kg/day. Start with IV administration for at least 3 days and continue with IM injections q 3 - 4 h.
Ampicillin Trihydrate	PRINCIPEN	Antibacterial	**Cpsl**: 250, 500 mg **Powd for Susp (per 5 mL)**: 125, 250 mg	Same dosages as for OMNIPEN above.
Amprenavir	AGENERASE	Antiviral	**Solution**: 15 mg/mL **Cpsl**: 50, 150 mg	1200 mg (eight 150 mg cpsls) bid po in combination with other antiretroviral agents. Drug may be taken with or without food, but high-fat meals should be avoided.
Amrinone Lactate	INOCOR	Inotropic Agent	**Inj**: 5 mg/mL	0.75 mg/kg IV bolus (over 2 - 3 minutes), then 5 - 10 μg/kg/min by IV infusion.
Anastrozole	ARIMIDEX	Antineoplastic	**Tab**: 1 mg	**Breast Cancer**: 1 mg once daily po.
Anistreplase	EMINASE	Thrombolytic	**Powd for Inj**: 30 units	30 units IV (over 2 to 5 minutes).
Anthralin	ANTHRA-DERM DRITHOCREME	Anti-Psoriasis Agent	**Oint**: 0.1, 0.25, 0.5, 1.0% **Cream**: 0.1, 0.25, 0.5, 1.0%	Begin with the 0.1% concentration and after at least 1 week gradually increase until the desired effect is obtained. Apply a thin layer to psoriatic areas once daily; rub in gently.
	DRITHO-SCALP		**Cream**: 0.25, 0.5%	Begin with the 0.25% concentration; apply to to the psoriatic lesions only once daily and rub in well. After at least 1 week, may increase dosage with the 0.5% strength.

Aprotinin	TRASYLOL	Systemic Hemostatic	**Inj**: 10,000 KIU (kallikrein Inhibitor Units)/mL (equivalent to 1.4 mg/mL)	Two dosage regimens (A and B) are suggested. Regimen A appears to be more effective in patients given aspirin preoperatively. The experience with Regimen B (reduced dosage) is limited (see table below).

Dosage Regimen	IV Test Dose (given at least 10 minutes before the loading dose is administered)	IV Loading Dose (given slowly over 20 - 30 minutes after induction of anesthesia but prior to sternotomy)	IV Pump Prime Dose	Constant IV Infusion Dose (continued until surgery is complete and patient leaves the operating room)
A	1 mL (10,000 KIU)	200 mL (2 million KIU)	200 mL (2 million KIU)	50 mL/h (500,000 KIU/h)
B	1 mL (10,000 KIU)	100 mL (1 million KIU)	100 mL (1 million KIU)	25 mL/h (250,000 KIU/h)

Ardeparin Sodium	NORMIFLO	Anticoagulant	**Inj**: 5,000; 10,000 anti-X_a Units/0.5 mL	50 anti-X_a Units/kg q 12 h by deep SC inject. Begin treatment the evening of the day of surgery or the following morning & continue for ≤ 14 days or the patient is fully ambulatory.
Asparaginase	ELSPAR	Antineoplastic	**Powd for Inj**: 10,000 IUnits	200 IU/kg/day IV (over a 30 minute period) for 28 days.
Aspirin	BAYER CHILDREN'S ASPIRIN ASPIRIN REGIMEN BAYER	Non-Opioid Analgesic, Antipyretic, Antiinflammatory	**Chewable Tab**: 81 mg **Enteric Coated Tab**: 81 mg **Enteric Coated Cplt**: 325 mg	**Usual Dosage**: 325 - 650 mg q 4 h po, prn. **Analgesic or Antiinflammatory**: the OTC maximum dosage is 4000 mg per day po in divided doses.
	BAYER ASPIRIN BAYER ASPIRIN, EXTRA STRENGTH	Drug for Suspected Acute MI	**Cplt & Tab**: 325 mg **Cplt & Tab**: 500 mg	**Transient Ischemic Attacks in Men**: 1300 mg daily po in divided doses (650 mg bid or 325 mg qid). **Suspected Acute Myocardial Infarction**: 160 to 162.5 mg po, as soon as the infarct is suspected & then daily for at least 30 days.
	BAYER 8-HOUR ASPIRIN		**Cplt**: 650 mg	
	ST. JOSEPH ADULT CHEWABLE ASPIRIN		**Chewable Cplt**: 81 mg	

[Continued on the next page]

GENERIC NAME	COMMON TRADE NAMES	THERAPEUTIC CATEGORY	PREPARATIONS	COMMON ADULT DOSAGE
Aspirin [Continued]	ECOTRIN	Non-Opioid Analgesic, Antiinflammatory	**Enteric Coated Tab**: 81, 325, 500 mg	Same dosages as for ASPIRIN REGIMEN BAYER above.
	ECOTRIN, BAYER ASPIRIN EXTRA-STRENGTH ARTHRITIS PAIN FORMULA	Non-Opioid Analgesic, Antiinflammatory	**Enteric Coated Cplt**: 500 mg	Same dosages as for ASPIRIN REGIMEN BAYER above.
	EASPRIN	Non-Opioid Analgesic, Antiinflammatory	**Enteric Coated Tab**: 975 mg	1 tab tid to qid po.
	HALFPRIN	Drug for Suspected Acute MI	**Tab**: 162 mg	162 mg po, taken as soon as the first infarct is suspected & then daily for at least 30 days.
Atenolol	TENORMIN	Antihypertensive, Antianginal, Post-MI Drug	**Tab**: 25, 50, 100 mg	**Hypertension & Angina**: Initially, 50 mg once daily po; dosage may be increased to 100 mg daily if necessary. **Acute Myocardial Infarction**: In patients who tolerate the full IV dose (10 mg), give 50 mg po 10 minutes after the last IV dose, followed by 50 mg po 12 h later. Thereafter, 100 mg daily po or 50 mg bid po for 6 - 9 days or until discharged from the hospital.
	TENORMIN I.V.	Post-MI Drug	**Inj**: 5 mg/10 mL	**Acute Myocardial Infarction**: 5 mg IV (over 5 to 10 minutes), followed by 5 mg IV 10 minutes later.
Atorvastatin Calcium	LIPITOR	Hypolipidemic	**Tab**: 10, 20, 40 mg	Initially, 10 mg daily po. After 2 - 4 weeks, adjust the dosage according to serum lipid levels.
Atovaquone	MEPRON	Antiprotozoal	**Susp**: 750 mg/5 mL	**Usual Dosage**: 750 mg bid po with food for 21 days. ***Pneumocystis carinii* Pneumonia Prophylaxis**: 1500 mg once daily po with food.

Atracurium Besylate	TRACRIUM INJECTION	Neuromuscular Blocker	**Inj**: 10 mg/mL	0.4 - 0.5 mg/kg IV bolus when used alone; 0.25 - 0.35 mg/kg IV bolus when used under steady state with certain general anesthetics. Doses of 0.08 - 0.10 mg/kg for maintenance during prolonged surgery.
Atropine Sulfate		Anticholinergic	**Tab**: 0.4, 0.6 mg **Inj**: 0.05 to 1.0 mg/mL	0.4 - 0.6 mg po. 0.4 - 0.6 mg IV, IM or SC.
	ISOPTO ATROPINE	Mydriatic - Cycloplegic	**Ophth Solution**: 0.5, 1% **Ophth Solution**: 2%	1 - 2 drops in eye(s) up to qid.
			Ophth Oint: 1%	Apply to eye(s) up to bid.
Attapulgite	DIASORB	Antidiarrheal	**Liquid**: 750 mg/5 mL **Tab**: 750 mg	20 mL or 4 tablets (3000 mg) po at the first sign of diarrhea, and repeat after each subsequent bowel movement. Maximum: 60 mL or 12 tablets per 24 hours.
	DONNAGEL		**Liquid**: 600 mg/15 mL (1.4% alcohol) **Chewable Tab**: 600 mg	30 mL or 2 chewable tablets (1200 mg) po at the first sign of diarrhea and after each subsequent loose bowel movement. Maximum: 7 doses per 24 hours.
	KAOPECTATE		**Liquid**: 750 mg/15 mL **Cplt**: 750 mg	30 mL or 2 caplets (1500 mg) po at the first sign of diarrhea and after each subsequent loose bowel movement. Maximum: 7 doses per 24 hours.
	RHEABAN		**Cplt**: 750 mg	2 caplets po after the initial bowel movement, and 2 caplets after each subsequent bowel movement. Max: 12 caplets per 24 hours.
Auranofin	RIDAURA	Antirheumatic	**Cpsl**: 3 mg	3 mg bid po or 6 mg daily po.

GENERIC NAME	COMMON TRADE NAMES	THERAPEUTIC CATEGORY	PREPARATIONS	COMMON ADULT DOSAGE
Aurothioglucose	SOLGANAL	Antiarthritic	**Inj**: 50 mg/mL	First dose: 10 mg IM; second and third doses: 25 mg IM; fourth and subsequent doses: 50 mg IM. The interval between doses is 1 week. The 50 mg dose is continued at weekly intervals until 0.8 - 1.0 g has been given. If the patient has improved and shows no sign of toxicity, the 50 mg dose may be continued for many months longer, at 3 - 4 week intervals.
Azathioprine	IMURAN	Immunosuppressant	**Tab**: 50 mg	**Renal Homotransplantation**: Initial dose is usually 3 - 5 mg/kg daily po or IV, beginning at the time of transplant. Usually given as a single daily dose. Therapy is often initiated with the IV administration of the sodium salt and continued with the tablets after the postoperative period. Dose reduction to maintenance levels of 1 - 3 mg/kg is usually possible. **Rheumatoid Arthritis**: Initially, 1 mg/kg (50 to 100 mg) as a single daily dose or on a bid schedule. May increase dose at 6 - 8 weeks and therafter by steps at 4-week intervals. Dose increments should be 0.5 mg/kg daily, up to a maximum dose of 2.5 mg/kg/day.
Azathioprine Sodium	IMURAN	Immunosuppressant	**Powd for Inj**: 100 mg	
Azelaic Acid	AZELEX	Anti-Acne Agent	**Cream**: 20%	Gently massage a thin film into affected areas bid, in the morning and evening.
Azelastine	ASTELIN	Antihistamine	**Nasal Spray**: 137 μg/spray	2 sprays in each nostril bid.
Azithromycin Dihydrate	ZITHROMAX	Antibacterial	**Cpsl**: 250 mg **Tab**: 250, 600 mg **Powd for Susp (per 5 mL)**: 100, 200 mg **Powd for Susp**: 1 g packets	**Usual Dosage**: 500 mg po as a single dose on the first day followed by 250 mg once daily on days 2 through 5. Administer Suspension on an empty stomach; tablets may be taken with or without food.

				Non-gonococcal Urethritis and Cervicitis due to *C. trachomatis*: 1 g po as a single dose. Administer Suspension on an empty stomach; tablets may be taken with or without food. **Gonococcal Urethritis and Cervicitis due to *N. gonorrhea***: 2 g po as a single dose. **Genital Ulcer Disease due to *H. ducreyi* (Chancroid)**: 1 g po as a single dose. **Prevention of Disseminated *Mycobacterium avium* Complex (MAC)**: 1200 mg po once weekly.
Aztreonam	AZACTAM	Antibacterial	**Powd for Inj**: 0.5, 1, 2 g **Inj (per 100 mL)**: 0.5, 1, 2 g	**Urinary Tract Infections**: 0.5 - 1.0 g q 8 or 12 h by IV infusion or IM. **Moderately Severe Systemic Infections**: 1 - 2 g q 8 or 12 h by IV infusion. **Severe Systemic or Life-Threatening Infections**: 2 g q 6 or 8 h by IV infusion.
Bacampicillin Hydrochloride	SPECTROBID	Antibacterial	**Tab**: 400 mg	**Upper Respiratory Tract Infections, Urinary Tract Infections, Skin and Skin Structure Infections**: 400 mg q 12 h po. **Lower Respiratory Tract Infections and Severe Infections**: 800 mg q 12 h po. **Gonorrhea, Acute Uncomplicated**: 1.6 g (plus 1 g of probenecid) as a single dose po.
Bacitracin		Antibacterial	**Ophth Oint**: 500 units/g	Apply to affected eye(s) 1 or more times daily.
			Oint: 500 units/g	Apply topically to the affected areas 1 - 3 times daily.
Baclofen	LIORESAL	Skeletal Muscle Relaxant	**Tab**: 10, 20 mg	5 mg tid po for 3 days; increase by 5 mg tid every 3 days (maximum 80 mg daily (20 mg qid)) until optimum effect is achieved.

GENERIC NAME	COMMON TRADE NAMES	THERAPEUTIC CATEGORY	PREPARATIONS	COMMON ADULT DOSAGE
Barley Malt Extract	MALTSUPEX	Bulk Laxative	**Liquid**: 16 grams/15 mL	30 mL bid po for 3 or 4 days, or until relief is noted; then 15 - 30mL daily po hs for maintenance, prn. Take a full glass (8 fl. oz.) of liquid with each dose.
			Powder: 8 grams/scoop	Up to 4 scoops bid po for 3 or 4 days, or until relief is noted; then 2 - 4 scoops daily po hs for maintenance, prn. Take a full glass (8 fl. oz.) of liquid with each dose.
			Tab: 750 mg	Initially 4 tablets qid po with meals and hs. Adjust dosage according to response. Drink a full glass of liquid (8 fl. oz.) with each dose.
Beclomethasone Dipropionate	BECLOVENT, VANCERIL	Corticosteroid	**Aerosol**: 42 μg/spray	2 inhalations tid - qid.
	VANCERIL DOUBLE STRENGTH		**Aerosol**: 84 μg/spray	2 inhalations bid.
	BECONASE, VANCENASE		**Nasal Aerosol**: 42 μg/spray	1 spray in each nostril bid - qid.
	BECONASE AQ, VANCENASE AQ		**Nasal Spray**: 0.042% (42 μg/spray)	1 or 2 inhalations in each nostril bid.
	VANCENASE AQ DOUBLE STRENGTH		**Nasal Spray**: 0.084% (84 μg/spray)	1 or 2 inhalations in each nostril once daily.
Benazepril Hydrochloride	LOTENSIN	Antihypertensive	**Tab**: 5, 10, 20, 40 mg	Initially, 10 mg once daily po. Maintenance dosage is 20 - 40 mg daily as a single dose or in two equally divided doses.

Bendroflumethiazide	NATURETIN	Diuretic, Antihypertensive	**Tab**: 5, 10 mg	**Diuresis**: 5 mg once daily po, preferably given in the morning. To initiate therapy, doses up to 20 mg may be given once daily or divided into two doses. For maintenance, 2.5 - 5 mg once daily should suffice. **Hypertension**: Initially, 5 - 20 mg daily po. Maintenance doses range from 2.5 - 15 mg daily.
Benzocaine	AMERICAINE	Local Anesthetic	**Lubricant Gel**: 20%	Apply evenly to exterior of tube or instrument prior to use.
			Spray: 20%	Apply liberally to affected areas not more than tid to qid.
	ANBESOL MAXIMUM STRENGTH		**Liquid & Gel**: 20%	Apply topically to the affected area on or around the lips, or within the mouth.
Benzoyl Peroxide	BREVOXYL-4 BREVOXYL-8	Anti-Acne Agent	**Gel**: 4% **Gel**: 8%	Cleanse affected area. Apply topically once or twice daily.
	BENZAC, BENZAGEL, PANOXYL		**Gel**: 5, 10%	Cleanse affected area. Apply topically once or twice daily.
	BENZAC W, PANOXYL AQ		**Water Base Gel**: 2.5, 5, 10%	Cleanse affected area. Apply topically once or twice daily.
	BENZAC W WASH		**Liquid**: 5, 10%	Wash face with product once or twice daily.
	DESQUAM-X		**Gel**: 5, 10%	Cleanse affected areas. Rub gently into all affected areas once or twice daily.
			Water Base Gel: 5, 10%	Wash affected areas with product once or twice daily. Rinse well.
	PANOXYL		**Bar**: 5, 10%	Wash entire area with fingertips for 1 or 2 minutes bid to tid. Rinse well.
Benzphetamine Hydrochloride (C-III)	DIDREX	Anorexiant	**Tab**: 50 mg	Initially, 25 - 50 mg once daily po with subsequent increase to tid according to the response. A single daily dose is preferably given in mid-morning or mid-afternoon.

GENERIC NAME	COMMON TRADE NAMES	THERAPEUTIC CATEGORY	PREPARATIONS	COMMON ADULT DOSAGE
Benzthiazide	EXNA	Diuretic, Antihypertensive	**Tab**: 50 mg	**Diuresis**: Initially, 50 - 200 mg daily po for several days, or until dry weight is attained. With 100 mg or more daily, it is preferable to administer in two doses following AM & PM meals. For maintenance, 50 - 150 mg daily po depending on patient's response. **Hypertension**: Initially, 50 - 100 mg daily po as a single dose or in two divided doses. For maintenance, adjust according to the patient's response. Max: 50 mg qid po.
Benztropine Mesylate	COGENTIN	Antiparkinsonian	**Tab**: 0.5, 1, 2 mg **Inj**: 1 mg/mL	0.5 - 2 mg daily or bid po. 0.5 - 2 mg daily or bid IM.
Bepridil Hydrochloride	VASCOR	Antianginal	**Tab**: 200, 300, 400 mg	200 mg once daily po. After 10 days, the dosage may be raised; most patients are maintained at 300 mg daily.
Betamethasone	CELESTONE	Corticosteroid	**Tab**: 0.6 mg **Syrup**: 0.6 mg/5mL	0.6 - 7.2 mg per day po.
Betamethasone Dipropionate, Regular	DIPROSONE, MAXIVATE	Corticosteroid	**Cream & Oint**: 0.05% (in a standard vehicle)	Apply a thin film to affected areas once or twice daily.
			Lotion: 0.05%	Massage a few drops into affected areas bid.
	DIPROSONE		**Topical Aerosol**: 0.1%	Apply sparingly to affected skin areas tid.
Betamethasone Dipropionate, Augmented	DIPROLENE	Corticosteroid	**Gel & Oint**: 0.05% (in an optimized vehicle) **Lotion**: 0.05%	Apply a thin film to affected areas once or twice daily. Massage a few drops into affected areas once or twice daily.
	DIPROLENE AF		**Cream**: 0.05%	Apply a thin film to affected areas once or twice daily.

Betamethasone Valerate	VALISONE	Corticosteroid	**Cream**: 0.1% **Lotion & Oint**: 0.1%	Apply topically 1 - 3 times daily. Apply topically 1 - 3 times daily.
	VALISONE REDUCED STRENGTH		**Cream**: 0.01%	Apply a thin film to affected areas 1 - 3 times daily.
	LUXIQ		**Foam**: 0.12%	Invert can and dispense a small amount of foam onto a clean saucer or other cool surface. Pick up a small amount of foam and massage into affected scalp areas until foam disappears; repeat until the entire affected area of scalp is treated. Use bid (AM and PM) for up to 2 weeks.
Betaxolol Hydrochloride	BETOPTIC BETOPTIC S	Anti-Glaucoma Agent	**Ophth Solution**: 0.5% **Ophth Suspension**: 0.25%	1 - 2 drops into affected eye(s) bid. 1 - 2 drops into affected eye(s) bid.
	KERLONE	Antihypertensive	**Tab**: 10, 20 mg	10 mg once daily po. If the desired response is not achieved, the dose can be doubled in 7 to 14 days.
Bethanechol Chloride	URECHOLINE	Cholinomimetic	**Tab**: 5, 10, 25, 50 mg **Inj**: 5 mg/mL	10 - 50 mg tid or qid po. 2.5 - 5 mg tid or qid SC.
	DUVOID		**Tab**: 10, 25, 50 mg	10 - 50 mg tid or qid po.
Bicalutamide	CASODEX	Antineoplastic	**Tab**: 50 mg	50 mg once daily po (morning or evening) in combination with an LHRH analog.
Biperiden Hydrochloride	AKINETON	Antiparkinsonian	**Tab**: 2 mg	2 mg tid - qid po.
Biperiden Lactate	AKINETON	Antiparkinsonian	**Inj**: 5 mg/mL	2 mg q 30 minutes IM or IV until symptoms resolve, not to exceed 4 doses in 24 hours.
Bisacodyl	DULCOLAX	Irritant Laxative	**Enteric-Coated Tab**: 5 mg **Rectal Suppos**: 10 mg	10 - 15 mg po once daily. Insert 1 rectally once daily.
	FLEET BISACODYL ENEMA		**Rectal Susp**: 10 mg/30 mL	Administer 30 mL rectally.

GENERIC NAME	COMMON TRADE NAMES	THERAPEUTIC CATEGORY	PREPARATIONS	COMMON ADULT DOSAGE
Bismuth Subsalicylate	PEPTO-BISMOL	Antidiarrheal	**Chewable Tab**: 262 mg **Cplt**: 262 mg **Liquid**: 262 mg/15 mL	2 tablets or caplets (or 30 mL of Liquid) po; repeat every 30 - 60 minutes prn, to a maximum of 8 doses in a 24 hour period.
	PEPTO-BISMOL MAXIMUM STRENGTH		**Liquid**: 525 mg/15 mL	30 mL po; repeat every 60 minutes prn, to a maximum of 4 doses in a 24 hour period.
Bisoprolol Fumarate	ZEBETA	Antihypertensive	**Tab**: 5, 10 mg	Initially 5 mg once daily po. The dose may be increased to 10 mg once daily and then to 20 mg once daily, if necessary.
Bitolterol Mesylate	TORNALATE	Bronchodilator	**Aerosol**: 370 μg/spray	**Acute Relief**: 2 inhalations at an interval of ≥ 1 - 3 minutes, followed by a third prn. **Prophylaxis**: 2 inhalations q 8 h.
			Solution for Inhalation: 0.2% (2.0 mg/mL)	**Intermittent Aerosol Flow Nebulizer (Patient Activated Nebulizer)**: 0.25 to 0.75 mL (0.5 to 1.5 mg) over 10 - 15 minutes tid. **Continuous Aerosol Flow Nebulizer**: 0.75 to 1.75 mL (1.5 to 3.5 mg) over 10 - 15 minutes tid.
Bleomycin Sulfate	BLENOXANE	Antineoplastic	**Powd for Inj**: 15, 30 units	0.25 - 0.50 units/kg (10 - 20 units/m^2) IV, IM or SC once or twice weekly.
Bretylium Tosylate		Antiarrhythmic	**Inj**: 50 mg/mL	**Life-Threatening Ventricular Arrhythmias**: Administer undiluted at 5 mg/kg by rapid IV. If the arrhythmia persists, the dosage may be increased to 10 mg/kg and repeated as necessary. **Other Ventricular Arrhythmias**: **IV**: Administer a diluted solution at 5 - 10 mg/kg by IV infusion over a period greater than 8 minutes. For maintenance, the same dosage may be administered q 6 h. **IM**: Administer undiluted at 5 - 10 mg/kg. Subsequent doses may be given at 1 - 2 hour intervals if the arrhythmia persists.

Brimonidine Tartrate	ALPHAGAN	Anti-Glaucoma Agent	**Ophth Solution**: 0.2%	1 drop into the affected eye(s) tid, approximately 8 h apart.
Brinzolamide	AZOPT	Anti-Glaucoma Agent	**Ophth Suspension**: 1%	1 drop into the affected eye(s) tid.
Bromocriptine Mesylate	PARLODEL	Antiparkinsonian	**Tab**: 2.5 mg **Cpsl**: 5 mg	Initially, 1.25 mg bid po with meals. If necessary, the dosage may be increased every 14 - 28 days by 2.5 mg per day.
Brompheniramine Maleate	DIMETAPP ALLERGY	Antihistamine	**Liqui-Gel**: 4 mg	4 mg q 4 - 6 h po.
Budesonide	RHINOCORT	Corticosteroid	**Aerosol**: 32 μg/spray	256 μg daily, given as either 2 sprays in each nostril in the morning and evening or 4 sprays in each nostril in the morning.
	PULMICORT TURBUHALER		**Aerosol**: 200 μg/spray	200 - 400 μg bid by oral inhalation.
Bumetanide	BUMEX	Diuretic	**Tab**: 0.5, 1, 2 mg **Inj**: 0.25 mg/mL	0.5 - 2 mg daily po. 0.5 - 1 mg IV (over 1 - 2 minutes) or IM; if necessary, repeat at 2 - 3 h intervals, not to exceed 10 mg/day.
Buprenorphine Hydrochloride (C-V)	BUPRENEX	Opioid Analgesic	**Inj**: 0.3 mg/mL	0.3 mg by deep IM or slow IV (over at least 2 minutes) at up to 6-hour intervals. Repeat once, if required, in 30 - 60 minutes.
Bupropion Hydrochloride	WELLBUTRIN	Antidepressant	**Tab**: 75, 100 mg	100 mg bid po. Dosage may be increased to 100 mg tid po no sooner than 3 days after beginning therapy.
	WELLBUTRIN SR	Antidepressant	**Sustained-Rel. Tab**: 100, 150 mg	Initially, 150 mg daily po in the AM. Dosage may be increased to 150 mg bid po (at least 8 h apart) as early as 4 days after beginning therapy.
	ZYBAN	Smoking Deterrent	**Sustained-Rel. Tab**: 150 mg	Initially, 150 daily po for the first 3 days, followed by 300 mg/day po in divided doses given at least 8 h apart. Continue treatment for 7 - 12 weeks.

GENERIC NAME	COMMON TRADE NAMES	THERAPEUTIC CATEGORY	PREPARATIONS	COMMON ADULT DOSAGE
Buspirone Hydrochloride	BUSPAR	Antianxiety Agent	**Tab**: 5, 10, 15 mg	7.5 mg bid po. Dosage may be increased 5 mg daily at 2 to 3 day intervals. Maximum: 60 mg per day.
Busulfan	MYLERAN	Antineoplastic	**Tab**: 2 mg	Daily dosage range is 4 - 8 mg po. Dosing on a weight basis is approximately 60 μg/kg daily or 1.8 mg/m^2 daily.
Butabarbital Sodium (C-III)	BUTISOL SODIUM	Sedative / Hypnotic	**Elixir**: 30 mg/5 mL (7% alcohol) **Tab**: 15, 30, 50, 100 mg	**Preoperative Sedation**: 50 - 100 mg po, 60 to 90 minutes before surgery. **Daytime Sedation**: 15 - 30 mg tid to qid po. **Bedtime Hypnosis**: 50 - 100 mg hs po.
Butamben Picrate	BUTESIN PICRATE	Local Anesthetic	**Oint**: 1%	Spread thinly on painful or denuded lesions of the skin, if these are small. Apply a loose bandage to protect the clothing.
Butenafine Hydrochloride	MENTAX	Antifungal	**Cream**: 1%	Apply to cover the affected area and the immediately surrounding skin once daily for 2 - 4 weeks.
Butoconazole Nitrate	FEMSTAT 3	Antifungal	**Vaginal Cream**: 2%	1 applicatorful intravaginally hs for 3 days. Treatment can be extended for another 3 days if necessary.
Butorphanol Tartrate (C-IV)	STADOL	Opioid Analgesic	**Inj (per mL)**: 1, 2 mg	**IM**: 2 mg. May be repeated q 3 - 4 h prn. **IV**: 1 mg. May be repeated q 3 - 4 h prn.
	STADOL NS		**Nasal Spray**: 10 mg/mL	1 spray in one nostril. If pain is not relieved in 60 - 90 minutes, an additional 1 spray may be given. The initial 2 dose sequence may be repeated in 3 - 4 h prn.
Caffeine	NO DOZ NO DOZ MAXIMUM STRENGTH	CNS Stimulant	**Chewable Tab**: 100 mg **Tab**: 200 mg	100 - 200 mg q 3 - 4 h po prn. 100 - 200 mg q 3 - 4 h po prn.

Calcifediol	CALDEROL	Vitamin D Analog	**Cpsl**: 20, 50 μg	300 - 350 μg weekly po, administered on a daily or alternate-day schedule. Most patients respond to doses of 50 - 100 μg daily or 100 - 200 μg on alternate days.
Calcipotriene	DOVONEX	Anti-Psoriasis Agent	**Cream**: 0.005%	Apply a thin layer to the affected skin bid and rub in gently and completely.
			Oint: 0.005%	Apply a thin layer to the affected skin once or twice daily and rub in gently and completely.
			Scalp Solution: 0.005%	Apply only to scalp lesions and rub in gently and completely, taking care to prevent the solution spreading onto the forehead.
Calcitonin-Salmon	CALCIMAR, MIACALCIN	Antiosteoporotic, Hypocalcemic	**Inj**: 200 IUnits/mL	**Paget's Disease**: 100 IUnits daily SC or IM. In many patients, 50 IUnits daily or every other day SC or IM is satisfactory. **Hypercalcemia**: Initially, 4 IUnits/kg q 12 h SC or IM. After 1 or 2 days the dosage may be increased to 8 IUnits/kg q 12 h SC or IM. **Postmenopausal Osteoporosis**: 100 IUnits daily SC or IM with calcium supplementation.
	MIACALCIN		**Nasal Spray**: 200 IUnits/spray	**Postmenopausal Osteoporosis**: 200 IUnits daily intranasally, alternating nostrils daily.
Calcitriol	ROCALTROL	Vitamin D Analog	**Cpsl**: 0.25, 0.5 μg **Solution**: 1.0 μg/mL	**Dialysis Patients**: 0.25 μg daily po. Dosage may be increased by 0.25 μg per day at 4 to 8 week intervals. Most patients respond to doses between 0.5 and 1 μg daily. **Predialysis Patients**: 0.25 μg daily po. Dosage may be increased to 0.5 μg daily if needed. **Hypoparathyroidism**: 0.25 μg daily po given in the AM. The dosage may be increased at 2 to 4 week intervals. Most patients respond to doses between 0.5 and 2 μg daily.

GENERIC NAME	COMMON TRADE NAMES	THERAPEUTIC CATEGORY	PREPARATIONS	COMMON ADULT DOSAGE
Calcium Carbonate	CALTRATE 600	Calcium Supplement	**Tab**: 600 mg (as calcium)	1 or 2 tab daily po.
	OS-CAL 500	Calcium Supplement	**Tab**: 500 mg (as calcium)	500 mg bid or tid po with meals.
	TUMS	Calcium Supplement, Antacid	**Chewable Tab**: 500 mg	**Calcium Supplement**: Chew 2 tablets bid. **Antacid**: Chew 2 - 4 tablets q h prn. Do not take more than 16 tablets in 24 h.
	TUMS E-X		**Chewable Tab**: 750 mg	**Calcium Supplement**: Chew 2 tablets bid. **Antacid**: Chew 2 - 4 tablets q h prn. Do not take more than 10 tablets in 24 h.
	TUMS ULTRA		**Chewable Tab**: 1000 mg	**Calcium Supplement**: Chew 2 tablets bid. **Antacid**: Chew 2 - 3 tablets q h prn. Do not take more than 8 tablets in 24 h.
	ROLAIDS, CALCIUM RICH/ SODIUM FREE	Antacid	**Chewable Tab**: 550 mg	Chew 1 or 2 tab prn, up to a maximum of 14 tab per day.
	MYLANTA SOOTHING LOZENGES	Antacid	**Lozenges**: 600 mg	Allow 1 lozenge to dissolve in the mouth. If necessary, follow with a second. Repeat prn, up to 12 lozenges per day.
	ALKA-MINTS	Antacid	**Chewable Tab**: 850 mg	Chew 1 or 2 tablets q 2 h.
	MAALOX CAPLETS	Antacid	**Cplt**: 1000 mg	1000 mg po prn. Do not take more than 8 caplets in 24 h.
Calcium Glubionate	NEO-CALGLUCON	Calcium Supplement	**Syrup**: 1.8 g/5 mL	**Dietary Supplement**: 15 mL tid po.
Calcium Polycarbophil	MITROLAN	Bulk Laxative	**Chewable Tab**: 625 mg	Chew and swallow 2 tablets qid or prn. A full glass of liquid (8 oz.) should be taken with each dose.
	FIBERCON		**Tab**: 625 mg	Swallow 2 tablets up to qid. A full glass of liquid (8 oz.) should be taken with each dose.

Candesartan Cilexetil	ATACAND	Antihypertensive	**Tab**: 4, 8, 16, 32 mg	Initially, 16 mg once daily po. May be given once daily or bid po with total doses ranging from 8 to 32 mg.
Capecitabine	XELODA	Antineoplastic	**Tab**: 150, 500 mg	2500 mg/m^2 daily po with food for 2 weeks, followed by a 1-week rest period given as 3 week cycles. Give the drug in 2 daily doses (approx. 12 h apart) at the end of a meal.
Capreomycin Sulfate	CAPASTAT SULFATE	Tuberculostatic	**Powd for Inj**: 1 g	1 g daily (not to exceed 20 mg/kg/day) IM or IV for 60 - 120 days, followed by 1 g IM or IV 2 or 3 times weekly.
Capsaicin	ZOSTRIX	Analgesic (Topical)	**Cream**: 0.025%	Apply to affected area tid or qid.
	ZOSTRIX-HP		**Cream**: 0.075%	Apply to affected area tid or qid.
	DOLORAC		**Cream**: 0.25%	Apply a thin film to the affected area bid.
Captopril	CAPOTEN	Antihypertensive, Heart Failure Drug, Post-MI Drug	**Tab**: 12.5, 25, 50, 100 mg	**Hypertension**: Initially, 25 mg bid or tid po. Dosage may be increased after 1 - 2 weeks to 50 mg bid or tid. **Diabetic Nephropathy**: 25 mg tid po. **Heart Failure**: Initially, 25 mg tid po. After a dose of 50 mg tid is reached, further increases in dosage should be delayed for at least 2 weeks. Most patients have a satisfactory response at 50 or 100 mg tid. **Left Ventricular Dysfunction after an MI**: Initiate therapy as early as 3 days following an MI. After a single 6.25 mg po dose, give 12.5 mg tid, then increase to 25 mg tid during the next several days and to a target of 50 mg tid over the next several weeks.
Carbachol	ISOPTO CARBACHOL	Anti-Glaucoma Agent	**Ophth Solution**: 0.75, 1.5, 2.25, 3%	1 - 2 drops into eye(s) up to tid.

GENERIC NAME	COMMON TRADE NAMES	THERAPEUTIC CATEGORY	PREPARATIONS	COMMON ADULT DOSAGE
Carbamazepine	TEGRETOL	Antiepileptic	**Susp**: 100 mg/5 mL **Chewable Tab**: 100 mg **Tab**: 200 mg	**Initial**: 100 mg qid po (Susp) or 200 mg bid po (Tabs or XR Tabs). Increase at weekly intervals by adding up to 200 mg per day using a tid or qid regimen (Susp or Tabs) or a bid regimen (XR Tabs). Maximum: 1000 mg daily (ages 12 to 15); 1200 mg daily (ages over 15). **Maintenance**: Adjust to minimum effective levels; usually 800 - 1200 mg daily po.
	TEGRETOL-XR		**Extended-Rel. Tab**: 100, 200, 400 mg	
Carbamide Peroxide	GLY-OXIDE	Antiseptic	**Liquid**: 10%	Apply several drops onto the affected mouth area; spit out after 2 minutes. Use up to qid pc & hs.
Carbenicillin Indanyl Sodium	GEOCILLIN	Antibacterial	**Tab**: 382 mg	**Urinary Tract Infections:** ***E. coli, Proteus* species, and *Enterobacter***: 382 - 764 mg qid po. ***Pseudomonas and Enterococcus***: 764 mg qid po. **Prostatitis**: 764 mg qid po.
Carboplatin	PARAPLATIN	Antineoplastic	**Powd for Inj**: 50, 150, 450 mg	360 mg/m^2 on day 1 every 4 weeks IV. Single intermittent doses should not be repeated until the neutrophil count is at least 2,000 and the platelet count is at least 100,000.
Carisoprodol	SOMA	Skeletal Muscle Relaxant	**Tab**: 350 mg	350 mg tid and hs po.
Carmustine	BiCNU	Antineoplastic	**Powd for Inj**: 100 mg	150 - 200 mg/m^2 IV q 6 weeks (given as a single dose or divided into daily injections on 2 successive days). A repeat course of drug should not be given until the leukocyte count is above 4,000/mm^3 and platelet count is above 100,000/mm^3.

Carteolol Hydrochloride	CARTROL	Antihypertensive	**Tab**: 2.5, 5 mg	Initially, 2.5 mg once daily po. Dosage may be gradually increased to 5 mg and 10 mg daily po.
	OCUPRESS	Anti-Glaucoma Agent	**Ophth Solution**: 1%	1 drop into affected eye(s) bid.
Carvedilol	COREG	Antihypertensive, Heart Failure Drug	**Tab**: 3.125, 6.25, 12.5, 25 mg	**Hypertension**: Initially, 6.25 mg bid po. After 7 - 14 days, the dosage may be increased to 12.5 mg bid po. After another 7 - 14 days, the dosage can be increased to 25 mg bid, if tolerated and required. **Congestive Heart Failure (in Conjunction with Digitalis, Diuretics, and ACE Inhibitors)**: Initially 3.125 mg bid po for 2 weeks. If tolerated, the dosage may be increased to 6.25 mg bid po. Dosing should then be doubled every 2 weeks to the highest level tolerated. The maximum dosage is 25 mg bid for patients weighing < 85 kg (187 lb) and 50 mg bid for patients weighing > 85 kg.
Cascara Sagrada		Irritant Laxative	**Tab**: 325 mg	325 mg po hs.
Castor Oil (Plain)		Irritant Laxative	**Liquid**: (pure)	15 - 30 mL po.
Castor Oil, Emulsified	NEOLOID	Irritant Laxative	**Liquid**: 36.4% w/w	30 - 60 mL po.
	FLEET FLAVORED CASTOR OIL EMULSION		**Liquid**: 67% v/v (10 mL of castor oil/15 mL)	**Laxative**: 45 mL po. **Purgative**: 90 mL po.
Cefaclor	CECLOR	Antibacterial	**Powd for Susp (per 5 mL)**: 125, 187, 250, 375 mg **Cpsl**: 250, 500 mg	**Usual Dosage**: 250 mg q 8 h po. For more severe infections or those caused by less susceptible organisms, the dosage may be doubled. **Secondary Bacterial Infections of Acute Bronchitis or Acute Bacterial Exacerabations of Chronic Bronchitis**: 500 mg q 12 h po for 7 days.

[Continued on the next page]

GENERIC NAME	COMMON TRADE NAMES	THERAPEUTIC CATEGORY	PREPARATIONS	COMMON ADULT DOSAGE
Cefaclor [Continued]	CECLOR			**Pharyngitis or Tonsillitis**: 375 mg q 12 h po for 10 days. **Skin and Skin Structure Infections, Uncompl.**: 375 mg q 12 h po for 7 to 10 days.
	CECLOR CD		**Extended-Rel. Tab**: 375, 500 mg	375 - 500 mg q 12 h po for 7 - 10 days.
Cefadroxil Monohydrate	DURICEF	Antibacterial	**Powd for Susp (per 5 mL)**: 125, 250, 500 mg **Cpsl**: 500 mg **Tab**: 1 g	**Urinary Tract Infections**: **Lower, Uncomplicated**: 1 - 2 g daily po in single or divided doses (bid). **Other**: 2 g daily po in divided doses (bid). **Skin and Skin Structure Infections**: 1 g daily po in single or divided doses (bid). **Pharyngitis and Tonsillitis**: 1 g daily po in single or divided doses (bid) for 10 days.
Cefazolin Sodium	ANCEF, KEFZOL	Antibacterial	**Powd for Inj**: 500 mg, 1 g	**Moderate to Severe Infections**: 500 mg - 1 g q 6 - 8 h IM or IV. **Mild Infections caused by susceptible Gram Positive Cocci**: 250 - 500 mg q 8 h IM or IV. **Urinary Tract Infect., Acute, Uncomplicated**: 1 g q 12 h IM or IV. **Pneumococcal Pneumonia**: 500 mg q 12 h IM or IV. **Severe, Life-Threatening Infections (e.g., Septicemia)**: 1 - 1.5 g q 6 h IM or IV.
Cefdinir	OMNICEF	Antibacterial	**Cpsl**: 300 mg	**Community-Acquired Pneumonia and Skin and Skin Structure Infections, Uncomplicated**: 300 mg q 12 h po for 10 days. **Acute Exacerbations of Chronic Bronchitis &** Acute Maxillary Sinusitis: 300 mg q 12 h po or 600 mg q 24 h po for 10 days. **Pharyngitis / Tonsillitis**: 300 mg q 12 h po for 5 - 10 days or 600 mg q 24 h po for 10 days.

Cefepime Hydrochloride	MAXIPIME	Antibacterial	**Powd for Inj**: 0.5, 1, 2 g	**Urinary Tract Infections:** **Mild to Moderate**: 0.5 - 1 g IM or IV (over 30 min.) q 12 h for 7 - 10 days. **Severe**: 2 g IV (over 30 min.) q 12 h for 10 days. **Pneumonia**: 1 - 2 g IV (over 30 min.) q 12 h for 10 days. **Skin & Skin Structure Infections**: 2 g IV (over 30 min.) q 12 h for 10 days. **Empiric Therapy for Febrile Neutropenic Patients**: 2 g IV (over 30 min.) q 8 h for 7 days or until resolution of neutropenia.
Cefixime	SUPRAX	Antibacterial	**Tab**: 200, 400 mg **Powd for Susp**: 100 mg/5 mL	**Usual Dosage**: 400 mg once daily or 200 mg q 12 h po. **Gonorrhea, Uncomplicated**: 400 mg once daily po.
Cefonicid Sodium	MONOCID	Antibacterial	**Powd for Inj**: 0.5, 1 g	**Usual Dosage**: 1 g daily IV or deep IM. **Urinary Tract Infections**: 0.5 g q 24 h IV or deep IM. **Mild to Moderate Infections**: 1 g q 24 h IV or deep IM. **Severe or Life-Threatening Infections**: 2 g q 24 h IV or deep IM in different large muscle masses. **Surgical Prophylaxis**: 1 g per day IV or deep IM preoperatively.
Cefoperazone Sodium	CEFOBID	Antibacterial	**Powd for Inj**: 1, 2 g	2 - 4 g daily in equally divided doses q 12 h IM or IV. In severe infections or infections caused by less susceptible organisms, the daily dosage may be increased.

GENERIC NAME	COMMON TRADE NAMES	THERAPEUTIC CATEGORY	PREPARATIONS	COMMON ADULT DOSAGE
Cefotaxime Sodium	CLAFORAN	Antibacterial	**Powd for Inj**: 0.5, 1, 2 g **Inj (per 50 mL)**: 1, 2 g	**Gonococcal Urethritis & Cervicitis (Males and Females**: 500 mg IM as a single dose. **Gonorrhea, Rectal**: **Females**: 500 mg IM as a single dose. **Males**: 1 g IM as a single dose. **Uncomplicated Infections**: 1 g q 12 h IM or IV. **Moderate to Severe Infections**: 1 - 2 g q 8 h IM or IV. **Infections Commonly Needing Antibiotics in Higher Dosage (e.g., Septicemia)**: 2 g q 6 - 8 h IV. **Life-Threatening Infections**: 2 g q 4 h IV.
Cefotetan Disodium	CEFOTAN	Antibacterial	**Powd for Inj**: 1, 2 g **Inj (per 50 mL)**: 1, 2 g	**Urinary Tract Infections**: 500 mg q 12 h IM or IV; or 1 - 2 g q 12 - 24 h IM or IV. **Skin and Skin Structure Infections**: **Mild to Moderate**: 2 g q 24 h IV or 1 g q 12 h IV or IM **Severe**: 2 g q 12 h IV. **Other Sites**: 1 - 2 g q 12 h IV or IM. **Severe Infections**: 2 g q 12 h IV. **Life-Threatening Infections**: 3 g q 12 h IV.
Cefoxitin Sodium	MEFOXIN	Antibacterial	**Inj (per 50 mL)**: 1, 2 g **Powd for Inj**: 1, 2 g	**Uncomplicated Infections (e.g., Pneumonia, Urinary Tract or Cutaneous Infections**: 1 g q 6 - 8 h IV. **Moderate to Severe Infections**: 1 g q 4 h IV or 2 g q 6 - 8 h IV. **Infections Commonly Needing Higher Dosage (e.g., Gas Gangrene)**: 2 g q 4 h IV or 3 g q 6 h IV.

Cefpodoxime Proxetil	VANTIN	Antibacterial	**Gran for Susp (per 5 mL):** 50, 100 mg **Tab**: 100, 200 mg	**Pharyngitis & Tonsillitis**: 100 mg q 12 h for 5 - 10 days. **Urinary Tract Infections, Uncomplicated**: 100 mg q 12 h po for 7 days. **Pneumonia**: 200 mg q 12 h po for 14 days. **Bacterial Exacerbation of Chronic Bronchitis:** 200 mg q 12 h po for 10 days. **Skin & Skin Structure Infections**: 400 mg q 12 h po for 7 - 14 days. **Gonococcal Infections**: 200 mg po as a single dose.
Cefprozil	CEFZIL	Antibacterial	**Powd for Susp (per 5 mL):** 125, 250 mg **Tab**: 250, 500 mg	**Paryngitis & Tonsillitis**: 500 mg q 24 h po for 10 days. **Acute Sinusitis**: 250 - 500 mg q 12 h po for 10 days. **Lower Respiratory Tract Infections**: 500 mg q 12 h po for 10 days. **Skin & Skin Structure Infections, Uncompl.:** 250 mg q 12 h po for 10 days or 500 mg q 12 - 24 h po for 10 days.
Ceftazidime	FORTAZ, TAZIDIME TAZICEF	Antibacterial	**Powd for Inj**: 0.5, 1, 2 g **Powd for Inj**: 1, 2 g	**Usual Dosage**: 1 g q 8 - 12 h IV or IM. **Urinary Tract Infections:** **Uncomplicated**: 250 mg q 12 h IV or IM. **Complicated**: 500 mg q 8 - 12 h IV or IM. **Bone & Joint Infections**: 2 g q 12 h IV. **Pneumonia, Skin & Skin Structure Infections:** 500 mg - 1 g q 8 h IV or IM. **Meningitis, Serious Gynecologic & Intra-Abdominal Infections, and Severe Life-Threatening Infections**: 2 g q 8 h IV.
Ceftazidime Sodium	FORTAZ	Antibacterial	**Inj (per 50 mL)**: 1, 2 g	Same dosages as for FORTAZ above.
Ceftibuten	CEDAX	Antibacterial	**Cpsl**: 400 mg **Powd for Susp (per 5 mL):** 90, 180 mg	400 mg once daily po at least 2 h before or 1 h after a meal for 10 days.

GENERIC NAME	COMMON TRADE NAMES	THERAPEUTIC CATEGORY	PREPARATIONS	COMMON ADULT DOSAGE
Ceftizoxime Sodium	CEFIZOX	Antibacterial	**Inj (per 20, 50, or 100 mL):** 1, 2 g	**Usual Dosage:** 1 -2 g q 8 - 12 h IM or IV. **Urinary Tract Infections:** 500 mg q 12 h IM or IV. **Pelvic Inflammatory Disease:** 2 g q 8 h IV. **Other Sites:** 1 g q 8 - 12 h IM or IV. **Severe or Refractory Infections:** 1 g q 8 h IM or IV; or 2 g q 8 - 12 h IM (divided dose in different large muscle masses) or IV. **Life-Threatening Infections:** 3 - 4 g q 8 h IV.
Ceftriaxone Sodium	ROCEPHIN	Antibacterial	**Powd for Inj:** 250, 500 mg; 1, 2 g	**Usual Dosage:** 1 - 2 g once daily (or in equally divided doses bid) IM or IV. **Gonococcal Infections, Uncomplicated:** 250 mg IM, one dose. **Meningitis:** 100 mg/kg/day in divided doses q 12 h IM or IV, with or without a loading dose of 75 mg/kg. **Surgical Prophylaxis:** 1 gram IV as a single dose 30 min - 2 h before surgery.
Cefuroxime Axetil	CEFTIN	Antibacterial	**Tab:** 125, 250, 500 mg **Powd for Susp (per 5 mL):** 125, 250 mg	**Pharyngitis & Tonsillitis:** 250 mg bid po for 10 days. **Urinary Tract Infections, Uncomplicated:** 125 - 250 mg bid po for 7 - 10 days. **Acute Bacterial Exacerbations of Chronic Bronchitis and Secondary Bacterial Infections of Acute Bronchitis:** 250 - 500 mg bid po for 10 days. **Skin or Skin Struct. Infections, Uncomplicated:** 250 - 500 mg bid po for 10 days. **Gonorrhea, Uncomplicated:** 1 g po as a single dose. **Early Lyme Disease:** 500 mg bid po for 20 days.

Cefuroxime Sodium	KEFUROX, ZINACEF	Antibacterial	**Powd for Inj**: 0.75, 1.5 g	**Usual Dosage**: 750 mg - 1.5 g q 8 h for 5 - 10 days IM or IV. **Bone & Joint Infections**: 1.5 g q 8 h IM or IV. **Life-Threatening Infections or Infections due to Less Susceptible Organisms**: 1.5 g q 6 h IV may be required. **Meningitis**: Up to 3.0 g q 8 h IM or IV. **Gonorrhea**: 1.5 g IM, single dose given at 2 different sites with 1.0 g of probenecid po.
Celecoxib	CELEBREX	Antiinflammatory	**Cpsl**: 100, 200 mg	**Osteoarthritis**: 200 mg once daily po or 100 mg bid po. **Rheumatoid Arthritis**: 100 - 200 mg bid po.
Cephalexin	KEFLEX	Antibacterial	**Powd for Susp (per 5 mL)**: 125, 250 mg **Cpsl**: 250, 500 mg	**Usual Dosage**: 250 mg q 6 h po. **Streptococcal Pharyngitis, Skin and Skin Structure Infections and Cystitis**: 500 mg may be used q 12 h po. For cystitis, continue therapy for 7 - 14 days.
Cephalexin Hydrochloride	KEFTAB	Antibacterial	**Tab**: 500 mg	Same dosage as for KEFLEX above.
Cephapirin Sodium	CEFADYL	Antibacterial	**Powd for Inj**: 1 g	**Usual Dosage**: 500 mg - 1 g q 4 - 6 h IV or IM. **Serious or Life-Threatening Infections**: Up to 12 g daily IV or IM. Use IV for high doses.
Cephradine	VELOSEF	Antibacterial	**Powd for Susp (per 5 mL)**: 125, 250 mg **Cpsl**: 250, 500 mg	**Respiratory Tract, Skin and Skin Structure Infections**: 250 mg q 6 h po or 500 mg q 12 h po. **Lobar Pneumonia**: 500 mg q 6 h po or 1 g q 12 h po. **Urinary Tract Infections**: 500 mg q 12 h po. In more serious urinary tract infections (including prostatitis), 500 mg q 6 h po or 1 g q 12 h po.
Cerivastatin Sodium	BAYCOL	Hypolipidemic	**Tab**: 0.2, 0.3, 0.4 mg	0.4 mg once daily po in the evening.

GENERIC NAME	COMMON TRADE NAMES	THERAPEUTIC CATEGORY	PREPARATIONS	COMMON ADULT DOSAGE
Cetirizine Hydrochloride	ZYRTEC	Antihistamine	**Syrup**: 5 mg/5 mL **Tab**: 5, 10 mg	5 - 10 mg once daily po depending on the severity of symptoms.
Chloral Hydrate (C-IV)		Sedative - Hypnotic	**Cpsl**: 500 mg **Syrup**: 500 mg/10 mL	**Sedative**: 250 mg tid po, pc. **Hypnotic**: 500 mg - 1 g po, 15 - 30 minutes before bedtime or 30 min. before surgery.
Chlorambucil	LEUKERAN	Antineoplastic	**Tab**: 2 mg	0.1 - 0.2 mg/kg daily po for 3 - 6 weeks.
Chloramphenicol		Antibacterial	**Cpsl**: 250 mg	50 mg/kg/day in divided doses at 6 h intervals po.
	CHLOROPTIC		**Ophth Solution**: 0.5%	2 drops in the affected eye(s) q 3 h. Continue administration day & night for 48 h, after which the dosing interval may be increased.
			Ophth Oint: 1%	Apply to affected eye(s) q 3 h day & night for 48 h, as above.
Chloramphenicol Sodium Succinate	CHLOROMYCETIN SODIUM SUCCINATE	Antibacterial	**Powd for Inj**: 100 mg/mL (when reconstituted)	50 mg/kg/day in divided doses at 6 h intervals IV.
Chlordiazepoxide Hydrochloride (C-IV)	LIBRIUM	Antianxiety Agent	**Cpsl**: 5, 10, 25 mg **Powd for Inj**: 100 mg	5 - 25 mg tid or qid po. 50 - 100 mg IM or IV initially; then 25 - 50 mg tid or qid, if necessary.
Chloroquine Hydrochloride	ARALEN HCL	Antimalarial	**Inj**: 50 mg salt (= to 40 mg of chloroquine base)/mL	160 - 200 mg of chloroquine base IM initially; repeat in 6 h if necessary.
Chloroquine Phosphate	ARALEN PHOSPHATE	Antimalarial	**Tab**: 500 mg salt (= to 300 mg of chloroquine base)	**Suppression**: 300 mg of chloroquine base once weekly po, on the same day each week. **Acute Attacks**: Initially, 600 mg of chloroquine base po, followed by 300 mg after 6 - 8 h and a single dose of 300 mg on each of two consecutive days.
Chlorothiazide	DIURIL	Diuretic, Antihypertensive	**Susp**: 250 mg/5 mL (0.5% alcohol) **Tab**: 250, 500 mg	**Diuresis**: 0.5 - 1.0 g once daily or bid po. **Hypertension**: 0.5 - 1.0 g po as a single dose or in divided doses.

Chlorothiazide Sodium	DIURIL	Diuretic	**Powd for Inj**: 500 mg	0.5 - 1.0 g once daily or bid IV.
Chloroxine	CAPITROL	Antibacterial	**Shampoo**: 2%	Massage thoroughly onto wet scalp. Leave lather on for 3 min., then rinse. Repeat the application once. Use twice per week.
Chlorpheniramine Maleate	CHLOR-TRIMETON ALLERGY 4 HOUR	Antihistamine	**Syrup**: 2 mg/5 mL (7% alcohol)	10 mL (4 mg) q 4 - 6 h po.
			Tab: 4 mg	4 mg q 4 - 6 h po.
	CHLOR-TRIMETON ALLERGY 8 HOUR		**Timed-Rel. Tab**: 8 mg	8 mg q 12 h po.
	CHLOR-TRIMETON ALLERGY 12 HOUR		**Timed-Rel. Tab**: 12 mg	12 mg q 12 h po.
			Inj: 10 mg/mL	10 - 20 mg IM, SC, or IV.
Chlorpromazine	THORAZINE	Antiemetic	**Suppos**: 25, 100 mg	50 - 100 mg rectally q 6 - 8 h.
Chlorpromazine Hydrochloride	THORAZINE	Antipsychotic, Antiemetic	**Syrup**: 10 mg/5 mL **Liquid Conc**: 30, 100 mg/mL **Tab**: 10, 25, 50, 100, 200 mg **Sustained-Rel. Cpsl**: 30, 75, 150 mg	**Psychoses (Hospitalized Patients, Less Acutely Disturbed)**: 25 mg tid po. Increase gradually until the effective dose is reached, usually 400 mg daily. **Psychoses (Outpatients)**: **Usual Dosage**: 10 mg tid or qid po; or 25 mg bid to tid po. **More Severe Cases**: 25 mg tid po. After 1 to 2 days, daily dosage may be raised by 20 - 50 mg at semiweekly intervals until patient becomes calm and cooperative. **Prompt Control of Severe Symptoms**: 25 mg IM. If necessary, repeat in 1 h. Subsequent doses should be oral, 25 - 50 mg tid. **Nausea & Vomiting**: 10 - 25 mg q 4 - 6 h po. **Presurgical Apprehension**: 25 - 50 mg po 2 - 3 h before the operation. **Intractable Hiccups**: 25 - 50 mg tid or qid po. If symptoms persist for 2 - 3 days, use injection [see dosage below].

[Continued on the next page]

GENERIC NAME	COMMON TRADE NAMES	THERAPEUTIC CATEGORY	PREPARATIONS	COMMON ADULT DOSAGE
Chlorpromazine Hydrochloride [Continued]	THORAZINE		**Inj**: 25 mg/mL	**Psychoses (Hospitalized Patients, Acutely Disturbed or Manic)**: 25 mg IM. If necessary, give additional 25 - 50 mg in 1 h. Increase subsequent IM doses gradually over several days (up to 400 mg q 4 - 6 h in severe cases) until patient is controlled. **Psychoses (Outpatients; Prompt Control of Severe Symptoms)**: 25 mg IM. If necessary, repeat in 1 h. Subsequent doses should be oral, 25 - 50 mg tid. **Nausea & Vomiting**: **Usual Dosage**: 25 mg IM. If no hypotension occurs, 25 - 50 mg q 3 - 4 h prn, until vomiting stops; then switch to oral dosage [above]. **During Surgery**: 12.5 mg IM. Repeat in 30 min. if necessary and if no hypotension occurs. May give 2 mg IV per fractional injection at 2 min. intervals. Dilute to 1 mg/mL and do not exceed 25 mg. **Presurgical Apprehension**: 12.5 - 25 mg IM 1 to 2 h before the operation. **Intractable Hiccups**: If symptoms persist for 2 or 3 days after oral dosing, give 25 - 50 mg IM. Should symptoms persist, use slow IV infusion with patient flat in bed: 25 - 50 mg in 500 - 1000 mL of saline.
Chlorpropamide	DIABINESE	Hypoglycemic Agent	**Tab**: 100, 250 mg	**Initial**: 250 mg daily po. After 5 - 7 days, dosage may be adjusted upward or downward by increments of not more than 50 - 125 mg at intervals of 3 - 5 days. **Maintenance**: ≤ 100 - 250 mg daily po.

Chlorthalidone	HYGROTON	Diuretic, Antihypertensive	**Tab**: 25, 50, 100 mg	**Edema**: Initially, 50 - 100 mg daily po or 100 mg on alternate days. Maintenance doses may be lower than initial doses. **Hypertension**: Initially, 25 mg daily po. May increase the dosage to 50 mg daily po and then to 100 mg daily po if necessary.
	THALITONE	Diuretic, Antihypertensive	**Tab**: 15, 25 mg	**Edema**: Initially, 30 - 60 mg daily po or 60 mg on alternate days. Maintenance doses may be lower than initial doses. **Hypertension**: Initially, 15 mg daily po. May increase the dosage to 30 mg daily po and then to 45 - 50 mg daily po if necessary.
Chlorzoxazone	PARAFON FORTE DSC	Skeletal Muscle Relaxant	**Cplt**: 500 mg	500 mg tid or qid po.
Cholestyramine	QUESTRAN	Hypolipidemic	**Powder**: 4 g drug/9 g powder	9 g 1 - 6 times daily po.
	QUESTRAN LIGHT		**Powder**: 4 g drug/5 g powder	5 g 1 - 6 times daily po.
Ciclopirox Olamine	LOPROX	Antifungal	**Cream & Lotion**: 1%	Gently massage into affected and surrounding skin areas bid, in the AM and PM.
Cidofovir	VISTIDE	Antiviral	**Inj**: 75 mg/mL	**Induction**: 5 mg/kg by IV infusion (see below) once weekly for 2 consecutive weeks. **Maintenance**: 5 mg/kg by IV infusion (see below) q 2 weeks. Cidofovir must be diluted in 100 mL of 0.9% NaCl solution prior to administration. The IV infusion is given at a constant rate over 1 h. Oral probenecid must be given with each dose: 2 g given 3 h prior to cidofovir and 1 g given at 2 h and 8 h after completion of the 1 h IV infusion (total probenecid dose = 4 g).
Cilostazol	PLETAL	Drug for Intermittant Claudication	**Tab**: 50, 100 mg	100 mg bid po taken ≥ 30 min before or 2 h after breakfast and dinner.

GENERIC NAME	COMMON TRADE NAMES	THERAPEUTIC CATEGORY	PREPARATIONS	COMMON ADULT DOSAGE
Cimetidine	TAGAMET HB 200	Histamine H_2-Blocker	**Tab**: 100 mg	**Heartburn, Acid Indigestion & Sour Stomach**: 200 mg po with water up to bid.
	TAGAMET	Histamine H_2-Blocker, Anti-Ulcer Agent	**Liquid**: 300 mg/5 mL (2.8% alcohol) **Tab**: 200, 300, 400, 800 mg	**Duodenal Ulcer:** **Active**: 800 mg hs po; or 300 mg qid po with meals & hs; or 400 mg bid po in the AM and PM. **Maintenance**: 400 mg hs po. **Active Benign Gastric Ulcer**: 800 mg hs po; or 300 mg qid po with meals & hs. **Erosive Gastroesophageal Reflux Disease**: 800 mg bid po; or 400 mg qid po for 12 weeks. **Pathological Hypersecretory Conditions**: 300 mg qid po with meals & hs.
			Inj: 300 mg/2 mL	**Pathological Hypersecretory Conditions or Intractable Ulcers**: 300 mg q 6 - 8 h IM or IV (infused over 15 - 20 minutes). For a Continuous IV Infusion: 37.5 mg/h (900 mg daily); may be preceded by a 150 mg loading dose by IV infusion (over 15 - 20 minutes).
Cinoxacin	CINOBAC	Urinary Tract Anti-infective	**Cpsl**: 250, 500 mg	1 g daily po, in 2 or 4 divided doses for 7 - 14 days.
Ciprofloxacin	CIPRO I.V.	Antibacterial	**Inj**: 200, 400 mg	**Urinary Tract Infections**: 200 mg q 12 h by IV infusion (over 60 minutes). For severe or complicated UTI, double the dose. **Lower Respiratory Tract, Bone & Joint, and Skin & Skin Structure Infections**: 400 mg q 12 h by IV infusion (over 60 minutes).

Ciprofloxacin Hydrochloride	CILOXAN	Antibacterial	**Ophth Solution**: 0.3%	**Corneal Ulcers**: 2 drops in affected eye(s) q 15 min. for the 1st 6 hours, then 2 drops q 30 min. for the rest of the 1st day. Second day: 2 drops q 1 h; 3rd - 14th day: 2 drops q 4 h. **Conjunctivitis**: 1 - 2 drops in affected eye(s) q 2 h while awake for 2 days, then 1 - 2 drops q 4 h while awake for the next 5 days.
			Ophth Oint: 0.3% (as the base)	Place 1/2 in strip into the conjunctival sac tid for 2 days, then bid for 5 days.
	CIPRO	Antibacterial	**Tab**: 100, 250, 500, 750 mg	**Urinary Tract Infections:** **Acute, Uncomplicated**: 100 mg q 12 h po for 3 days. **Mild to Moderate**: 250 mg q 12 h po for 7 to 14 days. **Severe/Complicated**: 500 mg q 12 h po for 7 - 14 days. **Lower Respiratory Tract and Skin & Skin Structure Infections**: 500 mg q 12 h po for 7 to 14 days. For severe or complicated infections, increase the dose to 750 mg q 12 h po for 7 - 14 days. **Bone & Joint Infections**: 500 mg q 12 h po for 4 - 6 weeks. For severe or complicated infections, increase the dose to 750 mg q 12 h po for 4 - 6 weeks. **Infectious Diarrhea**: 500 mg q 12 h po for 5 - 7 days. **Typhoid Fever**: 500 mg q 12 h po for 10 days. **Gonococcal Infections, Uncomplicated**: 250 mg po (as a single dose).
Cisapride	PROPULSID	GI Stimulant	**Tab**: 10, 20 mg **Susp**: 1 mg/mL	Initially, 10 mg qid po, at least 15 min ac & hs. May increase to 20 mg qid po.

GENERIC NAME	COMMON TRADE NAMES	THERAPEUTIC CATEGORY	PREPARATIONS	COMMON ADULT DOSAGE
Cisplatin	PLATINOL PLATINOL AQ	Antineoplastic	**Powd for Inj**: 10, 50 mg **Inj**: 1 mg/mL	**Metastatic Testicular Tumors**: 20 mg/m^2 IV daily for 5 days. **Metastatic Ovarian Tumors**: 100 mg/m^2 IV once every 4 weeks. **Advanced Bladder Cancer**: 50 - 70 mg/m^2 IV q 3 - 4 weeks.
Citalopram Hydrobromide	CELEXA	Antidepressant	**Tab**: 20, 40 mg	20 mg once daily po in the AM or PM. Dose increases should usually occur in increments of 20 mg at intervals of no less than 1 week. Maximum: 40 mg daily.
Cladribine	LEUSTATIN	Antineoplastic	**Inj**: 1 mg/mL	0.09 mg/kg/day by IV infusion in 0.9% Sodium Chloride solution for 7 consecutive days.
Clarithromycin	BIAXIN	Antibacterial	**Granules for Susp (per 5 mL)**: 125, 250 mg **Tab**: 250, 500 mg	**Usual Dosage**: 250 - 500 mg q 12 h po for 7 - 14 days. ***Mycobacterium avium* Complex (MAC)**: 500 mg bid po. **Active Duodenal Ulcer Associated with *Helicobacter pylori* Infection**: 500 mg tid po for days 1 - 14 plus omeprazole 40 mg po each AM or ranitidine bismuth citrate 400 mg bid for days 1 - 14.
Clemastine Fumarate	TAVIST	Antihistamine	**Syrup**: 0.67 mg/5 mL (5.5% alcohol)	**Allergic Rhinitis**: 10 mL bid po. **Urticaria and Angioedema**: 20 mL bid po.
	TAVIST ALLERGY TAVIST		**Tab**: 1.34 mg **Tab**: 2.68 mg	1.34 mg q 12 h po. 2.68 mg bid or tid po.
Clindamycin Hydrochloride	CLEOCIN HCL	Antibacterial	**Cpsl**: 75, 150, 300 mg	**Serious Infections**: 150 - 300 mg q 6 h po. **More Severe Infections**: 300 - 450 mg q 6 h po.
Clindamycin Palmitate HCl	CLEOCIN PEDIATRIC	Antibacterial	**Powd for Susp**: 75 mg/5 mL	Same dosages as for CLEOCIN HCL above.

Clindamycin Phosphate	CLEOCIN PHOSPHATE	Antibacterial	**Inj**: 150 mg/mL	**Serious Infections**: 600 - 1200 mg/day IV or IM in 2, 3 or 4 equal doses. **More Severe Infections**: 1200 - 2700 mg/day IV or IM in 2, 3 or 4 equal doses. **Life-Threatening Infections**: Up to 4800 mg/day IV.
	CLEOCIN	Antibacterial	**Vaginal Cream**: 2%	Insert 1 applicatorful intravaginally, preferably hs, for 7 consecutive days.
	CLEOCIN-T	Anti-Acne Agent	**Topical Solution, Gel &: Lotion**: 10 mg/mL	Apply a thin film to affected areas bid.
Clobetasol Propionate	TEMOVATE	Corticosteroid	**Cream, Oint & Gel**: 0.05% **Scalp Application**: 0.05%	Apply topically to affected area bid. Apply to affected scalp areas bid, AM and PM.
Clocortolone Pivalate	CLODERM	Corticosteroid	**Cream**: 0.1%	Apply sparingly to the affected area tid. Rub in gently.
Clofazimine	LAMPRENE	Leprostatic	**Cpsl**: 50, 100 mg	100 mg daily with meals po.
Clofibrate	ATROMID-S	Hypolipidemic	**Cpsl**: 500 mg	500 mg qid po.
Clomiphene Citrate	CLOMID, SEROPHENE	Ovulation Stimulant	**Tab**: 50 mg	50 mg daily for 5 days po.
Clomipramine Hydrochloride	ANAFRANIL	Antidepressant	**Cpsl**: 25, 50, 75 mg	Initiate with 25 mg daily po with meals and gradually increase, as tolerated, to 100 mg a day during the first 2 weeks. Thereafter, the dosage may be increased gradually over the next several weeks, up to a maximum of 250 mg daily. After titration, the total daily dose may be given once daily hs.
Clonazepam (C-IV)	KLONOPIN	Antiepileptic, Drug for Panic Disorder	**Tab**: 0.5, 1, 2 mg	**Seizure Disorders**: Initially, 0.5 mg tid po. Dosage may be increased in increments of 0.5 - 1 mg every 3 days; maximum 20 mg per day. **Panic Disorder**: Initially, 0.25 mg bid po. An increase to the target dose of 1 mg daily may be made after 3 days.

GENERIC NAME	COMMON TRADE NAMES	THERAPEUTIC CATEGORY	PREPARATIONS	COMMON ADULT DOSAGE
Clonidine	CATAPRES-TTS	Antihypertensive	**Transdermal**: rate = 0.1, 0.2, 0.3 mg/24 hr	Apply to hairless area of intact skin on the upper arm or torso, once every 7 days.
Clonidine Hydrochloride	CATAPRES	Antihypertensive	**Tab**: 0.1, 0.2, 0.3 mg	Initially, 0.1 mg bid po (AM and hs). Further increments of 0.1 mg may be made until the desired response is achieved.
	DURACLON	Non-Opioid Analgesic	**Inj**: 100 μg/mL	30 μg/hr by continuous epidural infusion.
Clopidogrel Bisulfate	PLAVIX	Platelet Aggregation Inhibitor	**Tab**: 75 mg	75 mg once daily po.
Clorazepate Dipotassium (C-IV)	TRANXENE-T TAB	Antianxiety Agent, Antiepileptic, Drug for Alcohol Withdrawal	**Tab**: 3.75, 7.5, 15 mg	**Anxiety**: 15 - 60 mg daily in divided doses po; or 15 mg hs po. **Epilepsy**: The maximum recommended initial dose is 7.5 mg tid po. Dosage should be increased no more than 7.5 mg every week and should not exceed 90 mg per day. **Acute Alcohol Withdrawal**: Day 1 (1st 24 h): 30 mg po initially, followed by 30 - 60 mg po in divided doses. Day 2 (2nd 24 h): 45 - 90 mg po in divided doses. Day 3 (3rd 24 h): 22.5 - 45 mg po in divided doses. Day 4: 15 - 30 mg po in divided doses. Thereafter: gradually reduce the dose to 7.5 to 15 mg daily po.
	TRANXENE-SD	Antianxiety Agent	**Gradual-Rel. Tab**: 11.25, 22.5 mg	**Anxiety**: 11.25 or 22.5 mg as a single po dose q 24 h. Used as an alternative for patients stabilized on TRANXENE.

Clotrimazole	LOTRIMIN AF MYCELEX	Antifungal	**Cream, Lotion & Solution**: 1% **Cream**: 1%	Massage into affected and surrounding skin areas bid, AM and PM.
			Troche: 10 mg	**Treatment**: Slowly dissolve 1 in the mouth 5 times daily for 14 consecutive days. **Prophylaxis**: Slowly dissolve 1 in the mouth 3 times daily for the duration of therapy.
	MYCELEX-G		**Vaginal Cream**: 1%	One applicatorful daily intravaginally for 7 to 14 consecutive days.
			Vaginal Tab: 500 mg	Insert 1 tablet intravaginally once only hs.
	GYNE-LOTRIMIN, MYCELEX-7		**Vaginal Cream**: 1%	One applicatorful daily intravaginally for 7 consecutive days, preferably hs.
			Vaginal Insert: 100 mg	Place 1 insert daily intravaginally for 7 consecutive days, preferably hs.
Cloxacillin Sodium		Antibacterial	**Cpsl**: 250, 500 mg **Powd for Solution**: 125 mg/5 mL	**Mild to Moderate Infections**: 250 mg q 6 h po. **Severe Infections**: 500 mg q 6 h po.
Clozapine	CLOZARIL	Antipsychotic	**Tab**: 25, 100 mg	Initially, 12.5 mg once or twice daily po; then, be continued with daily dosage increments of 25 - 50 mg/day (if well-tolerated) to a target dose of 300 - 450 mg/day by the end of 2 weeks. Subsequent dosage increments should be made no more than 1 - 2 times a week in increments not to exceed 100 mg.
Cocaine Hydrochloride (C-II)		Local Anesthetic	**Topical Solution**: 4, 10%	1 - 4% applied topically by means of cotton applicators or packs, or as a spray.
Codeine Phosphate (C-II)		Opioid Analgesic	**Inj (per mL)**: 30, 60 mg	15 - 60 mg q 4 - 6 h IM, SC or IV.
Codeine Sulfate (C-II)		Opioid Analgesic, Antitussive	**Tab**: 15, 30, 60 mg	**Analgesia**: 15 - 60 mg q 4 - 6 h po. **Antitussive**: 10 - 20 mg q 4 - 6 h po.

GENERIC NAME	COMMON TRADE NAMES	THERAPEUTIC CATEGORY	PREPARATIONS	COMMON ADULT DOSAGE
Colchicine		Antigout Agent	**Tab**: 0.5, 0.6 mg	**Acute**: 1.0 - 1.2 mg po stat; then 0.5 - 1.2 mg q 1 - 2 h po, until pain is relieved, or nausea, vomiting or diarrhea occurs. **Prophylaxis**: 0.5 or 0.6 mg daily for 3 - 4 days a week.
			Inj: 1 mg/2 mL	**Acute**: 2 mg stat IV; then 0.5 mg q 6 h IV up to a maximum of 4 mg in 24 h. **Prophylaxis**: 0.5 - 1 mg once daily or bid IV.
Colestipol Hydrochloride	COLESTID	Hypolipidemic	**Tab**: 1 g	Initially, 2 g once or twice daily po. Dosage increases of 2 g once or twice daily po should occur at 1 - 2 month intervals. Dosage range: 2 - 16 g/day po given once daily or in divided doses.
			Granules for Oral Susp: 5 g packettes and 300, 500 g bottles (Unflavored); 7.5 g packettes and 450 g bottles (Orange Flavor)	Initially, 5 g daily or bid po with a daily increment of 5 g at 1 - 2 month intervals. Usual dose: 5 - 30 g/day po given once daily or in divided doses.
Colistimethate Sodium	COLY-MYCIN M PARENTERAL	Antibacterial	**Powd for Inj**: 150 mg (= to colistin base)	2.5 - 5.0 mg/kg per day in 2 - 4 divided doses IV or IM.
Cromolyn Sodium	GASTROCROM	Antiallergic, Oral	**Conc. Solution**: 100 mg/5 mL	200 mg qid po, 30 minutes ac & hs.
	INTAL	Drug for Asthma	**Solution for Nebulization**: 20 mg/2 mL	20 mg qid nebulized.
			Inhaler: 800 μg/spray	2 sprays qid inhaled.
	NASALCROM	Antiallergic, Nasal	**Nasal Solution**: 40 mg/mL	1 spray in each nostril 3 - 6 times daily.
	CROLOM	Antiallergic, Ophthalmic	**Ophth Solution**: 4%	1 or 2 drops in each eye 4 - 6 times daily at regular intervals.

Crotamiton	EURAX	Scabicide, Antipruritic	**Cream & Lotion**: 10%	**Scabies:** Massage into the skin from the chin to the toes including folds and creases. Reapply 24 hours later. A cleansing bath should be taken 48 h after the last application. **Pruritus:** Massage gently into affected areas until medication is completely absorbed. Repeat prn.
Cyanocobalamin	NASCOBAL	Vitamin	**Metered-Dose Gel**: 500 μg per actuation	500 μg (1 actuation) intranasally once a week.
			Tab: 25, 50, 100, 250 μg	**Deficiency**: 25 - 250 μg daily po.
Cyclizine Hydrochloride	MAREZINE	Antiemetic	**Tab**: 50 mg	50 mg q 4 - 6 h po, staring 30 minutes prior to travel.
Cyclobenzaprine Hydrochloride	FLEXERIL	Skeletal Muscle Relaxant	**Tab**: 10 mg	10 mg tid po.
Cyclophosphamide	CYTOXAN	Antineoplastic	**Tab**: 25, 50 mg **Powd for Inj**: 100, 200, 500 mg; 1, 2 g	1 - 5 mg/kg/day po. 40 - 50 mg/kg IV in divided doses over a period of 2 - 5 days; or 10 - 15 mg/kg IV q 7 - 10 days; or 3 - 5 mg/kg IV twice weekly.
Cyclosporine	SANDIMMUNE	Immunosuppressant	**Cpsl**: 25, 50, 100 mg **Solution**: 100 mg/mL (12.5% alcohol)	15 mg/kg po, 4 to 12 hours prior to transplantation. Continue dose postoperatively for 1 - 2 weeks, then taper by 5% per week to a maintenance level of 5 - 10 mg/kg/day.
			Inj: 50 mg/mL	5 - 6 mg/kg/day IV, 4 to 12 hours prior to transplantation. Give as a dilute solution (50 mg in 20 to 100 mL) and administer as a slow infusion over 2 - 6 hrs. Continue this single dose postoperatively until patient can tolerate oral dosage forms.
Cyproheptadine Hydrochloride	PERIACTIN	Antihistamine, Antipruritic	**Syrup**: 2 mg/5 mL (5% alcohol) **Tab**: 4 mg	4 mg tid po.

GENERIC NAME	COMMON TRADE NAMES	THERAPEUTIC CATEGORY	PREPARATIONS	COMMON ADULT DOSAGE
Cytarabine, Conventional	CYTOSAR-U	Antineoplastic	**Powd for Inj**: 100, 500 mg; 1, 2 g	100 mg/m^2/day by continuous IV infusion or 100 mg/m^2 IV q 12 h.
Cytarabine, Liposomal	DEPO-CYT	Antineoplastic	**Inj**: 10 mg/mL	50 mg intrathecally (intraventricular or lumbar puncture) q 14 days for 2 to 4 doses.
Dacarbazine	DTIC-DOME	Antineoplastic	**Inj**: 10 mg/mL	**Malignant Melanoma**: 2 - 4.5 mg/kg/day IV for 10 days; may repeat q 4 weeks. Alternate dosage: 250 mg/m^2/day IV for 5 days; may repeat q 3 weeks. **Hodgkin's Dosease**: 150 mg/m^2/day IV for 5 days, in combination with other effective drugs; may repeat q 4 weeks. Alternate dosage: 375 mg/m^2 on day 1, in combination with other drugs; repeat q 15 days.
Dalteparin Sodium	FRAGMIN	Anticoagulant	**Solution (per 0.2 mL)**: 2,500 (16 mg); 5,000 (32 mg); 10,000 (64 mg) anti-X_a Units	**Patients Undergoing Abdominal Surgery with Risk of Thromboembolic Complications**: 2,500 Units each day, SC only, starting 1 - 2 h prior to surgery and repeated once daily 5 to 10 days postoperatively. In patients with high risk of thromoembolic complications, use 5,000 Units SC only in the evening before surgery and repeated once daily for 5 to 10 days postoperatively. **Hip Replacement Surgery**: 2,500 Units SC within 2 h before surgery and 2,500 Units in the evening of the day of surgery (≥ 6 h after the first dose). On the first post-operative day administer 5,000 Units SC once daily for 5 - 10 days. **Systemic Anticoagulation**: 200 Units/kg SC daily or 100 Units/kg SC bid. **Unstable Angina/Non-Q-Wave MI**: 120 Units/kg (but not more than 10,000 Units) SC q 12 h with concurrent oral aspirin (75 to 165 mg per day) therapy. Continue until the patient is clinically stabilized (usually 5 - 8 days).

Danaparoid Sodium	ORGARAN	Anticoagulant	**Inj**: 750 anti-Xa units per 0.6 mL	750 anti-Xa units bid SC starting 1 - 4 h pre-operatively; then not sooner than 2 h after surgery. Continue therapy throughout post-operative care until the risk of deep vein thrombosis has diminished (e.g., 7-10 days).
Danazol	DANOCRINE	Gonadotropin Inhibitor	**Cpsl**: 50, 100, 200 mg	**Endometriosis**: 100 - 200 mg bid po (mild disease) or 400 mg bid po (moderate to severe). Continue therapy for 3 - 6 months. **Fibrotic Breast Disease**: 50 - 200 mg bid po. Therapy should begin during menstruation. **Hereditary Angioedema**: 200 mg bid or tid po. After a favorable initial response, determine continuing dosage by reducing the dosage by 50% or less at intervals of 1 - 3 months or longer. If an attack occurs, increase dosage by up to 200 mg/day.
Dantrolene Sodium	DANTRIUM	Skeletal Muscle Relaxant	**Cpsl**: 25, 50, 100 mg	**Chronic Spasticity**: 25 mg once daily po for 7 days; then 25 mg tid for 7 days; then 50 mg tid for 7 days; then 100 mg tid. Therapy in some patients may require qid dosing. **Malignant Hyperthermia**: **Preoperatively**: 4 - 8 mg/kg/day po in 3 - 4 divided doses for 1 or 2 days prior to surgery, with the last dose given approx. 3 - 4 h before scheduled surgery. **Post Crisis Follow Up**: 4 - 8 mg/kg/day po in 4 divided doses for 1 - 3 days.
	DANTRIUM INTRAVENOUS		**Powd for Inj**: 20 mg	**Malignant Hyperthermia**: **Acute Therapy**: Administer by continuous rapid IV push beginning at a minimum dose of 1 mg/kg, and continuing until the symptoms subside or the max. cumulative dose of 10 mg/kg has been reached. **Preoperatively**: 2.5 mg/kg IV starting approx. 1.25 hours before anticipated anesthesia and infused over 1 h. **Post Crisis Follow Up**: Individualize dose.

GENERIC NAME	COMMON TRADE NAMES	THERAPEUTIC CATEGORY	PREPARATIONS	COMMON ADULT DOSAGE
Dapsone	DAPSONE USP	Leprostatic	**Tab**: 25, 100 mg	100 mg daily po alone or in combination with other leprostatic drugs.
Delavirdine Mesylate	RESCRIPTOR	Antiviral	**Tab**: 100, 200 mg	400 mg tid po. Disperse the dose in 3 fl. oz. of water prior to consumption.
Demecarium Bromide	HUMORSOL	Anti-Glaucoma Agent	**Ophth Solution**: 0.125, 0.25%	1 - 2 drops in the affected eye. Usual dosage can vary from as much as 1 - 2 drops bid to as little as 1 - 2 drops twice a week; for most patients 0.125% used bid is preferred.
Demeclocycline Hydrochloride	DECLOMYCIN	Antibacterial	**Tab**: 150, 300 mg	150 mg qid po or 300 mg bid po.
Desipramine Hydrochloride	NORPRAMIN	Antidepressant	**Tab**: 10, 25, 50, 75, 100, 150 mg	100 - 200 mg daily po in a single dose or in divided doses.
Desmopressin Acetate	DDAVP NASAL SPRAY DDAVP RHINAL TUBE	Posterior Pituitary Hormone, Anti-Enuretic Agent	**Nasal Spray**: 0.1 mg/mL (delivers 0.1 mL (10 μg) per spray) **Nasal Solution**: 0.1 mg/mL (with rhinal tube applicators)	**Central Cranial Diabetes Insipidus**: 0.1 - 0.4 mL daily as a single dose or in 2 - 3 divided doses intranasally. **Primary Nocturnal Enuresis**: 0.2 mL intranasally hs. Dosage adjustment up to 0.4 mL may be made if necessary.
	DDAVP TABLETS		**Tab**: 0.1, 0.2 mg	**Central Cranial Diabetes Insipidus**: Initially, 0.05 mg bid po. Dosage adjustments may be made such that the total daily dosage is in the range of 0.1 - 1.2 mg divided tid or bid.
	DDAVP INJECTION		**Inj**: 4, 15 μg/mL	**Diabetes Insipidus**: 0.25 - 0.5 mL (1 - 2 μg) bid SC or IV (4 μg/mL injection only). **Hemophilia A and von Willebrand's Disease (Type I)**: 0.3 μg/kg diluted in 50 mL of sterile physiological saline; infuse IV slowly over 15 to 30 minutes. If used preoperatively, give 30 minutes prior to the procedure.

	STIMATE	Posterior Pituitary Hormone	**Nasal Spray**: 1.5 mg/mL (delivers 0.1 mL (150 μg) per spray)	**Hemophilia A and von Willebrand's Disease (Type I)**: 1 spray per nostril (300 μg) in patients weighing ≥ 50 kg; 1 spray only in patients weighing < 50 kg. If used preoperatively, give 2 hours prior to the procedure.
Desonide	DESOWEN	Corticosteroid	**Cream, Oint & Lotion**: 0.05%	Apply to the affected areas bid to tid.
	TRIDESILON		**Cream & Oint**: 0.05%	Apply to the affected areas bid to qid.
Desoximetasone	TOPICORT	Corticosteroid	**Cream**: 0.05, 0.25% **Oint**: 0.25% **Gel**: 0.05%	Apply a thin film to the affected areas bid. Rub in gently.
Dexamethasone	DECADRON	Corticosteroid	**Elixir**: 0.5 mg/5 mL (5% alcohol) **Tab**: 0.5, 0.75, 4 mg	Initial dosage varies from 0.75 - 9 mg daily po, depending on the disease being treated. This should be maintained or adjusted until the patient's response is satisfactory.
	MAXIDEX		**Ophth Susp**: 0.1%	1 - 2 drops in affected eye(s). In severe disease, may use hourly; taper to discontinuation as the inflammation subsides. In mild disease, may use up to 4 - 6 times daily.
Dexamethasone Acetate	DECADRON-LA	Corticosteroid	**Inj**: 8 mg/mL	**Intramuscular Inj**: 8 - 16 mg q 1 - 3 weeks. **Intralesional Inj**: 0.8 - 1.6 mg per inj. site. **Intra-articular & Soft Tissue Inj**: 4 - 16 mg q 1 - 3 weeks.
Dexamethasone Sodium Phosphate	DECADRON PHOSPHATE	Corticosteroid	**Inj**: 4 mg/mL **Inj**: 24 mg/mL [for IV use only]	**IV and IM Inj**: Initial dosage varies from 0.5 - 9 mg daily depending on the disease being treated. This dosage should be maintained or adjusted until the patient's response is satisfactory. **Intra-articular, Intralesional, and Soft Tissue Injection**: Varies from 0.2 - 6 mg given from once q 3 - 5 days to once q 2 - 3 weeks.

[Continued on the next page]

GENERIC NAME	COMMON TRADE NAMES	THERAPEUTIC CATEGORY	PREPARATIONS	COMMON ADULT DOSAGE
Dexamethasone Sodium Phosphate [Continued]	DECADRON PHOSPHATE		**Ophth Solution**: 0.1%	**Eye**: 1 - 2 drops into eye(s) q 1 h during the day & q 2 h at night, initially. When a favorable response occurs, reduce to 1 drop into eye(s) q 4 h. Later, 1 drop tid - qid. **Ear**: 3 - 4 drops into aural canal bid - tid. When a favorable response occurs, reduce dosage gradually and eventually discontinue.
	DECADRON PHOSPHATE, MAXIDEX		**Ophth Oint**: 0.05%	Apply to eye(s) tid or qid. When a favorable response occurs, reduce daily applications to 2, and later to 1 as maintenance therapy.
			Topical Cream: 0.1%	Apply a thin film to affected area tid or qid.
	DEXACORT TURBINAIRE		**Nasal Aerosol**: 84 μg/spray	2 sprays in each nostril bid or tid.
Dexchlorpheniramine Maleate	POLARAMINE	Antihistamine	**Syrup**: 2 mg/5 mL (6% alcohol) **Tab**: 2 mg **Repeat Action Tab**: 4, 6 mg	5 mL (2 mg) q 4 - 6 h po. 2 mg q 4 - 6 h po. 4 or 6 mg po hs or q 8 - 10 h during the day.
Dextroamphetamine Sulfate (C-II)	DEXEDRINE	CNS Stimulant	**Tab**: 5 mg **Sustained-Rel. Cpsl**: 5, 10, 15 mg	**Narcolepsy**: 5 - 60 mg per day in divided doses, depending on the patient response.
Dextromethorphan Hydrobromide	ROBITUSSIN PEDIATRIC COUGH SUPPRESSANT	Antitussive	**Liquid**: 7.5 mg/5 mL	20 mL q 6 - 8 h po.
	BENYLIN PEDIATRIC COUGH SUPPRESSANT		**Liquid**: 7.5 mg/5 mL	20 mL (30 mg) q 6 - 8 h po.
	BENYLIN ADULT FORMULA		**Liquid**: 15 mg/5 mL	10 mL (30 mg) q 6 - 8 h po.
	ROBITUSSIN MAXIMUM STRENGTH COUGH SUPPRESSANT		**Liquid**: 15 mg/5 mL	10 mL (30 mg) q 6 - 8 h po.

Dextromethorphan Polistirex	DELSYM	Antitussive	**Syrup**: equal to 30 mg of dextromethorphan HBr/5 mL	10 mL (60 mg) q 12 h po.
Dezocine	DALGAN	Opioid Analgesic	**Inj (per mL)**: 5, 10, 15 mg	**IM**: 5 - 20 mg q 3 - 6 h. **IV**: 2.5 - 10 mg q 2 - 4 h.
Diazepam (C-IV)	VALIUM	Antianxiety Agent, Anticonvulsant, Skel. Muscle Relax., Drug for Alcohol Withdrawal	**Tab**: 2, 5, 10 mg	**Anxiety & Adjunct in Convulsive Disorders**: 2 - 10 mg bid to qid po. **Muscle Spasms**: 2 - 10 mg tid to qid po.
			Inj: 5 mg/mL	**Anxiety (Moderate)**: 2 - 5 mg IM or IV. Repeat in 3 - 4 h, if necessary. **Anxiety (Severe) and Muscle Spasms**: 5 - 10 mg IM or IV. Repeat in 3 - 4 h, if necessary. **Preoperative Medication**: 10 mg IM (preferred route) before surgery. **Status Epilepticus and Severe Recurrent Convulsive Seizures**: 5 - 10 mg IV. Repeat at 10 - 15 minute intervals, if necessary, up to a maximum dose of 30 mg. **Acute Alcohol Withdrawal**: Initially 10 mg IM or IV, then 5 - 10 mg in 3 - 4 h, if needed. **Endoscopic Procedures**: Titrate IV dosage to desired sedative response. Generally 10 mg or less is adequate, but up to 20 mg IV may be given.
	DIASTAT	Antiepileptic	**Rectal Gel (Adult)**: 10, 15, 20 mg	Administer 0.2 mg/kg rectally. Calculate the recommended dose by rounding up to the next available unit dose. A second dose, when required, may be given 4 - 12 h after the first dose. Do not treat more than 5 episodes/month or more than 1 episode q 5 days.
Diazoxide	PROGLYCEM	Hyperglycemic Agent	**Susp**: 50 mg/mL **Cpsl**: 50 mg	3 - 8 mg/kg po, divided into 2 or 3 equal doses q 8 - 12 h.
	HYPERSTAT I.V.	Antihypertensive	**Inj**: 300 mg/20 mL	1 - 3 mg/kg IV repeated at intervals of 5 - 15 minutes (max.: 150 mg in a single injection).

GENERIC NAME	COMMON TRADE NAMES	THERAPEUTIC CATEGORY	PREPARATIONS	COMMON ADULT DOSAGE
Dibucaine	NUPERCAINAL	Local Anesthetic Antihemorrhoidal	**Oint**: 1%	Apply to affected areas AM and PM and after each bowel movement.
Dichlorphenamide	DARANIDE	Anti-Glaucoma Agent	**Tab**: 50 mg	Initially, a priming dose of 100 - 200 mg po, followed by 200 mg q 12 h po until the desired response occurs. The maintenance dosage is 25 - 50 mg once daily to tid po.
Diclofenac Potassium	CATAFLAM	Antiinflammatory, Non-Opioid Analgesic	**Tab**: 50 mg	**Osteoarthritis**: 100 - 150 mg/day po in divided doses (50 mg bid or tid). **Rheumatoid Arthritis**: 150 - 200 mg/day po in divided doses (50 mg tid or qid). **Ankylosing Spondylitis**: 100 - 125 mg/day po as: 25 mg qid with an extra 25 mg hs, prn. **Analgesia and Primary Dysmenorrhea**: 50 mg tid po or 100 mg initially, followed by 50 mg doses po. Except for the first day when the total dose may be 200 mg, do not exceed 150 mg daily.
Diclofenac Sodium	VOLTAREN	Antiinflammatory	**Delayed-Rel. Tab**: 25, 50, 75 mg	**Osteoarthritis**: 100 - 150 mg/day po in divided doses (50 mg bid or tid, or 75 mg bid). **Rheumatoid Arthritis**: 150 - 200 mg/day po in div. doses (50 mg tid or qid, or 75 mg bid). **Ankylosing Spondylitis**: 100 - 125 mg/day po as: 25 mg qid with an extra 25 mg hs, prn.
		Antiinflammatory (Topical)	**Ophth Solution**: 0.1%	**Following Cataract Surgery**: 1 drop into the affected eye(s) qid beginning 24 h after cataract surgery and continuing for the first 2 weeks of the postoperative period. **Corneal Refractive Surgery**: 1 or 2 drops into the affected eye within 1 h prior to surgery. Instill 1 - 2 drops within 15 min after surgery and continue qid for up to 3 days.
	VOLTAREN-XR	Antiinflammatory	**Extended-Rel. Tab**: 100 mg	**Osteoarthritis & Rheumatoid Arthritis**: 100 mg once daily po.

Dicloxacillin Sodium	DYNAPEN, PATHOCIL	Antibacterial	**Powd for Susp:** 62.5 mg/5 mL **Cpsl**: 250, 500 mg	**Mild to Moderate Infections**: 125 mg q 6 h po. **More Severe Infections**: 250 mg q 6 h po.
Dicyclomine Hydrochloride	BENTYL	Anticholinergic	**Syrup**: 10 mg/5 mL **Cpsl**: 10 mg **Tab**: 20 mg **Inj**: 10 mg/mL	Initially 80 mg/day po (in 4 equally divided doses). Dosage may be increased during the first week, if necessary, to 160 mg/day po. 80 mg daily IM (in 4 equally divided doses).
Didanosine	VIDEX	Antiviral	**Chewable/Dispersible Tab**: 25, 50, 100, 150 mg	< **60 kg**: 250 mg once daily po or 125 mg bid q 12 h po. ≥ **60 kg**: 400 mg once daily po or 200 mg bid q 12 h po. Take at least 2 of the appropriate strength tablets at each dose for adequate buffering buffering and to prevent degradation by gastric acid. Chew or crush and disperse the tablets in at least 1 fl. oz. of water prior to consumption. Take on an empty stomach.
			Powd for Solution: 100, 167, 250 mg packets	< **60 kg**: 167 mg bid q 12 h po. ≥ **60 kg**: 250 mg bid q 12 h po. Dissolve contents of packet in 4 fl. oz. of water and drink on an empty stomach.
Dienestrol	ORTHO DIENESTROL	Estrogen	**Cream**: 0.01%	1 - 2 applicatorfuls intravaginally daily for 1 - 2 weeks, then gradually reduce to 1/2 initial dosage for a similar period. Maintenance dosage is 1 appicatorful 1 - 3 times a week.
Diethylpropion Hydrochloride (C-IV)	TENUATE TENUATE DOSPAN	Anorexiant	**Tab**: 25 mg **Controlled-Rel. Tab**: 75 mg	25 mg tid, 1 h ac po. 75 mg daily po in the midmorning.
Diethylstilbestrol Diphosphate	STILPHOSTROL	Antineoplastic	**Tab**: 50 mg	**Prostatic Cancer**: Initially 50 mg tid po. Raise the dosage to 200 mg or more tid depending on the tolerance of the patient.
			Inj: 250 mg/5 mL	**Prostatic Cancer**: 500 mg (in 250 mL of saline or 5% dextrose) slowly infused IV on the first day; then, 1000 mg (in 250 - 500 mL of fluid) for approx. 5 days. Thereafter, 250 - 500 mg (IV infusion) once or twice a week.

GENERIC NAME	COMMON TRADE NAMES	THERAPEUTIC CATEGORY	PREPARATIONS	COMMON ADULT DOSAGE
Diflorasone Diacetate	FLORONE, MAXIFLOR	Corticosteroid	**Cream & Oint**: 0.05%	Apply to the affected area once daily to qid, depending on the severity of the condition.
	FLORONE E		**Emollient Cream**: 0.05%	Apply to the affected area once daily to tid, depending on the severity of the condition.
Diflunisal	DOLOBID	Non-Opioid Analgesic, Antiinflammatory	**Tab**: 250, 500 mg	**Analgesic:** Initially 1000 mg po, followed by 500 mg q 12 h; or initially 500 mg po, followed by 250 mg q 8 - 12 h may also be appropriate. **Rheumatoid Arthritis & Osteoarthritis**: 250 to 500 mg bid po.
Digitoxin	CRYSTODIGIN	Heart Failure Drug, Inotropic Agent	**Tab**: 0.05, 0.1 mg	**Slow Digitalization**: 0.2 mg bid po for 4 days, followed by maintenance dosage. **Rapid Digitalization**: 0.6 mg po, followed by 0.4 mg and then 0.2 mg at intervals of 4 - 6 h. **Maintenance Dosage**: Ranges from 0.05 - 0.3 mg daily po; commonly 0.15 mg daily.
Digoxin	LANOXIN ELIXIR PEDIATRIC LANOXIN	Heart Failure Drug, Inotropic Agent	**Elixir**: 50 μg/mL (10% alcohol) **Tab**: 125, 250, 500 μg **Inj**: 250 μg/mL	Variable; see Digoxin Dosage Tables, pp. 254 to 257.
	LANOXICAPS		**Cpsl**: 50, 100, 200 μg	Variable; see Digoxin Dosage Tables, pp. 254 to 257.
Dihydrotachysterol	DHT HYTAKEROL	Vitamin D Analog	**Tab**: 0.125, 0.2, 0.4 mg **Solution**: 0.2 mg/mL **Cpsl**: 0.125 mg	**Initial**: 0.8 - 2.4 mg daily po for several days. **Maintenance:** 0.2 - 1.75 mg daily po. The average dose is 0.6 mg daily po.
Diltiazem Hydrochloride	CARDIZEM	Antianginal	**Tab**: 30, 60, 90, 120 mg	Initially, 30 mg qid po ac & hs. Dosage should be increased gradually at 1 - 2 day intervals. Usual optimum dosage: 180 - 360 mg/day.
	CARDIZEM SR	Antihypertensive	**Sustained-Rel. Cpsl**: 60, 90, 120 mg	Initially, 60 - 120 mg bid po; dosage may be adjusted after 14 days. Usual dosage: 240 to 360 mg/day.

	CARDIZEM CD	Antihypertensive, Antianginal	**Extended-Rel. Cpsl**: 120, 180, 240, 300, 360 mg	**Hypertension**: Initially, 180 - 240 mg once daily po. Dosage may be increased up to 480 mg once daily po (over 14 days). Usual dosage: 240 - 360 mg once daily. **Angina**: Initially, 120 or 180 mg once daily po. Dosage may be increased up to 480 mg once daily po (over 7 - 14 days).
	DILACOR XR	Antihypertensive, Antianginal	**Extended-Rel. Cpsl**: 120, 180, 240 mg	**Hypertension**: 180 - 240 mg once daily po. **Angina**: Initially, 120 mg once daily po. May be titrated to doses of up to 480 mg once daily over a 7 - 14 day period.
	TIAZAC	Antihypertensive	**Extended-Rel. Cpsl**: 120, 180, 240, 300, 360, 420 mg	**Hypertension**: Initially, 120 - 240 mg once daily po. Usual dosage range: 120 - 540 mg once daily po.
	CARDIZEM	Antiarrhythmic	**Inj**: 5 mg/mL	**IV Bolus (given over 2 min)**: Initially, 0.25 mg/kg; if response is inadequate, in 15 min. give 0.35 mg/kg. Individualize subsequent IV bolus doses. **Continuous IV Infusion (following IV bolus)**: Initially, 5 - 10 mg/hr; rate may be increased in 5 mg/hr increments up to 15 mg/hr prn for up to 24 h.
Dimenhydrinate	DRAMAMINE	Antivertigo Agent, Antiemetic	**Liquid**: 12.5 mg/5 mL **Tab & Chewable Tab**: 50 mg **Inj**: 50 mg/mL	50 - 100 mg q 4 - 6 h po. 50 - 100 mg q 4 - 6 h po. 50 mg q 4 - 6 h IM or slow IV.
Diphenhydramine Hydrochloride	BENADRYL DYE-FREE	Antihistamine	**Liquid**: 12.5 mg/5 mL **Liqui-Gel Cpsl**: 25 mg	25 - 50 mg (10 - 20 mL) q 4 - 6 h po. 25 - 50 mg q 4 - 6 h po.
	BENADRYL ALLERGY	Antihistamine, Antiemetic, Antiparkinsonian	**Liquid**: 12.5 mg/5 mL **Chewable Tab**: 12.5 mg **Cpsl & Tab**: 25 mg	25 - 50 mg (10 - 20 mL) q 4 - 6 h po. 25 - 50 mg q 4 - 6 h po. 25 - 50 mg q 4 - 6 h po.
	BENADRYL		**Inj (per mL)**: 10, 50 mg	10 - 50 mg IV or deep IM.
	UNISOM SLEEPGELS	Sedative	**Cpsl**: 50 mg	50 mg po hs, prn.

GENERIC NAME	COMMON TRADE NAMES	THERAPEUTIC CATEGORY	PREPARATIONS	COMMON ADULT DOSAGE
Dipyridamole	PERSANTINE	Platelet Aggregation Inhibitor	**Tab**: 25, 50, 75 mg	75 - 100 mg qid po.
Dirithromycin	DYNABAC	Antibacterial	**Enteric-Coated Tab**: 250 mg	500 mg once daily po with for 7 - 14 days. Administer with food or within 1 h of eating.
Disopyramide Phosphate	NORPACE	Antiarrhythmic	**Cpsl**: 100, 150 mg	600 mg/day po given in divided doses, e.g., 150 mg q 6 h. For patients under 110 lbs, 400 mg/day po, e.g., 100 mg q 6 h.
	NORPACE CR		**Extended-Rel. Cpsl**: 100, 150 mg	600 mg/day po given in divided doses, e.g., 300 mg q 12 h. For patients under 110 lbs, 400 mg/day po, e.g., 200 mg q 12 h.
Disulfiram	ANTABUSE	Antialcoholic	**Tab**: 250, 500 mg	**Initial**: A maximum of 500 mg po, given as a single dose for 1 - 2 weeks. **Maintenance**: 250 mg daily po.
Divalproex Sodium	DEPAKOTE	Antiepileptic, Antimaniacal, Antimigraine Agent	**Delayed-Rel. Tab**: 125, 250, 500 mg	**Epilepsy**: Initially, 10 - 15 mg/kg/day po; increase at 1 week intervals by 5 - 10 mg/kg/day (Maximum: 60 mg/kg/day). If the total daily dosage exceeds 250 mg, it should be given in divided doses. **Acute Mania**: Initially, 750 mg daily po in divided doses. The dose should be increased as rapidly as possible to achieve the lowest therapeutic dose that produces the desired clinical effect or the desired range of plasma concentrations (trough = 50 - 125 μg/mL). Maximum dosage is 60 mg/kg/day. **Migraine**: 250 mg bid po.
	DEPAKOTE	Antiepileptic	**Sprinkle Cpsl**: 125 mg	**Epilepsy**: Initially, 10 - 15 mg/kg/day po; increase at 1 week intervals by 5 - 10 mg/kg/day (Maximum: 60 mg/kg/day). If the total daily dosage exceeds 250 mg, it should be given in divided doses.

Dobutamine Hydrochloride	DOBUTREX	Sympathomimetic	**Powd for Inj**: 250 mg	2.5 - 15 μg/kg/min by IV infusion.
Docusate Calcium	SURFAK LIQUIGELS	Stool Softener	**Cpsl**: 240 mg	240 mg daily po.
Docusate Sodium	COLACE	Stool Softener	**Syrup**: 20 mg/5 mL **Cpsl**: 50, 100 mg	50 - 200 mg daily po.
	EX-LAX STOOL SOFTENER		**Cplt**: 100 mg	100 mg once daily to tid po.
	PHILLIPS LIQUI-GELS		**Liqui-Gel**: 100 mg	100 mg once daily to tid po.
Dolasetron Mesylate	ANZEMET	Antiemetic	**Tab**: 50, 100 mg	**Prevention of Chemotherapy-Induced Nausea and Vomiting**: 100 mg po within 1 h before chemotherapy. **Prevention or Treatment of Postoperative Nausea and Vomiting**: 100 mg po 2 h before surgery.
			Inj: 20 mg/mL	**Prevention of Chemotherapy-Induced Nausea and Vomiting**: 1.8 mg/kg IV as a single dose about 30 min before chemotherapy. Alternatively, 100 mg IV (over 30 sec). **Prevention or Treatment of Postoperative Nausea and Vomiting**: 12.5 mg IV as a single dose about 15 min before the cessation of anesthesia or as soon as nausea or vomiting presents.
Donepezil Hydrochloride	ARICEPT	Drug for Alzheimer's Disease	**Tab**: 5, 10 mg	5 - 10 mg once daily po.
Dopamine Hydrochloride	INTROPIN	Sympathomimetic	**Inj (per mL)**: 40, 80, 160 mg	2 - 10 μg/kg/min by IV infusion.
Dorzolamide Hydrochloride	TRUSOPT	Anti-Glaucoma Agent	**Ophth. Solution**: 2%	1 drop in the affected eye(s) tid.

GENERIC NAME	COMMON TRADE NAMES	THERAPEUTIC CATEGORY	PREPARATIONS	COMMON ADULT DOSAGE
Doxacurium Chloride	NUROMAX	Neuromuscular Blocker	**Inj**: 1 mg/mL	Initially, 0.025 - 0.05 mg/kg IV (depending on duration of effect desired and other drugs given); then, 0.005 - 0.01 mg/kg IV prn.
Doxazosin Mesylate	CARDURA	Antihypertensive, Benign Prostatic Hyperplasia Drug	**Tab**: 1, 2, 4, 8 mg	**Hypertension**: Initially, 1 mg once daily po. After 24 hours, dosage may be increased to 2 mg and thereafter, if needed, to 4, 8, and 16 mg daily. **Benign Prostatic Hyperplasia**: Initially, 1 mg once daily po. Depending on the condition, dosage may then be increased to 2 mg and thereafter 4 and 8 mg once daily (suggested titration interval is 1 - 2 weeks).
Doxepin Hydrochloride	SINEQUAN	Antianxiety Agent, Antidepressant	**Cpsl**: 10, 25, 50, 75, 100, 150 mg **Oral Concentrate**: 10 mg/mL	75 mg daily po in single or divided doses. The usual optimum dosage range is 75 - 150 mg daily.
	ZONALON	Antihistamine	**Cream**: 5%	Apply a thin film to affected areas qid, with at least 3 or 4 hours between applications.
Doxorubicin Hydrochloride	ADRIAMYCIN PFS ADRIAMYCIN RDF	Antineoplastic	**Inj**: 2 mg/mL **Powd for Inj**: 10, 20, 50 mg	60 - 75 mg/m^2 as a single IV injection given at 21-day intervals. Alternative: 20 mg/m^2 IV at weekly intervals.
Doxorubicin Hydrochloride Liposome Injection	DOXIL	Antineoplastic	**Inj**: 2 mg/mL (encapsulated in liposomes)	20 mg/m^2 as a single IV injection (over 30 min.) once every 3 weeks.
Doxycycline Calcium	VIBRAMYCIN	Antibacterial, Antimalarial	**Syrup**: 50 mg/5 mL	**Usual Dosage**: 100 mg q 12 h po for the first day, followed by a maintenance dose of 100 mg/day given as 50 mg q 12 h or 100 mg once daily. **Urinary Tract Infections**: 100 mg q 12 h po. **Malaria Prophylaxis**: 100 mg once daily po.

Doxycycline Hyclate	VIBRAMYCIN VIBRA-TAB	Antibacterial, Antimalarial	**Cpsl**: 50, 100 mg **Tab**: 100 mg	Same dosages as for VIBRAMYCIN Syrup.
	DORYX		**Cpsl (with coated pellets)**: 100 mg	Same dosages as for VIBRAMYCIN Syrup.
	VIBRAMYCIN INTRAVENOUS	Antibacterial	**Powd for Inj**: 100, 200 mg	**Usual Dosage**: 200 mg on the first day given in 1 or 2 IV infusions, then 100 - 200 mg a day, with 200 mg given in 1 or 2 infusions. **Syphilis**: 300 mg daily by IV infusion for at least 10 days.
Doxycycline Monohydrate	VIBRAMYCIN	Antibacterial, Antimalarial	**Powd for Susp**: 25 mg/5 mL	Same dosages as for VIBRAMYCIN Syrup.
Doxylamine Succinate	UNISOM	Sedative	**Tab**: 25 mg	25 mg po, 30 minutes before retiring.
Dronabinol (C-III)	MARINOL	Antiemetic, Appetite Stimulant	**Cpsl**: 2.5, 5, 10 mg	**Emesis**: 5 mg/m^2 po, 1 - 3 h prior to chemotherapy, then q 2 - 4 h after chemotherapy for a total of 4 - 6 doses/day. **Anorexia in AIDS patients**: Initially, 2.5 mg bid po, before lunch and supper. For patients who cannot tolerate this dosage, reduce to 2.5 mg once daily with supper or hs. When adverse reactions are absent or minimal or for further therapeutic effect, increase to 2.5 mg before lunch and 5 mg before supper (or 5 mg at lunch and 5 mg after supper). Approx. 50% of patients tolerate 10 mg bid.
Droperidol	INAPSINE	Antianxiety Agent	**Inj**: 2.5 mg/mL	**Premedication**: 2.5 - 10 mg IM, 30 - 60 minutes preoperatively. **Adjunct to General Anesthesia**: **Induction**: 2.5 mg per 20 - 25 lb IV. **Maintenance**: 1.25 - 2.5 mg IV.
Dyphylline	LUFYLLIN	Bronchodilator	**Tab**: 200, 400 mg **Elixir**: 100 mg/15 mL (20% alcohol)	Variable: up to 15 mg/kg q 6 h po.

GENERIC NAME	COMMON TRADE NAMES	THERAPEUTIC CATEGORY	PREPARATIONS	COMMON ADULT DOSAGE
Econazole Nitrate	SPECTAZOLE	Antifungal	**Cream**: 1%	**Tinea Infections**: Apply topically to affected areas once daily. **Cutaneous Candidiaisis**: Apply to affected areas bid.
Edrophonium Chloride	ENLON, TENSILON	Cholinomimetic	**Inj**: 10 mg/mL	**Diagnosis of Myasthenia**: 2 mg IV; if no reaction occurs after 45 seconds, give 8 mg IV. Test may be repeated in 30 minutes. May also administer 10 mg IM. Subject who shows hyperreactivity (cholinergic reaction), retest after 30 minutes with 2 mg IM. **Evaluation of Treatment Requirements**: 1 - 2 mg IV, 1 hour after oral intake of the drug being used in treatment. **Curare Antagonism**: 10 mg IV, given slowly over 30 - 45 seconds. May be repeated prn, up to a maximum of 40 mg.
Efavirenz	SUSTIVA	Antiviral	**Cpsl**: 50, 100, 200 mg	600 mg once daily po in combination with a protease inhibitor or nucleoside analog reverse transcriptase inhibitor.
Eflornithine Hydrochloride	ORNIDYL	Antiprotozoal	**Inj**: 200 mg/mL	100 mg/kg/dose by IV infusion (over a minimum of 45 minutes) q 6 h for 14 days.
Emedastine Difumarate	EMADINE	Antihistamine	**Ophth Solution**: 0.05%	1 drop in the affected eye(s) up to qid.
Enalapril Maleate	VASOTEC	Antihypertensive, Heart Failure Drug	**Tab**: 2.5, 5, 10, 20 mg	**Hypertension**: 5 mg once daily po. Usual dosage range is 10 - 40 mg/day as a single dose or in 2 divided doses. **Heart Failure**: As adjunctive therapy with a diuretic or digoxin, use 2.5 mg once daily or bid po. Usual dosage range is 5 - 20 mg/day in 2 divided doses.
Enalaprilat	VASOTEC I.V.	Antihypertensive	**Inj**: 1.25 mg/mL	1.25 mg q 6 h IV (over 5 minutes).

Enoxacin	PENETREX	Antibacterial	**Tab**: 200, 400 mg	**Urinary Tract Infections (Uncomplicated)**: 200 mg q 12 h po for 7 days. **Urinary Tract Infections (Complicated)**: 400 mg q 12 h po for 14 days. **Gonorrhea (Uncomplicated)**: 400 mg po as a single dose.
Enoxaparin Sodium	LOVENOX	Anticoagulant	**Inj**: 30 mg/0.3 mL, 40 mg/0.4 mL, 60 mg/0.6 mL, 80 mg/0.8 mL, 100 mg/mL	**Deep Vein Thrombosis Prophylaxis:** **Hip or Knee Replacement Surgery**: 30 mg SC (within 12 - 24 h postoperatively provided hemostasis has been established), then 30 mg q 12 h SC for 7 - 14 days. For Hip Replacement Surgery, consider 40 mg once daily SC, given initially 9 - 15 h prior to surgery. Continue for 3 weeks. **Abdominal Surgery**: 40 mg once daily SC with the initial dose given 2 h prior to surgery. The usual duration is 7 - 10 days. **DVT Treatment**: **Deep Vein Thrombosis/Pulmonary Embolism:** **Outpatients (e.g., Acute DVT without PE):** 1 mg/kg SC q 12 h. **Inpatients (e.g., Acute DVT with PE):** 1 mg/kg SC q 12 h or 1.5 mg/kg SC once daily (at the same time each day).
Entacapone	COMTAN	Antiparkinsonian	**Tab**: 200 mg	200 mg po given concomitantly with each levodopa/carbidopa dose to a maximum of 8 times daily (1600 mg).
Ephedrine Sulfate		Bronchodilator	**Cpsl**: 25 mg	12.5 - 25 mg q 4 h po.
			Inj: 50 mg/mL	25 - 50 mg SC or IM.
Epinephrine	PRIMATENE MIST	Bronchodilator	**Aerosol**: 0.2 mg/spray	1 inhalation, then wait at least 1 minute. If not relieved, use once more. Do not use again for at least 3 h.
	SUS-PHRINE		**Inj**: 5 mg/mL (1:200)	0.1 - 0.3 mL SC. Do not use more often than q 6 h.

GENERIC NAME	COMMON TRADE NAMES	THERAPEUTIC CATEGORY	PREPARATIONS	COMMON ADULT DOSAGE
Epinephrine Bitartrate	ASTHMAHLER MIST	Bronchodilator	**Aerosol**: 0.35 mg/spray (equal to 0.16 mg of epinephrine)	1 inhalation, then wait at least 1 minute. If not relieved, use once more. Do not use again for at least 3 h.
Epinephrine Hydrochloride	ADRENALIN CHLORIDE	Sympathomimetic, Bronchodilator	**Solution**: 1:100 (10 mg/mL) **Inj**: 1:1000 (1 mg/mL)	Variable, by nebulizer. 0.2 - 1.0 mg SC or IM.
	EPIPEN, EPI E-Z PEN		**Auto-injector**: 1:1000 soln (0.3 mg delivered per injection of 0.3 mL)	0.3 mg IM.
Eprosartan Mesylate	TEVETEN	Antihypertensive	**Tab**: 400, 600 mg	Initially 600 mg once daily po. Usual range: 400 - 800 mg/day given as a single dose or in 2 divided doses.
Ergotamine Tartrate	ERGOMAR	Antimigraine Agent	**Sublingual Tab**: 2 mg	2 mg under tongue stat; repeat q 30 minutes, prn, for a maximum of 6 mg per 24 hours.
Erythromycin	A/T/S ERYCETTE T-STAT 2%	Anti-Acne Agent	**Solution & Gel**: 2% **Solution**: 2% **Solution & Pads**: 2%	Apply to affected areas bid.
	ERY-TAB ERYC ERYTHROMYCIN BASE FILMTAB PCE	Antibacterial	**Delayed-Rel. Tab**: 250, 333, 500 mg **Delayed-Rel. Cpsl**: 250 mg **Tab**: 250, 500 mg **Dispersable Tab**: 333, 500 mg	**Usual Dosage**: 250 mg qid po; 333 mg q 8 h po; or 500 mg bid (q 12 h) po. **Streptococcal Infections**: Administer the usual dosage for at least 10 days. **Primary Syphilis**: 20 - 40 g po in divided doses over a period of 10 - 15 days. **Acute Pelvic Inflammatory Disease due to *N. gonorrhoeae***: After initial treatment with erythromycin lactobionate, give 250 mg q 6 h po for 7 days or 333 mg q 8 h for 7 days. **Urogenital Infections during pregnancy and Uncomplicated Urethral, Endocervical, or Rectal Infections due to *C. trachomatis***: 500 mg qid po or 666 mg q 8 h po for at least 7 days.

				Dysenteric Amebiasis: 250 mg qid po or 333 mg q 8 h po for 10 - 14 days. **Legionnaires Disease**: 1 - 4 g daily po in divided doses.
Erythromycin Estolate	ILOSONE	Antibacterial	**Susp (per 5 mL)**: 125, 250 mg **Cpsl**: 250 mg **Tab**: 500 mg	**Usual Dosage**: 250 mg q 6 h po or 500 mg q 12 h po. **Streptococcal Infections**: Administer the usual dosage for at least 10 days. **Primary Syphilis**: 20 - 40 g po in divided doses over a period of 10 - 15 days. **Urogenital Infections during pregnancy and Uncomplicated Urethral, Endocervical, or Rectal Infections due to *C. trachomatis***: 500 mg qid po for at least 7 days. **Dysenteric Amebiasis**: 250 mg qid po for 10 to 14 days. **Legionnaires Disease**: 1 - 4 g daily po in divided doses.
Erythromycin Ethylsuccinate	E.E.S.	Antibacterial	**Gran for Susp (per 5 mL)**: 200 mg **Susp (per 5 mL)**: 200, 400 mg **Tab**: 400 mg	**Usual Dosage**: 400 mg q 6 h po or 800 mg q 12 h po. **Streptococcal Infections**: Administer the usual dosage for at least 10 days. **Primary Syphilis**: 48 - 64 g po in divided doses over a period of 10 - 15 days. **Urethritis due to *C. trachomatis* or *U. urealyticum***: 800 mg tid po for 7 days. **Intestinal Amebiasis**: 400 mg qid po for 10 to 14 days. **Legionnaires Disease**: 1.6 - 4 g daily po in divided doses.
	ERYPED		**Powd for Susp (per 5 mL)**: 200, 400 mg **Chewable Tab**: 200 mg	
Erythromycin Gluceptate	ILOTYCIN GLUCEPTATE	Antibacterial	**Powd for Inj**: 1 g	**Usual Dosage**: 5 - 20 mg/kg/day by continuous IV infusion or in divided doses q 6 h IV. **Acute Pelvic Inflammatory Disease due to *N. gonorrhoeae***: 500 mg q 6 h IV for at least 3 days, followed by 250 mg of oral erythromycin q 6 h for 7 days.

GENERIC NAME	COMMON TRADE NAMES	THERAPEUTIC CATEGORY	PREPARATIONS	COMMON ADULT DOSAGE
Erythromycin Lactobionate	ERYTHROCIN IV	Antibacterial	**Powd for Inj**: 500 mg; 1 g	**Severe Infections**: 15-20 mg/kg/day by contin. IV infusion or by intermittent IV infusion in 20 - 60 min periods at intervals of ≤ 6 h.
Erythromycin Stearate	ERYTHROCIN STEARATE	Antibacterial	**Tab**: 250, 500 mg	**Usual Dosage**: 250 mg q 6 h po or 500 mg q 12 h po on an empty stomach or ac. **Streptococcal Infections**: Administer the usual dosage for at least 10 days. **Acute Pelvic Inflammatory Disease due to *N. gonorrhoeae***: After initial treatment with erythromycin lactobionate, give 250 mg q 6 h po for 7 days. **Urogenital Infections during pregnancy and Uncomplicated Urethral, Endocervical, or Rectal Infections due to *C. trachomatis***: 500 mg qid po for at least 7 days. **Intestinal Amebiasis**: 250 mg qid po for 10 to 14 days. **Legionnaires Disease**: 1 - 4 g daily po in divided doses.
Esmolol Hydrochloride	BREVIBLOC	Antiarrhythmic	**Inj (per mL)**: 10, 250 mg	500 μg/kg/min IV for 1 minute followed by a 4-minute infusion of 50 μg/kg/min. If an adequate effect is not seen within 5 min., repeat loading dose followed by a 4-minute infusion of 100 μg/kg/min. Continue process as above, increasing maintenance infusion by increments of 50 μg/kg/min. As the desired effect is reached, omit loading dose & lower incremental dose in maintenance infusion from 50 μg/kg/min to 25 μg/kg/min or lower.
Estazolam (C-IV)	PROSOM	Hypnotic	**Tab**: 1, 2 mg	1 - 2 mg hs po.

Estradiol	ESTRACE	Estrogen	**Tab**: 0.5, 1, 2 mg	**Menopausal Symptoms**: 1 - 2 mg daily po. **Prostatic Cancer**: 1 - 2 mg tid po. **Breast Cancer**: 10 mg tid po for at least 3 mos. **Osteoporosis Prevention**: 0.5 mg daily po cyclically (23 days on, 5 days off) as soon as possible after menopause.
			Vaginal Cream: 0.01%	**Initial**: 2 - 4 g intravaginally daily for 1 - 2 weeks, then gradually reduce to 1/2 initial dose for a similar period. **Maintenance**: 1 g intravag. 1 - 3 times a week.
	ESTRING		**Vaginal Ring**: 2 mg	**Urogenital Symptoms associated with Post-menopausal Vaginal Atrophy**: Insert 1 ring as deeply as possible into the upper third of the vagina. Leave in place for 3 mos, then remove and replace if necessary.
	FEMPATCH		**Transdermal**: rate = 0.025 mg/24 h	**Vulval or Vaginal Atrophy, Hypoestrogenism, and Vasomotor Symptoms associated with Menopause**: Initially, apply 1 patch to the skin on the buttocks once a week. If symptoms are not relieved after 4 - 6 weeks, 2 patches may be applied weekly.
	ESTRADERM		**Transdermal**: rate = 0.05, 0.1 mg/24 h	**Vulval or Vaginal Atrophy, Hypoestrogenism, and Vasomotor Symptoms associated with Menopause**: Initially, apply 1 patch (0.05 mg) to the skin on the trunk of the body (including the abdomen and buttocks) once a week (CLIMARA) or twice a week (ALORA, ESTRADERM and VIVELLE). Adjust dosage as necessary (with the lowest dosage needed to control symptoms, especially in women with a intact uterus). **Prophylactic Therapy to Prevent Postmeno-pausal Bone Loss**: Initiate with 0.05 mg/day as soon as possible after menopause. Adjust dosage as necessary to control menopausal symptoms.
	ALORA		**Transdermal**: rate = 0.05, 0.075, 0.1 mg/24 h	
	CLIMARA		**Transdermal**: rate = 0.025, 0.05, 0.075, 0.1 mg/24 h	
	VIVELLE, VIVELLE-DOT		**Transdermal**: rate = 0.0375, 0.05, 0.075, 0.1 mg/24 h	

[Continued on the next page]

GENERIC NAME	COMMON TRADE NAMES	THERAPEUTIC CATEGORY	PREPARATIONS	COMMON ADULT DOSAGE
Estradiol [Continued]				**Therapeutic Regimen**: May give continuously to patients who do not have an intact uterus. In patients with an intact uterus, may give on a cyclic schedule (3 weeks on the drug, followed by 1 week off the drug).
Estradiol Cypionate	DEPO-ESTRADIOL	Estrogen	**Inj (per mL)**: 5 mg (in oil)	**Menopausal Symptoms**: 1 - 5 mg IM q 3 - 4 weeks. **Female Hypogonadism**: 1.5 - 2 mg IM monthly.
Estradiol Hemihydrate	VAGIFEM	Estrogen	**Vaginal Tab**: 25 μg	**Atrophic Vaginitis:** **Initial Dose**: Insert 1 tab vaginally once daily (at the same time each day) for 2 weeks. **Maintenance**: Insert 1 tab vaginally twice weekly.
Estradiol Valerate	DELESTROGEN	Estrogen	**Inj (per mL)**: 10, 20, 40 mg (in oil)	**Menopausal Symptoms**: 10 - 20 mg IM q 4 weeks. **Female Hypogonadism**: 10 - 20 mg IM q 4 weeks given cyclically.
Estramustine Phosphate	EMCYT	Antineoplastic	**Cpsl**: 140 mg	14 mg/kg/day (1 cpsl per 22 lb) in 3 or 4 divided doses po.
Estrogens, Conjugated	PREMARIN	Estrogen, Antineoplastic	**Tab**: 0.3, 0.625, 0.9, 1.25, 2.5 mg	**Female Hypogonadism**: 2.5 - 7.5 mg daily po in divided doses for 20 days, followed by a rest period of 10 days. If bleeding does not occur by the end of this period, the same dosage schedule is repeated. If bleeding occurs before the end of the 10 day period, begin a 20 day regimen with 2.5 - 7.5 mg daily po in divided doses; add an oral progestin during the last 5 days of therapy. If bleeding occur before before this regimen ends, therapy is discontinued and may be resumed on the 5th day of bleeding.

				Vasomotor Symptoms associated with Menopause: 1.25 mg daily po. Administer on a cyclic schedule (3 weeks on the drug, followed by 1 week off the drug). **Atrophic Vaginitis**: 0.3 - 1.25 mg daily po. Administer cyclically as noted above. **Osteoporosis**: 0.625 mg daily po, cyclically (3 weeks on, 1 week off). **Mammary Carcinoma**: 10 mg tid po for at least 3 months. **Prostatic Carcinoma**: 1.25 - 2.5 mg tid po.
		Estrogen	**Vaginal Cream**: 0.625 mg/g	2 - 4 g (1/2 - 1 applicatorful) intravaginally daily. Administration should be cyclic (3 weeks on, 1 week off).
Estrogens, A Synthetic Conjugated	CENESTIN	Estrogen	**Tab**: 0.625, 0.9 mg	**Vasomotor Symptoms associated with Menopause**: Initially, 0.625 mg daily po. Administer on a cyclic schedule (3 weeks on the drug, followed by 1 week off the drug).
Estrogens, Esterified	ESTRATAB, MENEST	Estrogen, Antineoplastic	**Tab**: 0.3, 0.625, 1.25, 2.5 mg	**Female Hypogonadism**: 2.5 - 7.5 mg daily po, in divided doses for 20 days, followed by a rest period of 10 days. If bleeding does not occur by the end of this period, the same dosage schedule is repeated. If bleeding occurs before the end of the 10 day period, begin a 20 day regimen with 2.5 - 7.5 mg daily po in divided doses; add an oral progestin during the last 5 days of therapy. If bleeding occur before before this regimen ends, therapy is discontinued and may be resumed on the 5th day of bleeding. **Vasomotor Symptoms**: 1.25 mg daily po. Administration should be cyclic (3 weeks on the drug, followed by 1 week off). **Atrophic Vaginitis and Kraurosis Vulvae**: 0.3 to 1.25 mg daily po. Administer cyclically.

[Continued on the next page]

GENERIC NAME	COMMON TRADE NAMES	THERAPEUTIC CATEGORY	PREPARATIONS	COMMON ADULT DOSAGE
Estrogens, Esterified [Continued]	ESTRATAB, MENEST			**Osteoporosis Prevention**: 0.3 mg daily po and increase to a maximum of 1.25 mg daily po, if necessary. **Prostatic Cancer**: 1.25 - 2.5 mg tid po. **Breast Cancer in Men and Postmenopausal Women**: 10 mg tid po for at least 3 months.
Estropipate	OGEN	Estrogen, Antiosteoporotic	**Tab**: 0.75, 1.5, 3 mg (equivalent to sodium estrone sulfate: 0.625, 1.25, 2.5 mg respectively)	**Female Hypogonadism**: 1.5 - 9 mg daily po for the first 3 weeks of a theoretical cycle, followed by a rest period of 8 - 10 days. If bleeding does not occur by the end of this period, the same dosage schedule is repeated. If bleeding does not occur, an oral progestin may be added during the third week of the cycle. **Vasomotor Symptoms and Vulval and Vaginal Atrophy**: 0.75 - 6 mg daily po. Administration should be cyclic (3 weeks on the drug, followed by 1 week off). **Prevention of Osteoporosis**: 0.75 mg daily po for 25 days of a 31 day cycle per month.
	ORTHO-EST		**Tab**: 0.75, 1.5 mg (equivalent to sodium estrone sulfate: 0.625, 1.25 mg respectively)	
	OGEN	Estrogen	**Vaginal Cream**: 1.5 mg/g	2 - 4 g intravaginally daily. Administration should be cyclic (3 weeks on, 1 week off).
Etanercept	ENBREL	Antirheumatic	**Powd for Inj**: 25 mg	25 mg twice weekly by SC injection.
Ethacrynate Sodium	SODIUM EDECRIN	Diuretic	**Powd for Inj**: 50 mg	0.5 - 1.0 mg/kg IV (maximum: 100 mg).
Ethacrynic Acid	EDECRIN	Diuretic	**Tab**: 25, 50 mg	50 - 100 mg daily po.
Ethambutol Hydrochloride	MYAMBUTOL	Tuberculostatic	**Tab**: 100, 400 mg	**Initial**: 15 mg/kg po as a single dose q 24 h. **Retreatment**: 25 mg/kg po as a single dose q 24 h. After 60 days, decrease dose to 15 mg/kg po as a single dose q 24 h.
Ethchlorvynol (C-IV)	PLACIDYL	Sedative - Hypnotic	**Cpsl**: 200, 500, 750 mg	500 mg hs po.

Ethinyl Estradiol	ESTINYL	Estrogen, Antineoplastic	**Tab**: 0.02, 0.05, 0.5 mg	**Vasomotor Symptoms associated with Menopause**: 0.02 - 0.05 mg daily po. Administration should be cyclic (3 weeks on, 1 week off). **Prostatic Cancer**: 0.15 - 2.0 mg daily po. **Breast Cancer**: 1.0 mg tid po.
Ethionamide	TRECATOR-SC	Tuberculostatic	**Tab**: 250 mg	0.5 - 1 g daily in divided doses po.
Ethotoin	PEGANONE	Antiepileptic	**Tab**: 250, 500 mg	**Initial**: 1 g or less daily po in 4 - 6 divided doses, with gradual increases over a period of several days. Take after meals. **Maintenance**: Usually 2 - 3 g daily po in 4 - 6 divided doses after food.
Etidronate Disodium	DIDRONEL	Bone Stabilizer	**Tab**: 200, 400 mg	**Paget's Disease**: Initially, 5 mg/kg daily po, not to exceed 6 months. May increase to 10 mg/kg daily po, not to exceed 6 months or to 11 - 20 mg/kg daily po, not to exceed 3 months. Take on an empty stomach 2 h ac.
	DIDRONEL I.V. INFUSION		**Inj**: 300 mg/6 mL	7.5 mg/kg daily by IV infusion (over at least 2 h) for 3 days. Daily dose must be diluted in at least 250 mL of sterile normal saline.
Etodolac	LODINE	Non-Opioid Analgesic, Antiinflammatory	**Cpsl**: 200, 300 mg **Tab**: 400, 500 mg	**Analgesia**: 200 - 400 mg q 6 - 8 h po. **Osteoarthritis & Rheumatoid Arthritis**: Initially, 300 mg bid or tid po, 400 mg bid po, or 500 mg bid po. Adjust dosage within 600 to 1200 mg/day po prn for maintenance.
	LODINE XL	Antiinflammatory	**Extended-Rel. Tab**: 400, 500, 600 mg	**Osteoarthritis & Rheumatoid Arthritis**: 400 to 1000 mg once daily po.

GENERIC NAME	COMMON TRADE NAMES	THERAPEUTIC CATEGORY	PREPARATIONS	COMMON ADULT DOSAGE
Etoposide	VEPESID	Antineoplastic	**Inj**: 100 mg/5 mL	**Testicular Cancer**: Ranges from 50 - 100 mg/m^2/day IV for days 1 - 5 to 100 mg/m^2/day IV for day 1, 3 and 5. Repeat at 3 - 4 week intervals. **Small Cell Lung Cancer**: Ranges from 35 mg/m^2/day IV for 4 days to 50 mg/m^2/day IV for 5 days. Repeat at 3 - 4 week intervals.
			Cpsl: 50 mg	**Small Cell Lung Cancer**: Twice the IV dose po, rounded to the nearest 50 mg.
Etretinate	TEGISON	Anti-Psoriasis Agent	**Cpsl**: 10, 25 mg	**Initial**: 0.75 - 1 mg/kg/day po in divided doses. **Maintenance**: 0.5 - 0.75 mg/kg/day po (after 8 to 16 weeks).
Exemestane	AROMASIN	Antineoplastic	**Tab**: 25 mg	25 mg once daily po pc.
Famciclovir	FAMVIR	Antiviral	**Tab**: 125, 250, 500 mg	**Herpes zoster**: 500 mg q 8 h po for 7 days. **Genital Herpes (Recurrent)**: 125 mg bid po for 5 days.
Famotidine	PEPCID	Histamine H_2-Blocker, Anti-Ulcer Agent	**Powd for Susp**: 40 mg/5 mL **Tab**: 20, 40 mg	**Duodenal Ulcer**: **Acute**: 40 mg hs po; or 20 mg bid po. **Maintenance**: 20 mg hs po. **Active Benign Gastric Ulcer**: 40 mg hs po. **Pathol. Hypersecr. Conditions**: 20 mg q 6 h po. **Gastroesophageal Reflux Disease**: 20 mg bid po for up to 6 weeks.
	PEPCID INJECTION		**Inj**: 10 mg/mL	20 mg q 12 h IV.
	PEPCID INJECTION PREMIXED		**Inj**: 20 mg/50 mL	20 mg q 12 h by IV infusion (over 15 - 30 minutes).
	PEPCID AC	Histamine H_2-Blocker	**Tab**: 10 mg **Chewable Tab**: 10 mg	**Heartburn, Acid Indigestion & Sour Stomach**: **Treatment**: 10 mg po with water up to bid. **Prevention**: 10 mg po 1 h prior to eating symptom-causing foods or drinks. Repeat up to bid.
	MYLANTA AR ACID REDUCER		**Tab**: 10 mg	

Felbamate	FELBATOL	Antiepileptic	**Tab**: 400, 600 mg **Susp**: 600 mg/5 mL	**Monotherapy**: Begin at 1200 mg/day po, in 3 to 4 divided doses. Titrate under close supervision, increasing the dosage in 600 mg increments q 2 weeks to 2400 mg/day, and thereafter to 3600 mg/day if indicated. **Adjunctive Therapy**: Add 1200 mg/day po (in 3 to 4 divided doses) while lowering the dose of present antiepileptic drug by 20%. Further reductions in these drug may be necessary to minimize adverse effects due to drug interactions. Raise the dosage of felbamate by 1200 mg/day increments at weekly intervals to 3600 mg/day if necessary.
Felodipine	PLENDIL	Antihypertensive	**Extended-Rel. Tab**: 2,5, 5, 10 mg	Initially, 5 mg once daily po. Dosage may be decreased to 2.5 mg or increased to 10 mg once daily po after 2 weeks.
Fenofibrate	TRICOR	Hypolipidemic	**Cpsl**: 67 mg	Initially 67 mg once daily po with meals. The maximum dose is 3 capsules (201 mg) daily.
Fenoprofen Calcium	NALFON	Non-Opioid Analgesic, Antiinflammatiory	**Cpsl**: 200, 300 mg **Tab**: 600 mg	**Analgesia**: 200 mg q 4 - 6 h po, prn. **Rheumatoid Arthritis and Osteoarthritis**: 300 to 600 mg tid to qid po.
Fentanyl (C-II)	DURAGESIC	Opioid Analgesic	**Transdermal**: rate = 25, 50, 75, 100 μg/hr	Individualize dosage. Each system may be worn for up to 72 h.
Fentanyl Citrate (C-II)	SUBLIMAZE	Opioid Analgesic	**Inj**: 50 μg/mL (as the base)	2 - 50 μg/kg IM or IV.
	FENTANYL ORALET	Opioid Analgesic	**Lozenge**: 100, 200, 300, 400 μg	Administer only in a hospital setting. Individualize dosage. Fentanyl transmucosal doses of 5 μg/kg (400 μg) provide effects similar to usual doses of fentanyl citrate given IM, i.e., 0.75 - 1.25 μg/kg. Oral administration should begin 20 - 40 minutes prior to anticipated need of desired effect.

[Continued on the next page]

GENERIC NAME	COMMON TRADE NAMES	THERAPEUTIC CATEGORY	PREPARATIONS	COMMON ADULT DOSAGE
Fentanyl Citrate (C-II) [Continued]	ACTIQ		**Lozenge on a Stick**: 200, 400, 600, 800, 1200, 1600 μg	Initial dose to treat episodes of breakthrough cancer pain should be 200 μg consumed over a 15-min. period. Prescribe an initial titration supply of six 200 μg units. Advise patients to use all units before increasing to a higher dose. Redosing should not occur more often than q 30 min. Dose increases may be occur after evaluation over several episodes of breakthrough cancer pain.
Ferrous Gluconate (11.6% iron)	FERGON	Hematinic	**Tab**: 320 mg	320 mg daily po.
Ferrous Sulfate (20% iron)	FEOSOL	Hematinic	**Elixir**: 220 mg/5 mL (5% alcohol)	5 - 10 mL tid po, preferably between meals.
	FER-IN-SOL		**Syrup**: 90 mg/5 mL (5% alc.)	5 mL daily po.
	FERO-GRADUMET		**Controlled-Rel. Tab**: 525 mg	525 mg once daily or bid po.
Ferrous Sulfate, Exsiccated (30% iron)	FEOSOL	Hematinic	**Tab**: 200 mg **Cpsl**: 159 mg	200 mg tid - qid po pc & hs. 159 - 318 mg daily po.
	FER-IN-SOL		**Cpsl**: 190 mg	1 capsule daily po.
	SLOW FE		**Slow Release Tab**: 160 mg	160 - 320 mg daily po.
Fexofenadine Hydrochloride	ALLEGRA	Antihistamine	**Cpsl**: 60 mg	60 mg bid po.
Finasteride	PROSCAR	Benign Prostatic Hyperplasia Drug	**Tab**: 5 mg	5 mg once daily po.
	PROPECIA	Hair Growth Stimulator	**Tab**: 1 mg	1 mg once daily po.
Flavoxate Hydrochloride	URISPAS	Urinary Tract Antispasmodic	**Tab**: 100 mg	100 - 200 mg tid or qid po.

Flecainide Acetate	TAMBOCOR	Antiarrhythmic	**Tab**: 50, 100, 150 mg	Initially, 100 mg q 12 h po. May increase in increments of 50 mg bid q 4 days.
Floxuridine	STERILE FUDR	Antineoplastic	**Powd for Inj**: 500 mg	0.1 - 0.6 mg/kg/day by intra-arterial infusion.
Fluconazole	DIFLUCAN	Antifungal	**Tab**: 50, 100, 150, 200 mg **Powd for Susp**: 10, 40 mg/mL **Inj**: 200 mg/100 mL, 400 mg/200 mL	**Oropharyngeal Candidiasis**: 200 mg on the first day, followed by 100 mg once daily po or IV. Continue treatment for at least 2 weeks. **Esophageal Candidiasis**: 200 mg on the first day, followed by 100 mg once daily po or IV. Doses up to 400 mg may be used based on the patient response. Continue treatment for a minimum of 3 weeks and at least 2 weeks following resolution of symptoms. **Systemic Candidiasis and Cryptococcal Meningitis**: 400 mg on the first day, followed by 200 mg once daily po or IV. **Vaginal Candidiasis**: 150 mg po as a single dose.
Flucytosine	ANCOBON	Antifungal	**Cpsl**: 250, 500 mg	50 - 150 mg/kg/day po in divided doses at 6-hour intervals.
Fludrocortisone Acetate	FLORINEF ACETATE	Mineralocorticoid	**Tab**: 0.1 mg	0.1 mg daily po. If transient hypertension develops, reduce dosage to 0.05 mg daily.
Flumazenil	ROMAZICON	Benzodiazepine Antagonist	**Inj**: 0.1 mg/mL	**Reversal of Conscious Sedation or in General Anesthesia**: Initially 0.2 mg IV (over 15 seconds). After 45 seconds, a further dose of 0.2 mg can be injected and repeated at 60-second intervals where necessary (up to a maximum of 4 additional times) to a maximum total dose of 1 mg. **Management of Suspected Benzodiazepine Overdose**: Initially 0.2 mg IV (over 30 seconds). After 30 seconds, a further dose of 0.3 mg can be injected (over 30 seconds). Further doses of 0.5 mg can be given (over 30 seconds) at 60-second intervals up to a cumulative dose of 3 mg.

GENERIC NAME	COMMON TRADE NAMES	THERAPEUTIC CATEGORY	PREPARATIONS	COMMON ADULT DOSAGE
Flunisolide	AEROBID	Corticosteroid	**Aerosol**: 250 μg/spray	2 inhalations bid AM and PM.
	NASALIDE, NASAREL		**Spray**: 25 μg/spray	2 sprays in each nostril bid.
Fluocinolone Acetonide	SYNALAR	Corticosteroid	**Cream**: 0.01, 0.025% **Oint**: 0.025% **Solution**: 0.01%	Apply as a thin film bid - qid.
	SYNALAR-HP		**Cream**: 0.2%	Apply as a thin film bid - qid.
Fluocinonide	LIDEX	Corticosteroid	**Cream, Oint, Gel & Solution**: 0.05%	Apply as a thin film bid - qid.
Fluorometholone	FML	Corticosteroid	**Ophth Susp**: 0.1%	1 drop into affected eye(s) bid - qid. During the initial 24 - 48 hours, the frequency of dosing may be increased if necessary.
	FML FORTE		**Ophth Susp**: 0.25%	1 drop into affected eye(s) bid - qid.
	FML		**Ophth Oint**: 0.1%	Apply 1/2 inch ribbon to eye(s) q 4 h for the 1st 24 - 48 h. When a favorable response is observed, reduce dosage to 1 - 3 times daily.
Fluorometholone Acetate	FLAREX	Corticosteroid	**Ophth Susp**: 0.1%	1 - 2 drops into affected eye(s) qid. May initiate with 2 drops q 2 h during the initial 24 - 48 hours; then, the frequency of dosing may be decreased.
Fluorouracil	FLUOROURACIL INJECTION	Antineoplastic	**Inj**: 500 mg/10 mL	12 mg/kg daily IV for 4 days. If no toxicity is observed, 6 mg/kg are given on days 6, 8, 10 and 12. May repeat course in 30 days.
	EFUDEX		**Cream**: 5% **Solution**: 2, 5%	**Actinic or Solar Keratosis**: Cover lesions bid; continue therapy for at least 2 - 4 weeks. **Superficial Basal Cell Carcinomas**: Use only 5% cream or solution. Cover lesions bid; continue therapy for at least 3 - 6 weeks.

	FLUOROPLEX		**Cream & Solution**: 1%	Cover all lesions bid. Continue therapy for 2 to 6 weeks.
Fluoxetine Hydrochloride	PROZAC	Antidepressant, Drug for Obsessive-Compulsive Disorder	**Cpsl**: 10, 20, 40 mg **Tab**: 10 mg **Liquid**: 20 mg/5 mL (0.23% alcohol)	20 mg daily po in the AM. May increase dose after several weeks to 20 mg bid po. Do not exceed maximum dose of 80 mg/day.
Fluoxymesterone (C-III)	HALOTESTIN	Androgen	**Tab**: 2, 5, 10 mg	**Male Hypogonadism**: 5 - 20 mg daily po as a single dose or in 3 - 4 divided doses. **Breast Cancer**: 10 - 40 mg daily po in 3 - 4 divided doses.
Fluphenazine Decanoate	PROLIXIN DECANOATE	Antipsychotic	**Inj**: 25 mg/mL	12.5 - 25 mg IM or SC.
Fluphenazine Enanthate	PROLIXIN ENANTHATE	Antipsychotic	**Inj**: 25 mg/mL	25 mg IM or SC q 2 weeks.
Fluphenazine Hydrochloride	PROLIXIN	Antipsychotic	**Tab**: 1, 2.5, 5, 10 mg **Elixir**: 2.5 mg/5 mL (14% alcohol)	2.5 - 10 mg daily po in divided doses at 6- to 8-hour intervals.
			Inj: 2.5 mg/mL	1.25 - 10 mg daily IM in divided doses at 6- to 8-hour intervals.
Flurandrenolide	CORDRAN	Corticosteroid	**Cream & Oint**: 0.025, 0.05% **Lotion**: 0.05% **Tape**: 4 mcg/cm^2	Apply as a thin film to affected areas bid - tid and rub in gently. Apply to affected areas; replace q 12 h.
Flurazepam Hydrochloride (C-IV)	DALMANE	Hypnotic	**Cpsl**: 15, 30 mg	15 - 30 mg hs po.
Flurbiprofen	ANSAID	Antiinflammatory	**Tab**: 50, 100 mg	200 - 300 mg daily, given bid, tid or qid po.
Flurbiprofen Sodium	OCUFEN	Antiinflammatory (Topical)	**Ophth Solution**: 0.03%	1 drop in eye q 30 minutes, beginning 2 h before surgery (total of 4 drops).
Flutamide	EULEXIN	Antineoplastic	**Cpsl**: 125 mg	250 mg tid po at 8-hour intervals.

GENERIC NAME	COMMON TRADE NAMES	THERAPEUTIC CATEGORY	PREPARATIONS	COMMON ADULT DOSAGE
Fluticasone Propionate	CUTIVATE	Corticosteroid	**Oint**: 0.005% **Cream**: 0.05%	Apply a thin film to affected skin areas bid. Rub in gently.
	FLONASE	Corticosteroid	**Nasal Spray**: 50 µg/spray	Initially, 2 sprays in each nostril once daily or 1 spray in each nostril twice daily (morning and evening). May decrease to 1 spray in each nostril once daily based on response. **For Adolescents over 12 yrs**: Initially, 1 spray in each nostril once daily; may increase to 2 sprays in each nostril once daily, then may decrease to 1 spray in each nostril once daily based on response.
	FLOVENT 44 mcg FLOVENT 110 mcg FLOVENT 220 mcg	Corticosteroid	**Aerosol**: 44 µg/spray **Aerosol**: 110 µg/spray **Aerosol**: 220 µg/spray	**Patients Previously Using Bronchodilators Only**: 88 µg bid. **Patients Previously Using Inhaled Corticosteroids**: 88 - 220 µg bid. **Patient Previously Using Oral Corticosteroids**: 880 µg bid.
Fluvastatin Sodium	LESCOL	Hypolipidemic	**Cpsl**: 20, 40 mg	20 - 40 mg once daily po hs.
Fluvoxamine Maleate	LUVOX	Drug for Obsessive-Compulsive Disorder	**Tab**: 25, 50, 100 mg	Initially, 50 mg hs po. Increase dose in 50 mg increments q 4 - 7 days, as tolerated, until maximum therapeutic benefit occurs. Daily dosages over 100 mg should be given in divided doses (bid). Maximum: 300 mg/day.
Folic Acid		Vitamin	**Tab**: 0.4, 0.8, 1 mg	**Usual Therapeutic Dose**: up to 1 mg daily po.
Foscarnet Sodium	FOSCAVIR	Antiviral	**Inj**: 24 mg/mL	**CMV Retinitis**: **Initial**: 60 mg/kg IV (at a constant rate over a minimum of 1 h) q 8 h for 2 - 3 weeks. **Maintenance**: 90 mg/kg/day by IV infusion (over 2 h).

				***Herpes Simplex* Infection:** **Initial:** 40 mg/kg by IV infusion (over at least 1 h) q 8 or 12 h for 2 - 3 weeks or until healed. **Maintenance:** 90 mg/kg/day by IV infusion (over 2 h).
Fosfomycin Tromethamine	MONUROL	Urinary Ant-Infective	**Granules:** 3 g	**Women > 18 yrs:** Pour the contents of 1 packet into 3 - 4 fl. oz. of water; stir to dissolve. Drink immediately.
Fosinopril Sodium	MONOPRIL	Antihypertensive, Heart Failure Drug	**Tab:** 10, 20, 40 mg	**Hypertension:** Initially, 10 mg once daily po. May increase dosage to usual range: 20 to 40 mg daily. **Heart Failure:** Initially, 10 mg once daily po. Increase dosage over several weeks to a maximal and tolerated dose not to exceed 40 mg once daily.
Fosphenytoin Sodium	CEREBYX	Antiepileptic	**Powd for Inj:** 150 mg (100 mg of phenytoin sodium), 750 mg (500 mg of phenytoin sodium)	Dosages given as phenytoin sodium equivalent units (PE). **Status Epilepticus:** Loading Dose of 15 - 20 mg PE/kg IV given at 100 - 150 mg PE/min. **Nonemergent and Maintenance Dosing:** **Loading Dose:** 10 - 20 mg PE/kg IM or IV (at a rate ≤ 150 mg PE/min). **Maintenance Dose:** 4 - 6 mg PE/kg/day.
Furazolidone	FUROXONE	Antibacterial	**Liquid:** 50 mg/15 mL **Tab:** 100 mg	100 mg qid po.
Furosemide	LASIX	Diuretic, Antihypertensive	**Solution:** 10 mg/mL (11.5% alcohol) **Tab:** 20, 40, 80 mg	**Diuresis:** 20 - 80 mg daily po. May repeat in 6 to 8 h if needed. **Hypertension:** 40 mg bid po.
		Diuretic	**Inj:** 10 mg/mL	**Diuresis:** 20 - 40 mg IM or IV (over 1 - 2 min). **Acute Pulmonary Edema:** 40 mg IV (over 1 - 2 min). If response is not adequate after 1 h, dose may be doubled.

GENERIC NAME	COMMON TRADE NAMES	THERAPEUTIC CATEGORY	PREPARATIONS	COMMON ADULT DOSAGE
Gabapentin	NEURONTIN	Antiepileptic	**Cpsl**: 100, 300, 400 mg	Titrate with 300 mg po on day 1, 300 mg bid po on day 2, and 300 mg tid po on day 3. If necessary, the dosage may be increased by using 300 - 400 mg tid up to 1800 mg/day.
Gallium Nitrate	GANITE	Hypocalcemic	**Inj**: 25 mg/mL	200 mg/m^2 daily by IV infusion (over 24 h) for 5 consecutive days.
Ganciclovir	CYTOVENE	Antiviral	**Cpsl**: 250 mg	**CMV Retinitis (Maintenance)**: Following the IV induction treatment with CYTOVENE-IV (see below), 1000 mg tid po with food. Alternatively, 500 mg 6 times daily po (q 3 h during waking hours) with food. **Prevention of CMV in Patients with Advanced HIV Infection**: 1000 mg tid po with food.
Ganciclovir Sodium	CYTOVENE-IV	Antiviral	**Powd for Inj**: 500 mg	**CMV Retinitis**: **Induction**: 5 mg/kg IV (at a constant rate over 1 hour), q 12 h for 14 - 21 days. **Maintenance**: 5 mg/kg IV (at a constant rate over 1 hour), once daily 7 days each week, or 6 mg/kg IV once daily on 5 days each week. **Prevention of CMV in Transplant Recipients**: Initially, 5 mg/kg IV (at a constant rate over 1 hour), q 12 h for 7 - 14 days; then, 5 mg/kg IV once daily 7 days each week, or 6 mg/kg IV once daily on 5 days each week.
Gatifloxacin Sesquihydrate	TEQUIN	Antibacterial	**Tab**: 200, 400 mg **Inj**: 10 mg/mL	**Complicated Urinary Tract Infections, Bronchitis, Pyelonephritis**: 400 mg once daily po or by slow IV infusion for 7 - 10 days. **Pneumonia**: 400 mg once daily po or by slow IV infusion for 7 - 14 days. **Sinusitis**: 400 mg once daily po or by slow IV infusion for 10 days. **Gonorrhea**: 400 mg po or by slow IV infusion as a single dose.

Gemfibrozil	LOPID	Hypolipidemic	**Tab**: 600 mg	600 mg bid po 30 minutes before the morning and evening meal.
Gentamicin Sulfate	GARAMYCIN	Antibacterial	**Cream & Oint**: 0.1% **Ophth Solution**: 3 mg/mL	Apply to affected areas tid to qid. 1 - 2 drops into affected eye(s) q 4 h. In severe infections, dosage may be increased to as much as 2 drops once every hour.
			Ophth Oint: 3 mg/g	Apply to affected eye(s) bid or tid.
			Inj: 40 mg/mL	**Usual Dosage**: 3 mg/kg/day IM or IV divided in 3 doses at 8-hour intervals. **Life-Threatening Infections**: Up to 5 mg/kg/day may be administered in 3 or 4 equal doses.
Glatiramer Acetate	COPAXONE	Multiple Sclerosis Drug	**Powd for Inj**: 20 mg	20 mg daily SC.
Glimepiride	AMARYL	Hypoglycemic Agent	**Tab**: 1, 2, 4 mg	**Initial**: 1 - 2 mg once daily po, given with breakfast or the first main meal. **Maintenance**: 1 - 4 mg once daily po. After a dose of 2 mg is reached, increase the dose at increments of ≤ 2 mg at 1 - 2 week intervals based on patient's blood glucose.
Glipizide	GLUCOTROL	Hypoglycemic Agent	**Tab**: 5, 10 mg	**Initial**: 5 mg daily po before breakfast. **Titration**: As determined by blood glucose response, increase dosage in increments of 2.5 - 5 mg. At least several days should elapse between titration steps. **Maintenance**: Total daily doses above 15 mg should ordinarily be divided, e.g., bid.
	GLUCOTROL XL		**Extended-Rel. Tab**: 2.5, 5, 10 mg	Initially, 5 mg daily po with breakfast. Usual dosage range: 5 - 10 mg daily po.
Glyburide	DIAβETA, MICRONASE	Hypoglycemic Agent	**Tab**: 1.25, 2.5, 5 mg	**Initial**: 1.25 - 5 mg daily po with breakfast. **Maintenance**: 1.25 - 20 mg daily po as a single dose or in divided doses.

GENERIC NAME	COMMON TRADE NAMES	THERAPEUTIC CATEGORY	PREPARATIONS	COMMON ADULT DOSAGE
Glyburide Micronized	GLYNASE PRESTAB	Hypoglycemic Agent	**Tab**: 1.5, 3, 6 mg	**Initial**: 0.75 - 3 mg daily po with breakfast. **Maintenance**: 0.75 - 12 mg daily po as a single dose or in divided doses.
Glycopyrrolate	ROBINUL	Anticholinergic	**Tab**: 1 mg	**Initial**: 1 mg tid po (in the morning, early afternoon, and hs. **Maintenance**: 1 mg bid po is often adequate.
	ROBINUL FORTE		**Tab**: 2 mg	2 mg bid or tid po at equally spaced intervals.
Gold Sodium Thiomalate		Antirheumatic	**Inj (per mL)**: 50 mg	Weekly IM injections as follows: 1st– 10 mg; 2nd– 25 mg; 3rd and subsequent– 25 - 50 mg until toxicity or major improvement. Maintenance doses: 25 - 50 mg every other week for 2 - 20 weeks. If condition remains stable, give 25 - 50 mg every 3rd week.
Goserelin Acetate	ZOLADEX	Antineoplastic	**Powd for Inj**: 3.6 mg	3.6 mg q 28 days by SC injection into the upper abdominal wall.
Granisetron Hydrochloride	KYTRIL	Antiemetic	**Tab**: 1.12 mg (1 mg as the base)	1 mg bid po. The 1st dose is given up to 1 h before chemotherapy and the 2nd dose 12 h after the 1st, only on the days chemotherapy is given.
			Inj: 1.12 mg/mL (1 mg/mL as the base)	10 μg/kg, infused IV over 5 minutes, beginning within 30 minutes before initiation of chemotherapy, and only on the days that chemotherapy is given.
Griseofulvin Microsize	FULVICIN U/F	Antifungal	**Tab**: 250, 500 mg	500 mg daily po as a single dose or in divided doses.
	GRIFULVIN V		**Susp**: 125 mg/5 mL **Tab**: 250, 500 mg	500 mg daily po.
	GRISACTIN 500		**Tab**: 500 mg	500 mg daily po as a single dose or in divided doses, e.g., 250 mg bid.

Griseofulvin Ultramicrosize	FULVICIN P/G	Antifungal	**Tab**: 125, 165, 250, 330 mg	330 - 375 mg daily po as a single dose or in divided doses.
	GRISACTIN ULTRA		**Tab**: 250, 330 mg	330 mg daily po as a single dose or in divided doses.
	GRIS-PEG		**Tab**: 125, 250 mg	375 mg daily po (single dose or in div. doses).
Guaifenesin	ROBITUSSIN	Expectorant	**Syrup**: 100 mg/5 mL	10 - 20 mL (100 - 400 mg) q 4 h po.
	NALDECON SENIOR EX		**Liquid**: 200 mg/5 mL	200 mg q 4 h po.
	ORGANIDIN NR		**Liquid**: 100 mg/5 mL **Tab**: 200 mg	200 - 400 mg q 4 h po. 200 - 400 mg q 4 h po.
	HUMIBID SPRINKLE HUMIBID L.A.		**Sustained-Rel. Cpsl**: 300 mg **Sustained-Rel. Tab**: 600 mg	600 - 1200 mg q 12 h po.
	DURATUSS G		**Long-Acting Tab**: 1200 mg	1200 mg q 12 h po.
Guanabenz Acetate	WYTENSIN	Antihypertensive	**Tab**: 4, 8 mg	Initially, 4 mg bid po. May increase dosage in increments of 4 - 8 mg/day q 1 - 2 weeks.
Guanadrel Sulfate	HYLOREL	Antihypertensive	**Tab**: 10, 25 mg	Initially, 5 mg bid po. Adjust dosage weekly; most require 20 - 75 mg/day (given bid).
Guanethidine Monosulfate	ISMELIN	Antihypertensive	**Tab**: 10, 25 mg	**Ambulatory Patients**: Initially, 10 mg daily po. Dosage should be increased gradually, no more often than every 5 - 7 days. Average daily dose is 25 - 50 mg po. **Hospitalized Patients**: Initially, 25 - 50 mg po. May increase by 25 or 50 mg daily or every other day.
Guanfacine Hydrochloride	TENEX	Antihypertensive	**Tab**: 1, 2 mg	1 mg daily po hs. Dose may be increased after 3 - 4 weeks to 2 mg if necessary.
Halcinonide	HALOG	Corticosteroid	**Cream, Oint & Solution**: 0.1%	Apply to affected areas bid to tid.

GENERIC NAME	COMMON TRADE NAMES	THERAPEUTIC CATEGORY	PREPARATIONS	COMMON ADULT DOSAGE
Halobetasol Propionate	ULTRAVATE	Corticosteroid	**Cream & Oint**: 0.05%	Apply a thin layer to affected skin once or twice daily. Rub in gently and completely.
Halofantrine Hydrochloride	HALFAN	Antimalarial	**Tab**: 250 mg	**Non-Immune Patients**: 500 mg q 6 h po for 3 doses, with a repeat course of therapy given 7 days after the first. **Semi-Immune Patients**: 500 mg q 6 h po for 3 doses. A second course of therapy given 7 days after the first is optional. Give on an empty stomach at least 1 h ac or 2 h pc.
Haloperidol	HALDOL	Antipsychotic	**Tab**: 0.5, 1, 2, 5, 10, 20 mg	0.5 - 5 mg bid to tid po.
Haloperidol Decanoate	HALDOL DECANOATE 50 HALDOL DECANOATE 100	Antipsychotic	**Inj**: 70.5 mg/mL (50 mg/mL as the base) **Inj**: 141.0 mg/mL (100 mg/mL as the base)	Administer once q 4 wks by deep IM injection. For patients previously maintained on anti-psychotics, the recommended initial dose is 10 - 15 times the previous daily dose in oral haloperidol equivalents. The initial dose should not exceed 100 mg.
Haloperidol Lactate	HALDOL	Antipsychotic	**Liquid Conc**: 2 mg/mL **Inj**: 5 mg/mL	0.5 - 5 mg bid to tid po. 2 - 5 mg q 4 - 8 h IM.
Heparin Sodium		Anticoagulant	**Inj**: 1,000 - 40,000 units/mL	**Deep SC**: 5000 units IV, followed by 10,000 to 20,000 units SC. Then 8,000 - 10,000 units q 8 h or 15,000 - 20,000 units q 12 h. **Intermittent IV**: 10,000 units undiluted or in 50 - 100 mL of 0.9% sodium chloride injection. Then 5,000 - 10,000 units undiluted or in sodium chloride injection q 4 - 6 h. **IV Infusion**: 5,000 units IV; then 20,000 to 40,000 units/24 h in 1,000 mL of 0.9% NaCl injection by continuous IV infusion.

Homatropine Hydrobromide	ISOPTO HOMATROPINE	Mydriatic - Cycloplegic	**Ophth Solution**: 2, 5%	**Refraction**: Instill 1 - 2 drops in the eye(s). May be repeated in 5 - 10 min, if necessary. **Uveitis**: Instill 1 - 2 drops in the eye(s) q 3 - 4 h.
Hydralazine Hydrochloride	APRESOLINE	Antihypertensive	**Tab**: 10, 25, 50, 100 mg	Initiate therapy in gradually increasing doses: 10 mg qid po for 2 - 4 days, increase to 25 mg qid for the rest of the week. For the 2nd and subsequent weeks, raise to 50 mg qid.
			Inj: 20 mg/mL	20 - 40 mg IM or IV, repeated as necessary.
Hydrochlorothiazide	MICROZIDE	Antihypertensive	**Cpsl**: 12.5 mg	12.5 mg once daily po.
	ESIDRIX, HYDRODIURIL	Diuretic, Antihypertensive	**Tab**: 25, 50, 100 mg	**Diuresis**: 25 - 100 mg daily or bid po. **Hypertension**: 50 - 100 mg daily po in the AM.
Hydrocortisone	HYDROCORTONE	Corticosteroid	**Tab**: 10 mg	Initial dosage varies from 20 - 240 mg daily po depending on the disease being treated and the patient's response.
	CORTEF		**Tab**: 5, 10, 20 mg	
	CORTENEMA		**Retention Enema**: 100 mg/60 mL	Use 1 enema rectally nightly for 21 days or until patient comes into remission.
	ANUSOL-HC 2.5%, PROCTOCREAM-HC 2.5%		**Cream**: 2.5%	Apply as a thin film to affected areas bid - qid.
	CORT-DOME		**Cream**: 0.5, 1%	Apply as a thin film to affected areas bid - qid.
	HYTONE		**Cream, Oint & Lotion**: 2.5%	Apply as a thin film to affected areas bid - qid.
Hydrocortisone Acetate	HYDROCORTONE ACETATE	Corticosteroid	**Inj (per mL)**: 25, 50 mg [low solubility; provides a prolonged effect]	**Only for Intra-articular, Intralesional and Soft Tissue Injection**: Dose and frequency of injection are variable and must be individualized on the basis of the disease and the response of the patient. The initial dosage varies from 5 - 75 mg a day.

[Continued on the next page]

GENERIC NAME	COMMON TRADE NAMES	THERAPEUTIC CATEGORY	PREPARATIONS	COMMON ADULT DOSAGE
Hydrocortisone Acetate [Continued]	ANUSOL HC-1 ANUSOL-HC		**Oint**: 1% **Rectal Suppos**: 25 mg	Apply as a thin film to affected areas bid - qid. Insert 1 rectally AM and PM for 2 weeks. In more severe cases, 1 rectally tid or 2 bid.
	CORTICAINE		**Cream**: 0.5, 1%	Apply as a thin film to affected areas up to qid.
	CORTIFOAM		**Aerosol**: 10% (with rectal applicator)	1 applicatorful rectally once or twice daily for 2 - 3 weeks, and every 2nd day thereafter.
Hydrocortisone Buteprate	PANDEL	Corticosteroid	**Cream**: 1%	Apply a thin film to affected areas once or twice daily.
Hydrocortisone Butyrate	LOCOID	Corticosteroid	**Cream, Oint & Solution**: 0.1%	Apply to affected area as a thin film bid to tid.
Hydrocortisone Sodium Phosphate	HYDROCORTONE PHOSPHATE	Corticosteroid	**Inj**: 50 mg/mL [water soluble; rapid onset, short duration]	**For IV, IM & SC Injection**: Dose requirements vary and must be individualized on the basis of the disease and the response of the patient. Initial daily dose: from 15 - 240 mg.
Hydrocortisone Sodium Succinate	SOLU-CORTEF	Corticosteroid	**Powd for Inj**: 100, 250, 500, 1000 mg	100 - 500 mg IM, IV, or by IV infusion. Repeat at intervals of 2, 4, or 6 h.
Hydrocortisone Valerate	WESTCORT	Corticosteroid	**Cream & Oint**: 0.2%	Apply to affected areas as a thin film bid to tid.
Hydroflumethiazide	DIUCARDIN, SALURON	Diuretic, Antihypertensive	**Tab**: 50 mg	**Diuresis**: 50 mg once or twice daily po. **Hypertension**: 50 mg bid po.
Hydromorphone Hydrochloride (C-II)	DILAUDID	Opioid Analgesic	**Tab**: 1, 2, 3, 4, 8 mg	2 mg q 4 - 6 h po, prn. More severe pain may require 4 mg or more q 4 - 6 h po.
			Oral Liquid: 5 mg/5 mL **Inj**: 1, 2, 4 mg/mL	2.5 - 10 mg (2.5 - 10 mL) q 3 - 6 h po. 1 - 2 mg q 4 - 6 h SC or IM, prn. For IV use, give dose slowly over at least 2 - 3 minutes.
			Rectal Suppos: 3 mg	Insert 1 suppository rectally q 6 - 8 h.
	DILAUDID-HP	Opioid Analgesic	**Inj**: 10 mg/mL **Powd for Inj**: 250 mg	1 - 2 mg q 4 - 6 h SC or IM.

Hydroxyurea	HYDREA	Antineoplastic	**Cpsl**: 500 mg	**Solid Tumors:** **Intermittent Therapy**: 80 mg/kg po as a single dose every 3rd day. **Continuous Therapy**: 20 - 30 mg/kg po as a single dose daily. **Resistant Chronic Myelocytic Leukemia**: 20 to 30 mg/kg po as a single dose daily.
Hydroxyzine Hydrochloride	ATARAX	Sedative, Antipruritic, Antianxiety Agent	**Syrup**: 10 mg/5 mL (0.5% alcohol) **Tab**: 10, 25, 50, 100 mg	**Sedation**: 50 - 100 mg po. **Pruritis**: 25 mg tid or qid po. **Anxiety**: 50 - 100 mg qid po.
	VISTARIL	Antiemetic, Antipruritic, Antianxiety Agent, Sedative	**Inj (per mL)**: 25, 50 mg	**Nausea & Vomiting**: 25 - 100 mg IM. **Pruritis**: 25 mg tid or qid IM. **Anxiety**: 50 - 100 mg qid IM. **Sedation**: 50 - 100 mg IM.
Hydroxyzine Pamoate	VISTARIL	Sedative, Antipruritic, Antianxiety Agent	**Susp**: 25 mg/5 mL **Cpsl**: 25, 50, 100 mg	**Sedation**: 50 - 100 mg po. **Pruritis**: 25 mg tid or qid po. **Anxiety**: 50 - 100 mg qid po.
Hyoscyamine Sulfate	LEVSIN	Anticholinergic, Antispasmodic	**Solution**: 0.125 mg/mL (5% alcohol) **Elixir**: 0.125 mg/5 mL (20% alcohol) **Tab & Subling Tab**: 0.125 mg **Inj**: 0.5 mg/mL	0.125 - 0.25 mg q 4 h po. 0.125 - 0.25 mg q 4 h po. 0.125 - 0.25 mg q 4 h po or sublingually. 0.25 - 0.5 mg SC, IM, or IV up to qid at 4-hour intervals.
	LEVSINEX TIMECAPS	Anticholinergic, Antispasmodic	**Timed-Rel. Cpsl**: 0.375 mg	0.375 - 0.750 mg q 12 h po.
	LEVBID	Anticholinergic, Antispasmodic	**Extended-Rel. Tab**: 0.375 mg	0.375 - 0.750 mg q 12 h po.

GENERIC NAME	COMMON TRADE NAMES	THERAPEUTIC CATEGORY	PREPARATIONS	COMMON ADULT DOSAGE
Ibuprofen	ADVIL, MOTRIN IB, NUPRIN	Non-Opioid Analgesic, Antipyretic	**Tab**: 200 mg	200 - 400 mg q 4 - 6 h po.
	MOTRIN	Non-Opioid Analgesic, Antiinflammatory	**Susp**: 100 mg/5 mL **Tab**: 400, 600, 800 mg	**Analgesia**: 400 mg q 4 - 6 h po prn pain. **Dysmenorrhea**: 400 mg q 4 h po prn pain. **Rheumatoid Arthritis and Osteoarthritis**: 1200 to 3200 mg daily po in divided doses (300 mg qid or 400, 600, or 800 mg tid or qid).
Ibutilide Fumarate	CORVERT	Antiarrhythmic	**Inj**: 0.1 mg/mL	**≥ 60 kg**: Infuse 1 mg (1 vial) IV over 10 mins. If the arrhythmia does not terminate within 10 minutes after the initial infusion, a second infusion of equal strength may be given 10 minutes after completion of the first infusion. **< 60 kg**: Infuse 0.1 mL/kg (0.01 mg/kg) IV over 10 minutes. If the arrhythmia does not terminate within 10 minutes after the initial infusion, a second infusion of equal strength may be given 10 minutes after completion of the first infusion.
Idarubicin Hydrochloride	IDAMYCIN	Antineoplastic	**Powd for Inj**: 5, 10, 20 mg	12 mg/m^2 daily for 3 days by slow IV (10 - 15 minutes) in combination with cytarabine.
Imipramine Hydrochloride	TOFRANIL	Antidepressant	**Tab**: 10, 25, 50 mg	**Outpatients**: Initially, 75 mg/day po in divided doses, increased to 150 mg/day. **Hospitalized Patients**: Initially, 100 mg/day po in divided doses, gradually increased to 200 mg/day po as required.
Imipramine Pamoate	TOFRANIL-PM	Antidepressant	**Cpsl**: 75, 100, 125, 150 mg	**Outpatients**: Initially, 75 mg/day po; may raise dosage to 150 mg/day (dosage at which the optimum response usually occurs). The usual maintenance dosage is 75 - 150 mg daily as a single dose hs or in divided doses. **Hospitalized Patients**: Initially, 100 - 150 mg daily po; may increase to 200 mg/day. If no response in 2 weeks, give 250 - 300 mg/day.

Indapamide	LOZOL	Diuretic, Antihypertensive	**Tab**: 1.25, 2.5 mg	**Edema of CHF**: 2.5 mg daily po as a single dose in the AM. If response is not satisfactory, may double dose in 1 week. **Hypertension**: 1.25 mg daily po as a single dose in the AM. If response is not satisfactory, may double dose in 4 weeks.
Indinavir Sulfate	CRIXIVAN	Antiviral	**Cpsl**: 200, 333, 400 mg	800 mg (two 400 mg cpsls) q 8 h po, 1 h before or 2 h after a meal.
Indomethacin	INDOCIN	Antiinflammatory	**Susp**: 25 mg/5 mL **Cpsl**: 25, 50 mg **Rectal Suppos**: 50 mg	**Rheumatoid Arthritis**: 25 mg bid or tid po pc; if well tolerated, increase the daily dosage by 25 or 50 mg. In persistent night pain or AM stiffness, giving a large portion of the daily dose (up to 100 mg) hs po or by suppository may be helpful. **Acute Painful Shoulder**: 75 - 150 mg daily po pc in 3 - 4 divided doses for 7 - 14 days. **Acute Gout**: 50 mg tid po pc until pain is tolerable.
	INDOCIN SR		**Sustained-Rel. Cpsl**: 75 mg	75 mg daily po.
Insulin	ILETIN, HUMULIN, etc.	Hypoglycemic Agent	**Inj**: 100 units/mL	Variable: inject SC. See the Insulin Table, pp. 264 to 266 for preparations.
Insulin Lispro	HUMALOG	Hypoglycemic Agent	**Inj**: 100 units/mL	Variable: inject SC. See pp. 264.
Interferon alfa-2a	ROFERON-A	Antineoplastic	**Inj (per mL)**: 3, 6, 9, 36 million IUnits **Powd for Inj**: 6 million IUnits	**Hairy Cell Leukemia**: For Induction- 3 million IUnits daily for 16 - 24 weeks SC or IM. For Maintenance- 3 million IUnits 3 times a week SC or IM. **Kaposi's Sarcoma**: For Induction- 36 million IUnits daily for 10 - 12 weeks SC or IM. For Maintenance- 36 million IUnits 3 times a week SC or IM. **Chronic Myelogenous Leukemia**: 9 milion IUnits daily SC or IM.

GENERIC NAME	COMMON TRADE NAMES	THERAPEUTIC CATEGORY	PREPARATIONS	COMMON ADULT DOSAGE
Interferon alfa-2b	INTRON A	Antineoplastic	**Powd for Inj**: 3, 5, 10, 18, 25, 50 million IUnits/vial **Inj (per vial)**: 3, 5, 10 million IUnits	**Hairy Cell Leukemia**: 2 million IUnits/m^2 IM or SC 3 times a week. **Kaposi's Sarcoma**: 30 million IUnits/m^2 IM or SC 3 times a week. **Chronic Hepatitis B**: 30 - 35 million IUnits per week SC or IM, either as 5 million IUnits daily or 10 million IUnits 3 times a week for 16 weeks. **Chronic Hepatitis C**: 3 million IUnits 3 times per week SC or IM. At 16 weeks of therapy, extend treatment to 18 - 24 months at 3 million IUnits 3 times a week. **Chronic Hepatitis Non-A, Non-B/C**: 3 million IUnits 3 times a week SC or IM. **Condylomata Acuminata (10 million IU vial)**: 1 million IUnits into the base of each wart SC 3 times a week on alternate days, for 3 weeks. To reduce side effects, administer in the evening if possible. **Malignant Melanoma**: Initially, 20 million IUnits/m^2 IV on 5 consecutive days per week for 4 weeks. Maintenance dose is 10 million IUnits/m^2 SC 3 times weekly for 48 weeks.
Interferon alfa-n1 Lymphoblastoid	WELLFERON	Antiviral	**Inj**: 3 million IUnits/mL	**Chronic Hepatitis C Virus Infection**: 3 million IUnits SC or IM three times per week for 48 weeks (12 months).
Interferon alfa-n3	ALFERON N	Antineoplastic	**Inj**: 5 million IUnits/vial of 1 mL	**Condylomata Acuminata**: 250,000 IUnits per per wart. Max. dose per treatment session is 2.5 million IUnits SC at base of each wart. Use twice weekly for up to 8 weeks.
Interferon alfacon-1	INFERGEN	Antiviral	**Inj**: 9, 15 μg	**Chronic Hepatitis C Infection**: 9 μg SC as a single dose 3 times weekly for 24 weeks. At least 48 h should elapse between doses.

Interferon beta-1a	AVONEX	Multiple Sclerosis Drug	**Powd for Inj**: 6.6 million IUnits (33 μg)	6 million IUnits (30 μg) IM once a week.
Interferon beta-1b	BETASERON	Multiple Sclerosis Drug	**Powd for Inj**: 9.6 million IUnits (0.3 mg)	8 million IUnits (0.25 mg) SC every other day.
Iodoquinol	YODOXIN	Amebicide	**Tab**: 210, 650 mg	630 - 650 mg tid po after meals for 20 days.
Ipratropium Bromide	ATROVENT	Bronchodilator	**Aerosol**: 18 μg/spray **Solution**: 500 μg/2.5 mL	2 inhalations (36 μg) qid. 500 μg by nebulization tid - qid (q 6 - 8 h).
			Nasal Spray: 0.03, 0.06% (21, 42 μg/spray, respectively)	**0.03%**: 2 sprays (42 μg) per nostril bid - tid. **0.06%**: 2 sprays (84 μg) per nostril tid - qid.
Irbesartan	AVAPRO	Antihypertensive	**Tab**: 75, 150, 300 mg	Initially 150 mg once daily po. May increase to 300 mg once daily po.
Isocarboxazid	MARPLAN	Antidepressant	**Tab**: 10 mg	10 mg bid po. If tolerated, increase dosage by 10 mg q 2 - 4 days to achieve a dosage of 40 mg by the end of the 1st week. Increase dosage by increments of up to 20 mg/week, if needed and tolerated, to a maximum dosage of 60 mg per day. Daily dosage should be divided into 2 - 4 doses.
Isoetharine		Bronchodilator	**Solution for Inhalation**: 1%	**Hand Nebulizer**: 4 inhalations, up to q 4 h. **Oxygen Aerosolization**: 0.5 mL, diluted 1:3 with saline or other diluent, administered with O_2 flow adjusted to 4 - 6 L/min, over 15 - 20 minutes. **IPPB**: 0.5 mL, diluted 1:3 with saline or other diluent (with an inspiratory flow rate of 15 L/min at a cycling pressure of 15 cm H_2O).

GENERIC NAME	COMMON TRADE NAMES	THERAPEUTIC CATEGORY	PREPARATIONS	COMMON ADULT DOSAGE
Isoniazid	INH	Tuberculostatic	**Tab**: 300 mg	300 mg daily po.
	NYDRAZID		**Inj**: 100 mg/mL	**Treatment:** 5 mg/kg (up to 300 mg daily) IM in a single dose. **Preventive Therapy**: 300 mg daily IM in a single dose.
Isoproterenol Hydrochloride	ISUPREL MISTOMETER	Bronchodilator	**Aerosol**: 103 μg/spray	1 - 2 inhalations up to 5 times daily.
	ISUPREL		**Solution**: 1:200 (0.5%), 1:100 (1.0%)	**Acute Bronchial Asthma (Hand-Bulb Nebulizer)**: 5 - 15 inhalations (of 1:200) or 3 - 7 inhalations (of 1:100) up to 5 times daily. **Bronchospasm in COPD**: **Hand-Bulb Nebulizer**: Same dosage as for Acute Bronchial Asthma above. **Nebulization by Compressed Air or Oxygen**: 0.5 mL (of 1:200) diluted to 2 - 2.5 mL with water or isotonic saline. Flow rate is regulated to deliver over 10 - 20 minutes. Breath in mist up to 5 times daily. **IPPB**: 0.5 mL (of 1:200) diluted to 2 - 2.5 mL with water or isotonic saline. The IPPB treatments are usually given for 15 - 20 minutes, up to 5 times daily.
Isosorbide	ISMOTIC	Osmotic Diuretic	**Solution**: 100 g/220 mL (45%)	Initially 1.5 g/kg po, followed by 1 - 3 g/kg bid - qid po as indicated.
Isosorbide Dinitrate	ISORDIL	Antianginal	**Sublingual Tab**: 2.5, 5, 10 mg	2.5 - 10 mg q 2 - 3 h sublingually.
			Oral Tab: 5, 10, 20, 30, 40 mg	Initially, 5 - 20 mg po. For maintenance, 10 - 40 mg q 6 h po.
			Controlled-Rel. Cpsl & Tab: 40 mg	Initially, 40 mg po. For maintenance, 40 - 80 mg q 8 - 12 h po.

	SORBITRATE		**Sublingual Tab**: 2.5, 5 mg **Chewable Tab**: 5, 10 mg **Oral Tab**: 5, 10, 20, 30, 40 mg	2.5 - 5 mg q 2 - 3 h sublingually. 5 - 10 mg q 2 - 3 h po. Initially, 5 - 20 mg po. For maintenance, 10 - 40 mg q 6 h po.
	DILATRATE-SR		**Sustained-Rel. Cpsl**: 40 mg	Initially, 40 mg po. For maintenance, 40 - 80 mg q 8 - 12 h po.
Isosorbide Mononitrate	ISMO	Antianginal	**Tab**: 20 mg	20 mg bid po, with the doses given 7 h apart.
	MONOKET		**Tab**: 10, 20 mg	20 mg bid po, with the doses given 7 h apart.
	IMDUR		**Extended-Rel. Tab**: 30, 60, 120 mg	Initially, 30 - 60 mg once daily po. May increase to 120 mg once daily po.
Isotretinoin	ACCUTANE	Anti-Cystic Acne Agent	**Cpsl**: 10, 20, 40 mg	0.5 - 2 mg/kg/day divided in 2 doses po for 15 - 20 weeks.
Isradipine	DYNACIRC	Antihypertensive	**Cpsl**: 2.5, 5 mg	Initially, 2.5 mg bid po. May increase in increments of 5 mg/day at 2 - 4 week intervals to a maximum of 20 mg/day.
	DYNACIRC CR		**Controlled-Rel. Tab**: 5, 10 mg	Initially, 5 mg once daily po. May increase in increments of 5 mg at 2 - 4 week intervals to a maximum of 20 mg/day.
Itraconazole	SPORANOX	Antifungal	**Cpsl**: 100 mg	**Blastomycosis and Histoplasmosis**: 200 mg once daily po with food. May increase the dosage in 100 mg increments to a maximum of 400 mg daily. Doses over 200 mg/day should be given in 2 divided doses. **Aspergillosis**: 200 - 400 mg daily po. **Onychomycosis:** **Toenails with or without Fingernail Involvement**: 200 mg once daily po for 12 consecutive weeks. **Fingernails Only**: 200 mg bid po for 1 week. After 3 weeks without the drug, repeat the dosage.

[Continued on the next page]

GENERIC NAME	COMMON TRADE NAMES	THERAPEUTIC CATEGORY	PREPARATIONS	COMMON ADULT DOSAGE
Itraconazole [Continued]	SPORANOX		**Oral Solution**: 10 mg/mL	Vigorously swish solution in the mouth (10 mL at a time) for several seconds and swallow. **Oropharyngeal Candidiasis**: 200 mg daily po for 1 - 2 weeks. **Esophageal Candidiasis**: 100 mg daily po for a minimum of 3 weeks. Continue for 2 weeks following resolution of symptoms.
			Injection: 10 mg/mL	**Blastomycosis, Histoplasmosis, & Aspergillosis**: 200 mg by IV infusion over 1 h) bid for 4 doses, followed by 200 mg per day by IV infusion. Continue injection for a maximum of 14 days; then continue with capsules for minimum of 3 months until the infection has subsided.
Ivermectin	STROMECTOL	Anthelmintic	**Tab**: 6 mg	See Table below. Take tablets with water.

Dosage for Strongyloidiasis		Dosage for Onchocerciasis	
Body Weight (kg)	Number of Tablets	Body Weight (kg)	Number of Tablets
15 to 24	0.5	15 to 25	0.5
25 to 35	1	26 to 44	1
36 to 50	1.5	45 to 64	1.5
51 to 65	2	65 to 84	2
66 to 79	2.5	≥ 85	[150 μg/kg]
≥ 80	[200 μg/kg]		

GENERIC NAME	COMMON TRADE NAMES	THERAPEUTIC CATEGORY	PREPARATIONS	COMMON ADULT DOSAGE
Ketoconazole	NIZORAL	Antifungal	**Tab**: 200 mg	200 mg once daily po. In very severe infections, 400 mg once daily po.
			Cream: 2% **Shampoo**: 2%	Apply topically once daily. Shampoo twice a week for 4 weeks with at least 3 days between shampooing; then shampoo intermittently prn.

	NIZORAL A-D	Antidandruff Shampoo	**Shampoo**: 1%	Shampoo twice a week for up to 8 weeks with at least 3 days between shampooing; then shampoo intermittently prn.
Ketoprofen	ORUDIS KT	Non-Opioid Analgesic, Antiinflammatory	**Tab**: 12.5 mg	12.5 - 25 mg q 4 - 6 h po prn.
	ORUDIS		**Cpsl**: 25, 50, 75 mg	**Analgesia & Dysmenorrhea**: 25 - 50 mg q 6 - 8 h po. **Rheumatoid Arthritis & Osteoarthritis**: 75 mg tid po or 50 mg qid po.
	ORUVAIL	Antiinflammatory	**Extended-Rel. Cpsl**: 100, 150, 200 mg	**Rheumatoid Arthritis & Osteoarthritis**: 200 mg once daily po.
Ketorolac Tromethamine	ACULAR	Antiinflammatory (Topical)	**Ophth Solution**: 0.5%	1 drop into affected eye(s) qid.
	TORADOL IV/IM	Non-Opioid Analgesic	**Inj (per mL)**: 15, 30 mg	**Single-Dose Treatment (IM or IV*)**: < **65 yrs**: 1 dose of 60 mg IM or 30 mg IV. ≥ **65 yrs, renally impaired, or under 50 kg (110 lbs)**: 1 dose of 30 mg IM or 15 mg IV. **Multiple-Dose Treatment (IM or IV*)**: < **65 yrs**: 30 mg q 6 h IM or IV, not to exceed 120 mg per day. ≥ **65 yrs, renally impaired, or under 50 kg (110 lbs)**: 15 mg q 6 h IM or IV, not to exceed 60 mg per day. * The IV bolus dose must be given over no less than 15 seconds.

[Continued on the next page]

GENERIC NAME	COMMON TRADE NAMES	THERAPEUTIC CATEGORY	PREPARATIONS	COMMON ADULT DOSAGE
Ketorolac Tromethamine [Continued]	TORADOL ^{ORAL}		**Tab**: 10 mg	Indicated only as continuation therapy to TORADOL $^{IV/IM}$. The maximum combined duration of use (parenteral and oral) is 5 days. < **65 yrs**: 20 mg po as a first dose for those who received 60 mg IM (single dose), 30 mg IV (single dose), or 30 mg (multiple dose) of TORADOL $^{IV/IM}$, followed by 10 mg q 4 - 6 h po, not to exceed 40 mg/day. **≥ 65 yrs, renally impaired, or under 50 kg (110 lbs)**: 10 mg po as a first dose for those who received 30 mg IM or 15 mg IV (single dose), or 15 mg (multiple dose) of TORADOL $^{IV/IM}$, followed by 10 mg q 4 - 6 h po, not to exceed 40 mg/day.
Ketotifen Fumarate	ZADITOR	Antihistamine	**Ophth Solution**: 0.025%	1 drop into the affected eye(s) q 8 - 12 h.
Labetalol Hydrochloride	NORMODYNE, TRANDATE	Antihypertensive	**Tab**: 100, 200, 300 mg	**Initial**: 100 mg bid po. Titrate dosage upward in increments of 100 mg bid q 2 - 3 days. **Maintenance**: Usually, 200 - 400 mg bid po.
			Inj: 5 mg/mL	**Repeated IV**: 20 mg IV (over 2 minutes). May give additional injections of 40 - 80 mg at 10-minute intervals (maximum: 300 mg). **IV Infusion**: 200 mL of a diluted solution (1 mg/mL) given at a rate of 2 mL/min.
Lactulose	DUPHALAC	Laxative	**Syrup**: 10 g/15 mL	15 - 30 mL (10 - 20 g) daily po. Dose may be increased to 60 mL daily if necessary.
Lamivudine	EPIVIR	Antiviral	**Oral Solution**: 10 mg/mL **Tab**: 150 mg	**HIV Infection**: 150 mg bid po in combination with other antiretroviral agents.
	EPIVIR-HBV		**Oral Solution**: 5 mg/mL **Tab**: 100 mg	**Chronic Hepatitis B**: 100 mg once daily po.

Lamotrigine	LAMICTAL	Antiepileptic	**Tab**: 25, 100, 150, 200 mg	**Patients on Enzyme-Inducing Antiepileptic Drugs, but not Valproate:** Initially, 50 mg once daily po for 2 weeks, followed by 100 mg/day po in 2 divided doses for 2 weeks. Thereafter, 300 - 500 mg/day po in 2 divided doses. **Patients on Enzyme-Inducing Antiepileptic Drugs and Valproate:** Initially, 25 mg every other day po for 2 weeks, followed by 25 mg once daily po for 2 weeks. Thereafter, 100 - 150 mg/day po in 2 divided doses.
Lansoprazole	PREVACID	Gastric Acid Pump Inhibitor, Anti-Ulcer Agent	**Delayed-Rel. Cpsl**: 15, 30 mg	**Duodenal Ulcer:** **Treatment of**: 15 mg once daily po for 4 weeks. **Maintenance of Healed Ulcer**: 15 mg once daily po. **Associated with *H. pylori***: 30 mg of lansoprazole + 500 mg of clarithromycin + 1 g of amoxicillin bid po for 14 days, or 30 mg of lansoprazole + 1 g of amoxicillin tid for 14 days for those intolerant to or resistant to clarithromycin. **Gastric Ulcer, Treatment of**: 30 mg once daily po for up to 8 weeks. **Erosive Esophagitis:** **Treatment of**: 30 mg once daily po for up to 8 weeks. **Maintenance of Healing Esophagitis**: 15 mg once daily po. **Pathological Hypersecretory Conditions including Zollinger-Ellison Syndrome**: The recommended starting dose is 60 mg once a day po. Adjust to individual patient needs and continue for as long as indicated.
Latanoprost	XALATAN	Anti-Glaucoma Agent	**Ophth Solution**: 0.005% (50 μg/mL)	1 drop into affected eye(s) once daily in the evening.

GENERIC NAME	COMMON TRADE NAMES	THERAPEUTIC CATEGORY	PREPARATIONS	COMMON ADULT DOSAGE
Leflunomide	ARAVA	Antirheumatic	**Tab**: 10, 20, 100 mg	Initiate with a loading dose of one 100 mg tab po per day for 3 days. Then, 20 mg once daily po.
Letrozole	FEMARA	Antineoplastic	**Tab**: 2.5 mg	2.5 mg once daily po.
Levalbuterol Hydrochloride	XOPENEX	Bronchodilator	**Solution for Inhalation:** (0.73 mg/3 mL, equal to 0.63 mg/3 mL of base) **Solution for Inhalation:** (1.44 mg/3 mL, equal to 1.25 mg/3 mL of base)	0.63 mg (base) tid (q 6 - 8 h) by nebulization. For those patients with more severe asthma or for those who do not respond adequately to a lower dose, 1.26 mg (base) tid may be used with close monitoring for adverse effects.
Levetiracetam	KEPPRA	Antiepileptic	**Tab**: 250, 500, 750 mg	Initially 1000 mg/day, given as 500 mg bid po. Doses may be increased by 1000 mg/day q 2 weeks to a maximum of 3000 mg per day.
Levobunolol Hydrochloride	BETAGAN LIQUIFILM	Anti-Glaucoma Agent	**Ophth Solution**: 0.25, 0.5%	**0.25%**: 1 - 2 drops into the affected eye(s) bid daily. **0.5%**: 1 - 2 drops into the affected eye(s) once daily.
Levocabastine Hydrochloride	LIVOSTIN	Antiallergic, Ophthalmic	**Ophth Solution**: 0.05%	1 drop into affected eye(s) qid for up to 2 weeks.
Levodopa	LARODOPA	Antiparkinsonian	**Tab**: 100, 250, 500 mg	Initially, 500 mg to 1 g daily po divided in 2 or more doses with food. May increase dosage gradually in increments not more than 750 mg q 3 - 7 days. Maximum 8 g daily.
Levofloxacin	LEVAQUIN	Antibacterial	**Tab**: 250, 500 mg **Inj**: 25 mg/mL	**Bronchitis:** 500 mg once daily po or by IV infusion (over 60 min) for 7 days. **Pneumonia**: 500 mg once daily po or by IV infusion (over 60 min) for 7 - 14 days. **Sinusitis**: 500 mg once daily po or by IV infusion (over 60 min) for 10 - 14 days.

				Skin & Skin Structure Infections: 500 mg once daily po or by IV infusion (over 60 min) for 7 - 10 days. **Urinary Tract Infections (Complicated) and Pyelonephritis:** 250 mg once daily po or by IV infusion (over 60 min) for 10 days. **Urinary Tract Infections (Uncomplicated):** 250 mg once daily po for 3 days.
Levonorgestrel	NORPLANT SYSTEM	Implant Contraceptive	**Kit:** 6 cpsls (each with 36 mg levonorgestrel) plus trocar, scalpel, forceps, syringe, 2 syringe needles, package of skin closures, gauze sponges, stretch bandages, surgical drapes	Total implanted dose is 216 mg. Perform implantation of all 6 capsules during the first 7 days of the onset of menses. Insertion is subdermal in the mid-portion of the upper arm; distribute capsules in a fan-like pattern, about 15 degrees apart, for a total of 75 degrees.
	PLAN B	Emergency Contraceptive	**Tab:** 0.75 mg	0.75 mg po within 72 h after unprotected intercourse; follow with 0.75 mg 12 h later.
Levorphanol Tartrate (C-II)	LEVO-DROMORAN	Opioid Analgesic	**Tab:** 2 mg	2 mg po q 6 - 8 h prn. May be increased to 3 mg q 6 - 8 h if needed.
			Inj: 2 mg/mL	1 - 2 mg IM or SC q 6 - 8 prn.
Levothyroxine Sodium	LEVOTHROID	Thyroid Hormone	**Tab:** 25, 50, 75, 88, 100, 112, 125, 137, 150, 175, 200, 300 μg	**Usual Dosage:** 50 μg daily po with increases of 25 - 50 μg at 2 - 4 week intervals until the patient is euthyroid or symptoms preclude further dose increases. The usual maintenance dosage is 100 - 200 μg daily po. **Myxedema Coma or Hypothyroid Patients with Angina:** Starting dose should be 25 μg daily po with increases of 25 - 50 μg at 2 - 4 week intervals as determined by response.
	SYNTHROID		**Tab:** 25, 50, 75, 88, 100, 112, 125, 150, 175, 200, 300 μg	
			Powd for Inj: 200, 500 μg	**Myxedema Coma:** Initially, 200 - 500 μg (100 μg/mL) IV. Then, 100 - 200 μg daily IV. After evaluation of thyroid state, 50 - 100 μg daily IV is usually sufficient.

GENERIC NAME	COMMON TRADE NAMES	THERAPEUTIC CATEGORY	PREPARATIONS	COMMON ADULT DOSAGE
Lidocaine	XYLOCAINE	Local Anesthetic	**Oint**: 2.5% **Oint**: 5%	Apply topically prn. Apply topically. Maximum single application- 5 g (≈ 6 inches of ointment). Maximum daily application- 1/2 tube (≈ 17 - 20 g).
	LIDODERM		**Adhesive Patch**: 5%	Apply to intact skin, covering the most painful area. To adjust dose, cut patches before removing release liner. May apply up to 3 patches at once for up to 12 hours of a 24-hour period.
	XYLOCAINE		**Oral Spray**: 10%	2 metered doses per quadrant are advised as the upper limit.
Lidocaine Hydrochloride	XYLOCAINE	Antiarrhythmic	**Inj (per mL)**: 10 mg (1%), 20 mg (2%)	**IV Injection**: 50 - 100 mg IV bolus (at a rate of 25 - 50 mg/min). May repeat dose in 5 min. **IV Infusion**: Following bolus administration, give at a rate of 1 - 4 mg/min.
	4% XYLOCAINE-MPF	Local Anesthetic	**Inj**: 40 mg/mL (4%)	**Retrobulbar Injection**: 3 - 5 mL/70 kg (1.7 - 3 mg/kg. **Transtracheal Injection**: 2 - 3 mL injected rapidly through a large needle. **Topical**: Spray pharynx with 1 - 5 mL.
	XYLOCAINE 2% VISCOUS	Local Anesthetic	**Solution**: 2%	**Mouth**: 15 mL swished around mouth and spit out. Readminister q 3 - 8 h prn. **Pharynx**: 15 mL gargled & may be swallowed. Readminister q 3 - 8 h prn.

Lincomycin Hydrochloriae	LINCOCIN	Antibacterial	**Cpsl**: 500 mg	**Serious Infections**: 500 mg tid (q 8 h) po. **More Severe Infections**: 500 mg or more qid (q 6 h) po.
			Inj: 300 mg/mL	**Serious Infections**: 600 mg q 24 h IM or 600 to 1000 mg (diluted in 100 mL of fluid) q 8 to 12 h by IV infusion (over 1 hour). **More Severe Infections**: 600 mg q 12 h IM or up to 8 g daily by IV infusion (at a rate of 1 g/100 mL/hour).
Lindane		Antiparasitic, Scabicide	**Lotion**: 1%	**Scabies**: Apply to dry skin as a thin layer and rub in thoroughly. Leave on for 8 - 12 h, then remove by thorough washing.
			Shampoo: 1%	**Head & Crab Lice**: Apply 30 - 60 mL to dry hair. Work thoroughly into hair and allow to remain in place for 4 minutes. Add small amounts of water to form a good lather. Rinse thoroughly and towel dry.
Liothyronine Sodium	CYTOMEL	Thyroid Hormone	**Tab**: 5, 25, 50 μg	**Usual Dosage**: 25 μg daily po. Daily dosage may be increased by 12.5 - 25 μg q 1 - 2 weeks. Usual maintenance dose is 25 - 75 μg daily po. **Myxedema**: Starting dose is 5 μg daily po. May increase by 5 - 10 μg daily q 1 - 2 weeks. When 25 μg daily is reached, dosage may be increased by 12.5 - 25 μg q 1 - 2 weeks. Usual maintenance dose is 50 - 100 μg daily.
	TRIOSTAT		**Inj**: 10 μg/mL	**Myxedema Coma**: Initially, 25 - 50 μg IV. The dosage may be repeated at least 4 h and no more than 12 h apart.

GENERIC NAME	COMMON TRADE NAMES	THERAPEUTIC CATEGORY	PREPARATIONS	COMMON ADULT DOSAGE
Lisinopril	PRINIVIL, ZESTRIL	Antihypertensive, Heart Failure Drug, Post-MI Drug	**Tab**: 2.5, 5, 10, 20, 30, 40 mg	**Hypertension**: Initially, 10 mg once daily po. Usual dosage range is 20 - 40 mg as a single daily dose. **Heart Failure**: Initially, 5 mg once daily po with diuretics and digitalis. Usual dosage range is 5 - 20 mg once daily. **Acute Myocardial Infarction**: 5 mg po within 24 h of the onset of acute MI symptoms, followed by 5 mg po after 24 h, 10 mg po after 48 h, and then 10 mg once daily po. Continue dosing for 6 weeks.
Lithium Carbonate	ESKALITH	Antimaniacal	**Cpsl**: 300 mg	**Usual Dosage**: 300 mg tid or qid po. **Acute Mania**: 900 mg bid po or 600 mg tid po. **Long-Term Control**: 900 - 1200 mg daily po in 2 or 3 divided doses.
	ESKALITH CR		**Controlled-Rel. Tab**: 450 mg	**Usual Dosage**: 450 mg bid po.
	LITHOBID		**Slow-Rel. Tab**: 300 mg	**Acute Mania**: 900 mg bid po or 600 mg tid po. **Long-Term Control**: 900 - 1200 mg daily po in 2 or 3 divided doses.
	LITHONATE		**Cpsl**: 300 mg	**Acute Mania**: 600 mg tid po. **Long-Term Control**: 300 mg tid or qid po.
	LITHOTAB		**Tab**: 300 mg	Same dosages as for LITHONATE above.
Lithium Citrate		Antimaniacal	**Syrup**: 8 mEq (= 300 mg of lithium carbonate)/5 mL	**Acute Mania**: 10 mL (16 mEq) tid po. **Long-Term Control**: 5 mL (8 mEq) tid or qid po.
Lodoxamide Tromethamine	ALOMIDE	Antiallergic, Ophthalmic	**Ophth Solution**: 0.1%	1 - 2 drops in each affected eye qid for up to 3 months.

Lomefloxacin Hydrochloride	MAXAQUIN	Antibacterial	**Tab**: 400 mg	**Lower Respiratory Tract and Urinary Tract Infections (Uncomplicated)**: 400 mg once daily po for 10 days. **Urinary Tract Infections, Complicated**: 400 mg once daily po for 14 days.
Lomustine	CeeNU	Antineoplastic	**Cpsl**: 10, 40, 100 mg	130 mg/m^2 po as a single dose q 6 weeks. Dosage adjustments are made in 6 weeks based on platelet and leukocyte counts.
Loperamide Hydrochloride	IMODIUM	Antidiarrheal	**Cpsl**: 2 mg	4 mg po followed by 2 mg after each unformed stool. Maximum daily dosage- 16 mg.
	IMODIUM A-D, PEPTO DIARRHEA CONTROL		**Liquid**: 1 mg/5 mL (5.25% alcohol) **Cplt**: 2 mg	4 mg po followed by 2 mg after each unformed stool. Maximum daily dosage- 8 mg.
Loracarbef	LORABID	Antibacterial	**Powd for Susp (per 5 mL)**: 100, 200 mg **Cpsl**: 200, 400 mg	**Lower Resp. Tract Infect. (Except Pneumonia)**: 200 - 400 mg q 12 h po for 7 days. **Pneumonia**: 400 mg q 12 h po for 14 days. **Upper Respiratory Tract Infections**: 200 - 400 mg q 12 h po for 10 days. **Skin and Skin Structure Infections**: 200 mg q 12 h po for 7 days. **Urinary Tract Infections (Uncomplicated Cystitis)**: 200 mg q 24 h po for 7 days. **Urinary Tract Infections (Uncomplicated Pyelonephritis)**: 400 mg q 12 h po for 14 days.
Loratadine	CLARITIN	Antihistamine	**Syrup**: 1 mg/mL **Tab**: 10 mg	10 mL (10 mg) once daily po. 10 mg once daily po.
Lorazepam (C-IV)	ATIVAN	Antianxiety Agent	**Tab**: 0.5, 1, 2 mg	**Anxiety**: 2 - 3 mg daily po given bid or tid. **Insomnia due to Anxiety**: 2 - 4 mg hs po.
			Inj (per mL): 2, 4 mg	**Premedicant**: 0.05 mg/kg (maximum 4 mg) IM. **Anxiety**: 0.044 mg/kg (maximum 2 mg) IV.

GENERIC NAME	COMMON TRADE NAMES	THERAPEUTIC CATEGORY	PREPARATIONS	COMMON ADULT DOSAGE
Losartan Potassium	COZAAR	Antihypertensive	**Tab**: 25, 50, 100 mg	Usual starting dose is 50 mg once daily po. For patients treated with a diuretic, start with 25 mg once daily po. The drug can be given once or twice daily with the total daily dose range of 25 - 100 mg.
Loteprednol Etabonate	ALREX	Corticosteroid	**Ophth Suspension**: 0.2%	1 drop into the affected eye(s) qid.
	LOTEMAX		**Ophth Suspension**: 0.5%	**Steroid Responsive Disease**: 1 - 2 drops into the affected eye(s) qid. During the initial treatment within the first week, the dosing may be increased up to 1 drop every hour. **Postoperative Inflammation**: 1 - 2 drops into operated eye(s) qid, beginning 24 h after surgery & continuing for 2 weeks.
Lovastatin	MEVACOR	Hypolipidemic	**Tab**: 10, 20, 40 mg	Initially, 20 mg once daily po with the evening meal. Dosage adjustments may be made at 4 week intervals. Usual dosage range is 10 to 80 mg/day po in single or divided doses.
Loxapine Hydrochloride	LOXITANE C	Antipsychotic	**Conc Liquid**: 25 mg/mL	Initially, 10 mg bid po. Dosage should be increased rapidly over 7 - 10 days; usual maintenance range is 60 - 100 mg daily, but many patients do well at 20 - 60 mg daily.
	LOXITANE IM		**Inj**: 50 mg/mL	12.5 - 50 mg q 4 - 6 h IM.
Loxapine Succinate	LOXITANE	Antipsychotic	**Cpsl**: 5, 10, 25, 50 mg	Same dosage as for LOXITANE C above.
Mafenide Acetate	SULFAMYLON	Burn Preparation	**Cream**: 85 mg/g	Apply to the clean and debrided wound with a sterile gloved hand, once or twice daily, to a thickness of about 1/16 in.
Magaldrate	RIOPAN	Antacid	**Susp**: 540 mg/5 mL	5 - 10 mL po, between meals & hs.

Magnesium Hydroxide	MILK OF MAGNESIA	Antacid, Saline Laxative	**Susp**: 400 mg/5 mL	**Antacid**: 5 - 15 mL with water, up to qid po. **Laxative**: 30 - 60 mL followed by 8 oz. of fluid.
	MILK OF MAGNESIA CONCENTRATED	Saline Laxative	**Susp**: 800 mg/5 mL	**Laxative**: 15 - 30 mL followed by 8 oz. of fluid.
Magnesium Sulfate		Anticonvulsant	**Inj**: 12.5, 50%	**IM**: 4 - 5 g of a 50% solution q 4 h prn. **IV**: 4 g of a 10 - 20% solution (not exceeding 1.5 mL/min of a 10% solution). **IV Infusion**: 4 - 5 g in 250 mL of 5% Dextrose or Sodium Chloride Solution (not exceeding 3 mL/min).
Maprotiline Hydrochloride	LUDIOMIL	Antidepressant	**Tab**: 25, 50, 75 mg	**Outpatients**: Initially, 75 mg daily po as a single dose or in divided doses. May increase dosage gradually after 2 weeks in increments of 25 mg. Usual maintenance dosage is 75 to 150 mg daily po. **Hospitalized Patients**: Initially, 100 - 150 mg daily po as a single dose or in divided doses. May increase dosage gradually, if needed, up to a maximum dose of 225 mg daily.
Mazindol (C-IV)	SANOREX	Anorexiant	**Tab**: 1, 2 mg	1 mg tid po 1 hour ac or 2 mg once daily po 1 hour before lunch.
Mebendazole	VERMOX	Anthelmintic	**Chewable Tab**: 100 mg	**Pinworm**: 100 mg daily po (1 dose). **Common Roundworm, Whipworm, Hookworm**: 100 mg bid AM & PM for 3 days po.
Mechlorethamine Hydrochloride	MUSTARGEN	Antineoplastic	**Powd for Inj**: 10 mg	0.4 mg/kg IV either as a single dose or in divided doses of 0.1 - 0.2 mg/kg/day.
Meclizine Hydrochloride	ANTIVERT	Antivertigo Agent	**Tab**: 12.5, 25, 50 mg	**Vertigo**: 25 - 100 mg daily po in divided doses. **Motion Sickness**: 25 - 50 mg po, 1 hour prior to embarkation; repeat dose q 24 h prn.
	BONINE		**Chewable Tab**: 25 mg	**Motion Sickness**: 25 - 50 mg po, 1 hour before travel starts, for up to 24 h protection.

GENERIC NAME	COMMON TRADE NAMES	THERAPEUTIC CATEGORY	PREPARATIONS	COMMON ADULT DOSAGE
Meclocycline Sulfosalicylate	MECLAN	Anti-Acne Agent	**Cream**: 1%	Apply to affected area bid, AM and PM.
Meclofenamate Sodium		Non-Opioid Analgesic, Antiinflammatory	**Cpsl**: 50, 100 mg	**Analgesia**: 50 - 100 mg q 4 - 6 h po. **Dysmennorhea**: 100 mg tid po, for up to 6 days, starting at the onset of menses. **Rheumatoid Arthritis & Osteoarthritis:** 200 to 400 mg daily po in 3 or 4 equal doses.
Medroxyprogesterone Acetate	PROVERA, CYCRIN	Progestin	**Tab**: 2.5, 5, 10 mg	5 - 10 mg daily po for 5 - 10 days.
	DEPO-PROVERA	Antineoplastic	**Inj (per mL)**: 400 mg	Initially, 400 - 1000 mg weekly IM. If improvement is noted within a few weeks, patient may be maintained with as little as 400 mg per month.
		Injectable Contraceptive	**Inj**: 150 mg/mL	150 mg q 3 months by deep IM injection in the gluteal or deltoid muscle.
Medrysone	HMS	Corticosteroid	**Ophth Susp**: 1%	1 drop into affected eye(s) up to q 4 h.
Mefenamic Acid	PONSTEL	Non-Opioid Analgesic	**Cpsl**: 250 mg	500 mg po, then 250 mg q 6 h po with food.
Mefloquine Hydrochloride	LARIAM	Antimalarial	**Tab**: 250 mg	**Treatment**: 1250 mg po as a single dose with food and with at least 8 oz. of water. **Prophylaxis**: 250 mg once weekly po for 4 weeks, then 250 mg every other week. Take with food and at least 8 oz of water. Start 1 week prior to departure to endemic area.
Megestrol Acetate	MEGACE	Progestin	**Susp**: 40 mg/mL	**Appetite Stimulant in Patients with AIDS**: 800 mg/day (20 mL/day) po.
		Antineoplastic	**Tab**: 20, 40 mg **Susp**: 40 mg/mL	**Breast Cancer**: 40 mg qid po. **Endometrial Cancer:** 40 - 320 mg daily po in divided doses for at least 2 months.

Melphalan	ALKERAN	Antineoplastic	**Tab**: 2 mg	**Multiple Myeloma**: 6 mg daily po as a single dose. After 2 - 3 weeks, discontinue drug for up to 4 weeks; when WBC and platelet counts begin rising, maintenance dose of 2 mg daily po may be initiated. **Epithelial Ovarian Cancer**: 0.2 mg/kg daily for 5 days. Repeat q 4 - 5 weeks.
			Powd for Inj: 50 mg	Usual dose is 16 mg/m^2 given as a single IV infusion over 15 - 20 min. Administer at 2 week intervals for 4 doses, then, after recovery from toxicity, at 4 week intervals.
Meperidine Hydrochloride (C-II)	DEMEROL	Opioid Analgesic	**Tab**: 50, 100 mg **Syrup**: 50 mg/5 mL **Inj (per mL)**: 25, 50, 75, 100 mg	**Analgesia**: 50 - 150 mg q 3 - 4 h po, IM or SC. **Preoperatively**: 50 - 100 mg IM or SC, 30 - 90 minutes prior to anesthesia. **Obstetrical Analgesia**: 50 - 100 mg IM or SC when pain becomes regular; may repeat at 1 - 3 hour intervals.
Mephenytoin	MESANTOIN	Antiepileptic	**Tab**: 100 mg	Initially 50 - 100 mg daily po, increasing the daily dose by 50 - 100 mg at weekly intervals to a maintenance dose of 200 to 600 mg daily.
Mephobarbital (C-IV)	MEBARAL	Antiepileptic, Sedative	**Tab**: 32, 50, 100 mg	**Epilepsy**: 400 - 600 mg daily po. **Sedation**: 32 - 100 mg tid or qid po. Optimum dosage is 50 mg tid or qid po.
Meprobamate (C-IV)	EQUANIL, MILTOWN	Antianxiety Agent	**Tab**: 200, 400 mg	1200 - 1600 mg/day po in 3 - 4 divided doses.
Mercaptopurine	PURINETHOL	Antineoplastic	**Tab**: 50 mg	**Induction**: 2.5 mg/kg daily po. May increase after 4 weeks to 5 mg/kg daily po. **Maintenance**: 1.5 - 2.5 mg/kg daily po as a single dose.
Meropenem	MERREM IV	Antibacterial	**Powd for Inj**: 0.5, 1 g	1 g q 8 h by IV infusion (over 15 - 30 min) or as an IV bolus (5 - 20 mL) over 3 - 5 min.

GENERIC NAME	COMMON TRADE NAMES	THERAPEUTIC CATEGORY	PREPARATIONS	COMMON ADULT DOSAGE
Mesalamine	ASACOL	Bowel Antiinflammatory Agent	**Delayed-Rel. Tab**: 400 mg	800 mg tid po for 6 weeks.
	PENTASA		**Controlled-Rel. Cpsl**: 250 mg	1000 mg qid po for up to 8 weeks.
	ROWASA		**Rectal Susp**: 4 g/60 mL	One rectal instillation (4 g) once a day, preferably hs, and retained for approx. 8 h.
			Rectal Suppos: 500 mg	Insert 1 rectally bid, and retained for 1 - 3 h.
Mesoridazine Besylate	SERENTIL	Antipsychotic	**Tab**: 10, 25, 50, 100 mg **Conc Liquid**: 25 mg/mL (0.61% alcohol)	**Schizophrenia**: 50 mg tid po. **Behavioral Problems in Mental Deficiency and Chronic Brain Syndrome**: 25 mg tid po. **Alcoholism**: 25 mg bid po. **Psychoneurotic Manifestations**: 10 mg tid po.
			Inj: 25 mg/mL	25 mg IM. May repeat in 30 - 60 minutes.
Metaproterenol Sulfate	ALUPENT	Bronchodilator	**Syrup**: 10 mg/5 mL **Tab**: 10, 20 mg **Aerosol**: 650 μg/spray	20 mg tid or qid po. 20 mg tid or qid po. 2 - 3 inhalations q 3 - 4 h.
Metaraminol Bitartrate	ARAMINE	Sympathomimetic	**Inj**: 10 mg/mL (1%)	**IM or SC**: 2 - 10 mg. **IV Infusion**: 15 - 100 mg in 500 mL of Sodium Chloride Injection or 5% Dextrose Injection, adjusting the rate of infusion to maintain the blood pressure.
Metaxolone	SKELAXIN	Skeletal Muscle Relaxant	**Tab**: 400 mg	800 mg tid to qid po.
Metformin Hydrochloride	GLUCOPHAGE	Hypoglycemic Agent	**Tab**: 500, 850 mg	**500 mg**: Usual staring dose is 500 mg bid po, given with the morning and evening meals. Make dosage increases in increments of 500 mg every week, given in divided doses, up to a maximum of 2500 mg/day. Can be given bid up to 2000 mg/day; if 2500 mg per day is required, it may be better tolerated if given tid with meals.

				850 mg: Usual staring dose is 850 mg daily po, given with the morning meal. Make dosage increases in increments of 850 mg every other week, given in divided doses, up to a maximum of 2550 mg/day. The usual maintenance dose is 850 mg bid with the morning & evening meals. When necessary, may give 850 mg tid with meals.
Methadone Hydrochloride (C-II)	DOLOPHINE HYDROCHLORIDE	Opioid Analgesic	**Tab**: 5, 10 mg **Inj**: 10 mg/mL	2.5 - 10 mg q 3 - 4 h po, IM or SC prn pain.
Methamphetamine Hydrochloride (C-II)	DESOXYN	CNS Stimulant, Anorexiant	**Sustained-Rel. Tab**: 5, 10, 15 mg	**Attention Deficit Hyperactivity Disease**: Initially 5 mg once daily or bid po. Dosage may be raised in increments of 5 mg at weekly intervals until optimum response is achieved. Usual dosage 20 - 25 mg daily. **Exogenous Obesity**: 10 - 15 mg once daily po in the AM.
Methenamine Hippurate	HIPREX, UREX	Urinary Tract Anti-Infective	**Tab**: 1 g	1 g bid (morning and night) po.
Methenamine Mandelate	MANDELAMINE	Urinary Tract Anti-Infective	**Tab**: 0.5, 1 g **Susp**: 0.5 g/5 mL	1 g qid po, pc and hs. 1 g qid po, pc and hs.
Methimazole	TAPAZOLE	Antithyroid Drug	**Tab**: 5, 10 mg	**Initial**: 15 mg daily po (mild disease), 30 - 40 mg daily po (moderately severe), and 60 mg daily po (severe), divided into 3 doses q 8 h. **Maintenance**: 5 - 15 mg daily po.
Methocarbamol	ROBAXIN	Skeletal Muscle Relaxant	**Tab**: 500 mg	**Initial**: 1500 mg qid po. **Maintenance**: 1000 mg qid po.
	ROBAXIN-750		**Tab**: 750 mg	**Initial**: 1500 mg qid po. **Maintenance**: 750 mg q 4 h po or 1500 mg tid po.

GENERIC NAME	COMMON TRADE NAMES	THERAPEUTIC CATEGORY	PREPARATIONS	COMMON ADULT DOSAGE
Methotrexate Sodium		Anti-Psoriasis Agent	**Tab**: 2.5 mg **Powd for Injection**: 20 mg **Inj**: 25 mg/mL	Individualize dosage. A test dose may be given prior to therapy to detect extreme sensitivity. 10 - 25 mg once a week po, IM, or IV until response is achieved. For po use, may given 2.5 mg q 12 h for 3 doses, once a week. Do not exceed 30 mg per week.
Methsuximide	CELONTIN	Antiepileptic	**Cpsl**: 150, 300 mg	300 mg daily po for the 1st week. May raise dosage at weekly intervals by 300 mg/day for 3 weeks to a daily dosage of 1200 mg.
Methyclothiazide	ENDURON	Diuretic, Antihypertensive	**Tab**: 2.5, 5 mg	**Diuresis**: 2.5 - 10 mg once daily po. **Hypertension**: 2.5 - 5 mg once daily po.
Methylcellulose	CITRUCEL CITRUCEL (Sugar-Free)	Bulk Laxative	**Powder**: 2 g/heaping tablespoonful (19 g) **Powder**: 2 g/heaping tablespoonful (10.2 g)	1 heaping tablespoonful stirred into 8 fl. oz. of cold water 1 - 3 times daily po at the first sign of constipation.
Methyldopa	ALDOMET	Antihypertensive	**Susp**: 250 mg/5 mL (1% alcohol) **Tab**: 125, 250, 500 mg	**Initial**: 250 mg bid or tid po for the first 48 h. Adjust dosage at intervals of not less than 2 days. **Maintenance**: 500 mg - 2 g daily po in 2 - 4 divided doses.
Methyldopate Hydrochloride	ALDOMET	Antihypertensive	**Inj**: 50 mg/mL	250 - 500 mg q 6 h IV.
Methylergonovine	METHERGINE	Oxytocic	**Tab**: 0.2 mg **Inj**: 0.2 mg/mL	0.2 mg tid or qid po for a maximum of 1 week. 0.2 mg q 2 - 4 h IM.
Methylphenidate Hydrochloride (C-II)	RITALIN RITALIN SR	CNS Stimulant	**Tab**: 5, 10, 20 mg **Sustained-Rel. Tab**: 20 mg	10 - 30 mg daily po in divided dose 2 or 3 times daily, preferably 30 - 45 minutes ac. 20 mg q 8 h po, preferably 30 - 45 minutes ac.

Methylprednisolone	MEDROL	Corticosteroid	**Tab**: 2, 4, 8, 16, 24, 32 mg	Initial dosage varies from 4 - 48 mg daily po, depending on the disease being treated. This dosage should be maintained or adjusted until the patient's response is satisfactory.
Methylprednisolone Acetate	DEPO-MEDROL	Corticosteroid	**Inj (per mL)**: 40, 80 mg	Initial dosage varies from 20 - 80 mg weekly to monthly, depending on the disease being treated; the dosage may be given intra-articularly or IM. The dosage should be maintained or adjusted until the patient's response is satisfactory.
Methylprednisolone Sodium Succinate	SOLU-MEDROL	Corticosteroid	**Powd for Inj**: 40, 125, 500 mg; 1, 2 g	30 mg/kg IV (administered over at least 30 minutes) q 4 - 6 h for 48 hours.
Methyltestosterone (C-III)	ANDROID, TESTRED	Androgen, Antineoplastic	**Cpsl**: 10 mg	**Replacement Therapy in Males**: 10 - 50 mg daily po. **Breast Carcinoma in Females**: 50 - 200 mg daily po.
	ORETON METHYL		**Tab**: 10 mg	Same dosages as for ANDROID above.
Methysergide Maleate	SANSERT	Antimigraine Agent	**Tab**: 2 mg	4 - 8 mg daily with meals po.
Metipranolol Hydrochloride	OPTIPRANOLOL	Anti-Glaucoma Agent	**Ophth Solution**: 0.3%	1 drop into affected eye(s) bid.
Metoclopramide Hydrochloride	REGLAN	GI Stimulant, Antiemetic	**Inj**: 5 mg/mL	**Diabetic Gastroparesis (severe symptoms)**: 10 mg slow IV (over 1 - 2 minutes) for up to 10 days; then switch to oral therapy. **Nausea and Vomiting associated with Cancer Chemotherapy**: 1 - 2 mg/kg slow IV (over 15 minutes), 30 min before beginning cancer therapy; repeat q 2 h for 2 doses, then q 3 h for 3 doses. **Postoperative Nausea and Vomiting**: 10 mg IM. **Facilitate Small Bowel Intubation**: 10 mg slow IV (over 1 - 2 minutes).

[Continued on the next page]

GENERIC NAME	COMMON TRADE NAMES	THERAPEUTIC CATEGORY	PREPARATIONS	COMMON ADULT DOSAGE
Metoclopramide Hydrochloride [Continued]	REGLAN		**Syrup**: 5 mg/5 mL **Tab**: 5, 10 mg	**Gastroesophageal Reflux**: 10 - 15 mg po up to qid 30 minutes ac & hs. If symptoms are intermittent, single doses of up to 20 mg may be used prior to the provoking stimulus. **Diabetic Gastroparesis (early symptoms)**: 10 mg po 30 minutes ac & hs for 2 - 8 weeks.
Metocurine Iodide	METUBINE IODIDE	Neuromuscular Blocker	**Inj**: 2 mg/mL	0.2 - 0.4 mg/kg IV (over 30 - 60 seconds). Supplemental doses (average, 0.5 - 1 mg) may be made as required.
Metolazone	MYKROX	Antihypertensive	**Tab**: 0.5 mg	0.5 mg once daily po, usually in the morning. If necessary, the dosage may be increased to 1 mg daily po.
	ZAROXOLYN	Diuretic, Antihypertensive	**Tab**: 2.5, 5, 10 mg	**Diuresis**: 5 - 20 mg once daily po. **Hypertension**: 2.5 - 5 mg once daily po.
Metoprolol Succinate	TOPROL XL	Antihypertensive, Antianginal	**Extended-Rel. Tab**: 47.5, 95, 190 mg (equivalent to 50, 100, 200 mg of metoprolol tartrate, respectively)	**Hypertension**: Initially, 50 - 100 mg daily po in a single dose. May increase dosage at weekly (or longer) intervals up to a maximum of 400 mg daily. **Angina**: Initially 100 mg daily po in a single dose. May increase dosage at weekly intervals up to a maximum of 400 mg daily.
Metoprolol Tartrate	LOPRESSOR	Post-MI Drug	**Inj**: 1 mg/mL	**Post-Myocardial Infarction**: Start with 3 bolus IV injections of 5 mg each, at approximately 2-minute intervals. Then, switch to oral dosing as described below.
		Antihypertensive, Antianginal, Post-MI Drug	**Tab**: 50, 100 mg	**Hypertension and Angina**: Initially, 100 mg daily po in a single or divided doses. May increase at weekly intervals. The effective dosage range is 100 - 400 mg/day.

				Post-Myocardial Infarction: **Early Treatment**: In patients who tolerate the full IV dose (15 mg; see below), 50 mg po q 6 h, initiated 15 minutes after the last IV dose and continue for 48 h. Then give a maintenance dose of 100 mg bid po. In patients who do <u>not</u> tolerate the full IV dose, 25 - 50 mg po q 6 h, initiated 15 minutes after the last IV dose or as soon as their condition allows. **Late Treatment**: Patients who appear not to tolerate full Early Treatment or those with contraindications to treatment, 100 mg po bid, as soon as their condition allows.
Metronidazole	FLAGYL FLAGYL 375	Antitrichomonal, Amebicide, Antibacterial	**Tab**: 250, 500 mg **Cpsl**: 375 mg	**Trichomoniasis**: 250 mg tid po for 7 days; 375 mg bid po for 7 days; or 2 g as a single dose po. **Acute Intestinal Amebiasis**: 750 mg tid po for 5 - 10 days. **Amebic Liver Abscess**: 500 - 750 mg tid po for 5 - 10 days. **Anaerobic Bacterial Infections**: Following IV dosing (as described below), 7.5 mg/kg q 6 h for 7 - 10 days.
	FLAGYL ER	Antitrichomonal, Antibacterial	**Tab**: 750 mg	**Bacterial Vaginosis**: 750 mg once daily po for 7 days. Take at least 1 h ac or 2 h pc.
	METROGEL METROCREAM	Anti-Acne Agent	**Gel**: 0.75% **Cream**: 0.75%	Apply and rub in a thin film to affected areas bid, morning and evening.
	METROGEL VAGINAL	Antibacterial	**Vaginal Gel**: 0.75%	Insert 1 applicatorful intravaginally once daily hs or bid, morning and evening, for 5 days.

GENERIC NAME	COMMON TRADE NAMES	THERAPEUTIC CATEGORY	PREPARATIONS	COMMON ADULT DOSAGE
Metronidazole Hydrochloride	FLAGYL I.V. FLAGYL I.V. RTU	Antibacterial	**Powd for Inj**: 500 mg **Inj**: 500 mg/100 mL	**Treatment of Anaerobic Infections**: 15 mg/kg infused IV (over 1 h) as a loading dose; then, 7.5 mg/kg infused IV (over 1 h) q 6 h. **Surgical Prophylaxis**: 15 mg/kg infused IV (over 30 - 60 minutes) and completed 1 hour before surgery; then 7.5 mg/kg infused IV (over 30 - 60 minutes) at 6 and 12 h after the initial dose.
Metyrosine	DEMSER	Antihypertensive	**Cpsl**: 250 mg	250 mg qid po. This may be increased by 250 to 500 mg every day to a maximum of 4.0 g per day in divided doses.
Mexiletine Hydrochloride	MEXITIL	Antiarrhythmic	**Cpsl**: 150, 200, 250 mg	Initially, 200 mg q 8 h po with food or antacid. After 2 - 3 days, dosage may be adjusted in in 50 or 100 mg increments. For rapid control of arrhythmias, 400 mg po may be used as an initial loading dose.
Mezlocillin Sodium	MEZLIN	Antibacterial	**Powd for Inj**: 1, 2, 3, 4 g	**Urinary Tract Infections (Uncomplicated)**: 100 to 125 mg/kg as 1.5 - 2.0 g q 6 h IV or IM. **Urinary Tract (Complicated) and Lower Respiratory Tract Infections**: 150 - 200 mg/kg as 3.0 g q 6 h IV. **Intra-Abdominal, Gynecological, Skin & Skin Structure Infections and Septicemia**: 225 to 300 mg/kg as 3.0 g q 4 h IV or 4.0 g q 6 h IV.
Miconazole	MONISTAT I.V.	Antifungal	**Inj**: 10 mg/mL	200 - 1200 mg per IV infusion. The following daily doses may be divided over 3 infusions: **Candidiasis**: 600 - 1800 mg/day. **Cryptococcosis**: 1200 - 2400 mg/day. **Coccidioidomycosis**: 1800 - 3600 mg/day. **Pseudoallescheriosis**: 600 - 3000 mg/day. **Paracoccidioidomycosis**: 200 - 1200 mg/day.

Miconazole Nitrate	MICATIN	Antifungal	**Cream, Liquid, Powder & Spray Powder**: 2%	Apply to affected areas bid, AM and PM.
	MONISTAT-DERM		**Cream**: 2%	Apply to affected areas bid, AM and PM.
	MONISTAT 3		**Vaginal Suppos**: 200 mg	200 mg intravaginally once daily hs for 3 days.
	MONISTAT 7		**Vaginal Cream**: 2%	Insert 1 applicatorful intravaginally once daily hs for 7 days.
			Vaginal Suppos: 100 mg	100 mg intravaginally once daily hs for 7 days.
Midazolam Hydrochloride (C-IV)	VERSED	Sedative - Hypnotic	**Inj (per mL)**: 1, 5 mg	**Preoperative Sedation**: 0.07 - 0.08 mg/kg deep IM (approx. 5 mg) 1 h before surgery. **Conscious Sedation:** Titrate IV dose slowly to the desired effect. Give no more than 2.5 mg (over at least 2 minutes). Wait another 2 minutes to fully evaluate effect. If further titration is needed, use small increments.
Midodrine Hydrochloride	PRO-AMATINE	Drug for Orthostatic Hypotension	**Tab**: 2.5, 5 mg	10 mg tid po (during the daytime, e.g., at 4 hour intervals).
Miglitol	GLYSET	Hypoglycemic Agent	**Tab**: 25, 50, 100 mg	**Initial**: 25 mg tid po with the first bite of each main meal. **Maintenance**: After 4 - 8 weeks at the 25 mg dose, give 50 mg tid po with the first bite of each main meal.
Milrinone Lactate	PRIMACOR	Inotropic Agent	**Inj**: 1 mg/mL **Inj (Premixed)**: 200 μg/mL in 5% Dextrose Injection	**Loading Dose**: 50 μg/kg IV (over 10 minutes). **Maintenance**: 0.375 - 0.75 μg/kg/min by IV infusion. Total daily dosage: 0.59 - 1.13 mg/kg per 24 hours.
Mineral Oil	FLEET MINERAL OIL ENEMA	Emollient Laxative	**Rectal Liquid**: (pure)	Administer 1 bottle (118 mL) rectally as a single dose.

GENERIC NAME	COMMON TRADE NAMES	THERAPEUTIC CATEGORY	PREPARATIONS	COMMON ADULT DOSAGE
Minocycline Hydrochloride	MINOCIN	Antibacterial	**Susp**: 50 mg/5 mL (5% alc.) **Powd for Inj**: 100 mg	200 mg initially po or IV, followed by 100 mg q 12 h po or IV.
			Cpsl: 50, 100 mg	200 mg initially po, followed by 100 mg q 12 h po; or, 100 - 200 mg initially po, followed by 50 mg qid po.
	DYNACIN		**Cpsl**: 50, 75, 100 mg	
Minoxidil	LONITEN	Antihypertensive	**Tab**: 2.5, 10 mg	Initially, 5 mg once daily po. May increase to 10, 20 and then to 40 mg daily po as a single dose or in divided doses. Intervals between dosage adjustments should be at least 3 days.
	ROGAINE	Hair Growth Stimulator	**Solution**: 20 mg/mL (2%)	Apply 1 mL to the total affected areas of the scalp bid.
	ROGAINE EXTRA STRENGTH		**Solution**: 50 mg/mL (5%)	Apply 1 mL to the total affected areas of the scalp bid.
Mirtazapine	REMERON	Antidepressant	**Tab**: 15, 30, 45 mg	15 mg/day po, preferably in the evening prior to sleep.
Misoprostol	CYTOTEC	Anti-Ulcer Agent	**Tab**: 100, 200 μg	200 μg qid with food po.
Mivacurium Chloride	MIVACRON	Neuromuscular Blocker	**Inj (per mL)**: 0.5, 2 mg	**Initial**: 0.15 mg/kg IV (over 5-15 sec), or 0.20 mg/kg IV (over 30 sec), or 0.25 mg/kg IV (0.15 mg/kg followed in 30 sec by 0.10 mg/kg) for tracheal intubation. **Maintenance**: 0.1 mg/kg IV.
Modafinil	PROVIGIL	CNS Stimulant	**Tab**: 100, 200 mg	**Narcolepsy**: 200 mg once daily po in the AM.
Moexipril Hydrochloride	UNIVASC	Antihypertensive	**Tab**: 7.5, 15 mg	**Initial**: 7.5 mg once daily po, 1 h ac. **Maintenance**: 7.5 - 30 mg daily po in 1 or 2 divided doses, 1 h ac.

Molindone Hydrochloride	MOBAN	Antipsychotic	**Conc Liquid**: 20 mg/mL (alcohol) **Tab**: 5, 10, 25, 50, 100 mg	**Initial**: 50 - 75 mg/day po; increase to 100 mg/day in 3 - 4 days. **Maintenance**: 5 - 15 mg tid or qid po (mild); 10 - 25 mg tid or qid po (moderate); 225 mg/day may be needed (severe psychosis).
Mometasone Furoate	ELOCON	Corticosteroid	**Cream, Oint & Lotion**: 0.1%	Apply a thin film to affected areas once daily.
	NASONEX		**Nasal Spray**: 50 μg/spray	**Allergic Rhinitis:** 2 sprays in each nostril once daily. For prophylaxis, begin 2 - 4 weeks prior to anticipated start of pollen season.
Montelukast Sodium	SINGULAIR	Drug for Asthma	**Tab**: 5, 10 mg	10 mg daily po, taken in the evening.
Moricizine Hydrochloride	ETHMOZINE	Antiarrhythmic	**Tab**: 200, 250, 300 mg	600 - 900 mg/day po, given q 8 h in 3 equally divided doses. Within this range, the dosage can be adjusted in increments of 150 mg/day at 3-day intervals.
Morphine Sulfate (C-II)	ASTRAMORPH/PF, DURAMORPH	Opioid Analgesic	**Inj (per mL)**: 0.5, 1 mg	**IV**: 2 - 10 mg/70 kg. **Epidural**: Initially, 5 mg in the lumbar region; after 1 hour, incremental doses of 1 - 2 mg at interval sufficient to assess effectiveness may be given carefully. Max: 10 mg/24 h. **Intrathecal**: 0.2 - 1 mg in the lumbar area.
	INFUMORPH		**Inj (per mL)**: 10, 25 mg	**Intrathecal Infusion**: Initially, 0.2 - 1 mg/day (patients with no opioid tolerance) and 1 - 10 mg/day (opioid tolerance) in the lumbar area. **Epidural Infusion**: 3.5 - 7.5 mg/day (patients with no opioid tolerance) and 4.5 - 10 mg/day (opioid tolerance).
	KADIAN		**Sustained-Rel. Cpsl**: 20, 50, 100 mg	Variable po dosages based on patient tolerance to opioids and type of conversion, e.g., from oral morphine, parenteral morphine, or other opioid analgesics. Commonly used q 24 h.

[Continued on the next page]

GENERIC NAME	COMMON TRADE NAMES	THERAPEUTIC CATEGORY	PREPARATIONS	COMMON ADULT DOSAGE
Morphine Sulfate (C-II) [Continued]	MS CONTIN		**Controlled-Rel. Tab**: 15, 30, 60, 100, 200 mg	Variable po dosages based on patient tolerance to opioids and type of conversion, e.g., from oral morphine, parenteral morphine, or other opioid analgesics. Commonly used q 12 h.
	ORAMORPH SR		**Sustained-Rel. Tab**: 15, 30, 60, 100 mg	
	MSIR		**Solution (per 5 mL)**: 10, 20 mg **Conc Solution**: 20 mg/mL **Cpsl & Tab**: 15, 30 mg	5 - 30 mg q 4 h po prn pain.
	RMS		**Rectal Suppos**: 5, 10, 20, 30 mg	10 - 20 mg q 4 h rectally.
	ROXANOL		**Oral Solution**: 20 mg/mL	10 - 30 mg q 4 h po prn pain.
	ROXANOL 100		**Oral Solution**: 100 mg/5 mL	10 - 30 mg q 4 h po prn pain.
Moxifloxacin Hydrochloride	AVELOX	Antibacterial	**Tab**: 400 mg	**Acute Bacterial Exacerbation of Chronic Bronchitis**: 400 mg once daily po for 5 days. **Community-Acquired Pneumonia and Acute Bacterial Sinusitis**: 400 mg once daily po for 10 days.
Mupirocin	BACTROBAN	Antibacterial	**Oint**: 2%	Apply a small amount to affected area tid.
Mupirocin Calcium	BACTROBAN NASAL	Antibacterial	**Oint**: 2%	Apply approximately 1/2 of the ointment from the single-use tube into each nostril bid (morning & evening) for 5 days.
	BACTROBAN		**Cream**: 2%	Apply a small amount to affected area tid for 10 days.

Mycophenolate Mofetil	CELLCEPT	Immunosuppressant	**Cpsl**: 250 mg **Tab**: 500 mg **Powd for Inj**: 500 mg (as the HCl)	**Renal Transplantation**: 1 g po or IV (over ≥ 2 h) bid. **Cardiac Transplantation**: 1.5 g po of IV (over ≥ 2 h) bid. Give the initial oral dose as soon as possible following transplantation. Give on an empty stomach. IV administration is recommended for patients unable to take cpls or tabs. Use within 24 h of transplantation and for ≤ 14 days. Switch to the oral medication ASAP.
Nabumetone	RELAFEN	Antiinflammatory	**Tab**: 500, 750 mg	Initially 1000 mg po as a single dose with or without food. Dosage may be increased to 1500 - 2000 mg/day as a single dose or in 2 divided doses.
Nadolol	CORGARD	Antihypertensive, Antianginal	**Tab**: 20, 40, 80, 120, 160 mg	**Hypertension**: Initially, 40 mg once daily po. May increase dosage in increments of 40 to 80 mg until optimal response occurs. Usual maintenance dose is 40 - 80 mg once daily. **Angina**: Initially, 40 mg once daily po. May increase dosage in increments of 40 - 80 mg at 3 - 7 day intervals until optimal response occurs. Usual maintenance dosage is 40 to 80 mg once daily.
Nafcillin Sodium	UNIPEN	Antibacterial	**Cpsl**: 250 mg	**Mild to Moderate Infections**: 250 - 500 mg q 4 to 6 h po. **Severe Infections**: 1000 mg q 4 - 6 h po.
Naftifine Hydrochloride	NAFTIN	Antifungal	**Cream**: 1% **Gel**: 1%	Gently massage into affected areas once daily. Gently massage into affected areas bid, morning and evening.
Nalbuphine Hydrochloride	NUBAIN	Opioid Analgesic	**Inj (per mL)**: 10, 20 mg	10 mg/70 kg SC, IM, or IV; dose may be repeated q 3 - 6 h prn.

GENERIC NAME	COMMON TRADE NAMES	THERAPEUTIC CATEGORY	PREPARATIONS	COMMON ADULT DOSAGE
Nalidixic Acid	NEG-GRAM	Urinary Tract Anti-Infective	**Susp**: 250 mg/5 mL **Cplt**: 250, 500 mg; 1 g	Initially, 1 g qid po for 1 - 2 weeks. For prolonged therapy, may reduce dosage to 500 mg qid after the initial treatment period.
Nalmefene Hydrochloride	REVEX	Opioid Antagonist	**Inj (per mL)**: 100 μg, 1.0 mg	**Opioid Overdose (Known or Suspected)**: Use the **1.0 mg/mL** strength. **Non-Opioid Dependent Patients**: 0.5 mg/70 kg IM, SC, or IV. If needed, this may be followed by a 2nd dose of 1.0 mg/70 kg, 2 - 5 minutes later. **Suspected Opioid-Dependent Patients**: An initial challenge dose of 0.1 mg/70 kg should be used. If no evidence of withdrawal occurs, use the above dosage. **Postoperative Opioid Respiratory Depression**: Use the **100 μg/mL** strength. Initially 0.25 μg/kg IM, SC or IV, followed by 0.25 μg/kg incremental doses at 2 - 5 minute intervals, stopping as soon as the desired degree of opioid reversal occurs.
Naloxone Hydrochloride	NARCAN	Opioid Antagonist	**Inj (per mL)**: 0.4, 1 mg	**Opioid Overdose (Known or Suspected)**: Initially, 0.4 - 2 mg IV. Dose may be repeated at 2 - 3 min intervals. Max: 10 mg. **Postoperative Opioid Respiratory Depression**: 0.1 - 0.2 mg IV at 2 - 3 minute intervals. Doses may be repeated in 1 - 2 hours.
Naltrexone Hydrochloride	REVIA	Opioid Antagonist	**Tab**: 50 mg	50 mg once daily po for most patients.
Nandrolone Decanoate (C-III)	DECA-DURABOLIN	Anabolic Steroid	**Inj (per mL)**: 50, 100, 200 mg (in oil)	**Women**: 50 - 100 mg per week by deep IM. **Men**: 100 - 200 mg per week by deep IM.
Nandrolone Phenpropionate (C-III)	DURABOLIN	Anabolic Steroid	**Inj (per mL)**: 25, 50 mg (in oil)	50 - 100 mg weekly by deep IM.

Naphazoline Hydrochloride	PRIVINE	Nasal Decongestant	**Nasal Solution**: 0.05% **Nasal Spray**: 0.05%	2 drops in each nostril no more than q 3 h. 2 sprays in each nostril q 4 - 6 h.
	NAPHCON NAPHCON FORTE	Ocular Decongestant	**Ophth Solution**: 0.012% **Ophth Solution**: 0.1%	1 - 2 drops into the affected eye(s) up to qid. 1 - 2 drops into the affected eye(s) q 3 - 4 h.
Naproxen	NAPROSYN	Non-Opioid Analgesic, Antiinflammatory	**Susp**: 125 mg/5 mL **Tab**: 250, 375, 500 mg	**Analgesia, Dysmenorrhea, Acute Tendonitis and Bursitis**: 500 mg po, followed by 250 mg po q 6 - 8 h prn. **Acute Gout**: 750 mg po, followed by 250 mg po q 8 h until the attack has subsided. **Rheumatoid Arthritis, Osteoarthritis and Ankylosing Spondylitis**: 250 - 500 mg bid po, morning and evening. **Juvenile Arthritis**: 5 mg/kg bid po.
	EC-NAPROSYN	Antiinflammatory	**Delayed-Rel. Tab**: 375, 500 mg	**Rheumatoid Arthritis, Osteoarthritis and Ankylosing Spondylitis**: 375 - 500 mg bid po, morning and evening.
Naproxen Sodium	ALEVE	Non-Opioid Analgesic, Antipyretic	**Cplt, Tab & Gelcap**: 220 mg	**Analgesia & Fever**: 220 mg q 8 - 12 h po with a full glass of liquid, while symptoms persist or 440 mg initially, followed by 220 mg 12 h later.
	ANAPROX ANAPROX DS	Non-Opioid Analgesic, Antiinflammatory	**Tab**: 275 mg **Tab**: 550 mg	**Analgesia, Dysmenorrhea, Acute Tendonitis and Bursitis**: 550 mg po, followed by 275 mg po q 6 - 8 h prn. **Acute Gout**: 825 mg po, followed by 275 mg po q 8 h until the attack has subsided. **Rheumatoid Arthritis, Osteoarthritis and Ankylosing Spondylitis**: 275 or 550 mg bid po, morning and evening.

GENERIC NAME	COMMON TRADE NAMES	THERAPEUTIC CATEGORY	PREPARATIONS	COMMON ADULT DOSAGE
	NAPRELAN	Non-Opioid Analgesic, Antiinflammatory	**Controlled-Rel. Tab**: 412.5 550 mg (equivalent to 375 and 500 mg of naproxen, respectively)	**Analgesia, Dysmenorrhea, Acute Tendonitis and Bursitis**: 1000 mg once daily po. **Acute Gout**: 1000 - 1500 mg once daily po on the first day, followed by 1000 mg once daily until the attack has subsided. **Rheumatoid Arthritis, Osteoarthritis and Ankylosing Spondylitis**: 750 - 1000 mg once daily po.
Naratriptan Hydrochloride	AMERGE	Antimigraine Agent	**Tab**: 1, 2.5 mg	1 - 2.5 mg po taken with fluid. If the headache returns or if the patient has only a partial response, the dose may be repeated after 4 h. Do not exceed 5 mg within a 24 h period.
Natamycin	NATACYN	Antifungal	**Ophth Susp**: 5%	**Fungal Keratitis**: 1 drop into the affected eye(s) at 1 or 2 hour intervals. The frequency of application can usually be reduced to 1 drop 6 - 8 times daily after the first 3 or 4 days. **Fungal Blepharitis & Conjunctivitis**: 4 to 6 daily applications may be sufficient.
Nedocromil Sodium	TILADE	Drug for Asthma	**Aerosol**: 1.75 mg/spray	2 inhalations qid at regular intervals.
	ALOCRIL	Antiallergic, Ophthalmic	**Ophth Solution**: 2%	1 - 2 drops in each eye bid at regular intervals.
Nefazodone Hydrochloride	SERZONE	Antidepressant	**Tab**: 50, 100, 150, 200, 250 mg	Initially, 100 mg bid po. Effective dose range is 300 - 600 mg/day; therefore, increase dose in increments of 100 - 200 mg/day (given on a bid basis) at interval of no less than 1 week.
Nelfinavir Mesylate	VIRACEPT	Antiviral	**Tab**: 250 mg	750 mg (3 tablets) tid po, with meals or a light snack, in combination with nucleoside analogues.

Neostigmine Methylsulfate	PROSTIGMIN	Cholinomimetic	**Inj (per mL)**: 0.5, 1 mg	**Myastenia Gravis**: 0.5 mg SC or IM. Adjust subsequent doses based on response. **Postoperative Distension & Urinary Retention**: **Prevention**: 0.25 mg SC or IM as soon as possible after operation; repeat q 4 - 6 h for 2 - 3 days. **Treatment**: 0.5 mg SC or IM. **Reversal of Neuromuscular Blockade**: 0.5 - 2 mg by slow IV, repeated as required. Also administer IV atropine sulfate, 0.6 - 1.2 mg.
Netilmicin Sulfate	NETROMYCIN	Antibacterial	**Inj**: 100 mg/mL	**Urinary Tract Infections (Complicated)**: 1.5 - 2.0 mg/kg q 12 h IM or IV. **Serious Systemic Infections**: 1.3 - 2.2 mg/kg q 8 h IM or IV; or, 2.0 - 3.25 mg/kg q 12 h IM or IV.
Nevirapine	VIRAMUNE	Antiviral	**Tab**: 200 mg **Suspension**: 50 mg/5 mL	**Initial**: 200 mg once daily po for 14 days. **Maintenance**: 200 mg bid po in combination with a nucleoside analog antiretroviral drug.
Niacin	NICOLAR	Hypolipidemic	**Tab**: 500 mg	Start with 250 mg once daily po following the evening meal. Frequency of dosing and total daily dose can be increased q 4 - 7 days until the desired response is attained or the first-level therapeutic dose of 1.5 - 2 g daily is reached. If response is not adequate after 2 months, the dosage can be increased at 2 to 4 week intervals to 3 grams/day (1 g tid po). The usual dose is 1 - 2 g bid to tid po.
	NIASPAN		**Extended-Rel. Tab**: 375, 500, 750, 1000 mg	Take hs with a low-fat meal or snack. 375 mg once daily po for 1 week; then 500 mg once daily po for 1 week; then 750 mg once daily po for 1 week; then 1000 mg once daily po for weeks 4 - 7. May increase by 500 mg every 4 weeks until an adequate response is achieved. Maximum: 2 g/day.

GENERIC NAME	COMMON TRADE NAMES	THERAPEUTIC CATEGORY	PREPARATIONS	COMMON ADULT DOSAGE
Nicardipine Hydrochloride	CARDENE	Antianginal, Antihypertensive	**Cpsl**: 20, 30 mg	**Angina**: Initially, 20 mg tid po; may increase dosage after 3 days. Doses in the range of 20 - 40 mg tid are effective. **Hypertension**: Initially, 20 mg tid po. Doses in the range of 20 - 40 mg tid are effective.
	CARDENE SR	Antihypertensive	**Sustained-Rel. Cpsl**: 30, 45, 60 mg	Initially, 30 mg bid po. Effective doses range from 30 - 60 mg bid po.
	CARDENE I.V.	Antihypertensive	**Inj**: 2.5 mg/mL	**Initiation in a Drug-free Patient**: Administer by contin. IV infusion at a conc. of 0.1 mg/mL. **Titration**: For gradual reduction in blood pressure, start at 5 mg/h (50 mL/h); may increase rate by 2.5 mg/h (25 mL/h) q 15 min up to a max. of 15 mg/h (150 mL/h). For rapid reduction in blood pressure, begin at 5 mg/h (50 mL/h); may increase rate by 2.5 mg/h (25 mL/h) q 5 min up to a maximum of 15 mg/h (150 mL/h). In either case, after desired effect is achieved reduce infusion rate to 30 mL/h. **Maintenance**: Adjust infusion rate as needed. **Substitution for Oral Nicardipine**: Use the infusion rate as indicated in the table below:

Oral Dose	Equivalent IV Infusion Rate
20 mg q 8 h	0.5 mg/h
30 mg q 8 h	1.2 mg/h
40 mg q 8 h	2.2 mg/h

Nicotine	HABITROL, NICODERM CQ	Smoking Deterrent	**Transdermal**: rate = 7, 14, 21 mg/24 hr	Apply to clean, dry, non-hairy site on upper body or upper outer arm. Initially, one 21 mg/24 h patch daily for 6 weeks; then, one 14 mg/24 h patch daily for 2 - 4 weeks; then, one 7 mg/24 h patch daily for 2 - 4 weeks.
	NICOTROL		**Transdermal**: rate = 15 mg/16 hr	Apply to clean, dry, non-hairy site on upper body or upper outer arm. Apply one patch daily for 6 weeks.
	PROSTEP		**Transdermal**: rate = 11, 22 mg/24 hr	Apply to clean, dry, non-hairy site on upper body or upper outer arm. Initially, one 22 mg/24 h patch daily for 4 - 8 weeks; then, one 11 mg/24 h patch daily for 2 - 4 weeks.
	NICOTROL NS		**Nasal Spray**: 0.5 mg/spray	1 spray in each nostril. Start with 1 - 2 doses per hour, which may be increased up to a maximum of 5 doses per hour (40 doses per day).
Nicotine Polacrilex	NICORETTE	Smoking Deterrent	**Chewing Gum**: 2 mg/piece	**Less Dependent Smokers**: Chew 1 piece slowly and intermittently for 30 minutes. Most patients require 9 - 12 pieces of gum per day. Maximum: 30 pieces per day.
	NICORETTE DS		**Chewing Gum**: 4 mg/piece	**Highly Dependent Smokers**: Chew 1 piece slowly and intermittently for 30 minutes. Most patients require 9 - 12 pieces of gum per day. Maximum: 20 pieces per day.
Nifedipine	ADALAT, PROCARDIA	Antianginal	**Cpsl**: 10, 20 mg	Initially, 10 mg tid po; may increase dosage over a 7 - 14 day period. Usual effective dosage range is 10 - 20 mg tid po.
	ADALAT CC, PROCARDIA XL	Antianginal, Antihypertensive	**Extended-Rel. Tab**: 30, 60, 90 mg	Initially, 30 or 60 mg once daily po; adjust the dosage over a 7 - 14 day period.
Nilutamide	NILANDRON	Antineoplastic	**Tab**: 50 mg	300 mg (6 tablets) once daily po for 30 days, followed by 150 mg (3 tablets) once daily.

GENERIC NAME	COMMON TRADE NAMES	THERAPEUTIC CATEGORY	PREPARATIONS	COMMON ADULT DOSAGE
Nisoldipine	SULAR	Antihypertensive	**Extended-Rel. Tab**: 10, 20, 30, 40 mg	Initially 20 mg once daily po, then increase the dose by 10 mg per week, or longer intervals, to adequate control of blood pressure. The usual maintenance dosage is 20 - 40 mg once daily po.
Nitrofurantoin	FURADANTIN	Urinary Tract Anti-Infective, Antibacterial	**Oral Susp**: 25 mg/5 mL	50 - 100 mg qid po with food. For long-term suppressive therapy, reduce dosage to 50 - 100 mg po hs.
Nitrofurantoin Macrocrystals	MACRODANTIN	Urinary Tract Anti-Infective, Antibacterial	**Cpsl**: 25, 50, 100 mg	**Usual Dosage**: 50 - 100 mg qid po with food. **Urinary Tract Infections (Uncomplicated)**: 50 mg qid po with food.
Nitrofurantoin Monohydrate	MACROBID	Urinary Tract Anti-Infective	**Cpsl**: 100 mg	100 mg q 12 h po with food for 7 days.
Nitrofurazone	FURACIN	Burn Preparation	**Cream & Soluble Dressing**: 0.2%	Apply directly to the lesion or place on gauze. Reapply daily or every few days.
Nitroglycerin	DEPONIT	Antianginal	**Transdermal**: rate = 0.2, 0.4 mg/h	Apply a 0.2 mg/h or 0.4 mg/h patch for 12 to 14 h daily as a starting dose.
	MINITRAN		**Transdermal**: rate = 0.1, 0.2, 0.4, 0.6 mg/h	Same dosage as for DEPONIT above.
	NITRODISC		**Transdermal**: rate = 0.2, 0.3, 0.4 mg/h	Same dosage as for DEPONIT above.
	NITRO-DUR		**Transdermal**: rate = 0.1, 0.2, 0.3, 0.4, 0.6, 0.8 mg/h	Same dosage as for DEPONIT above.
	TRANSDERM-NITRO		**Transdermal**: rate = 0.1, 0.2, 0.4, 0.6 mg, 0.8 mg/h	Same dosage as for DEPONIT above.
	NITRO-BID		**Oint**: 2%	Apply 0.5 inch of ointment to a 1 x 3-inch area of skin q 8 h. Titrate upward (1 inch on a 2 x 3-in area q 8 h) until angina is controlled.

	NITROGARD		**Extended-Rel. Buccal Tab**: 1, 2, 3 mg	Place tablet under the upper lip or in the buccal pouch; allow tablet to dissolve slowly over a 3 - 5 hour period. Initial dose is 1 mg, with subsequent increases guided by symptoms and side effects.
	NITROLINGUAL SPRAY		**Aerosol**: 0.4 mg/dose	1 - 2 sprays onto or under tongue at onset of attack. No more than 3 sprays within a 15 minute period.
	NITRO-BID IV		**Inj (per mL)**: 5 mg	Initially, 5 μg/min by IV infusion. Titrate dosage based upon clinical situation; increases of 5 μg/min can be made at 3 - 5 min intervals. If no response occurs at 20 μg/min, increments of 10 and later 20 μg/min can be used.
Nizatidine	AXID	Histamine H_2-Blocker, Anti-Ulcer Agent	**Cpsl**: 150, 300 mg	**Active Duodenal Ulcer or Benign Gastric Ulcer**: 300 mg once daily po hs or 150 mg bid po. **Maintenance of Healed Duodenal Ulcer**: 150 mg once daily po hs. **Gastroesophageal Reflux Disease**: 150 mg bid po.
	AXID AR	Histamine H_2-Blocker	**Tab**: 75 mg	**Prevention of Heartburn, Acid Indigestion, and Sour Stomach**: 75 mg po with water 30 - 60 min. before consuming food and beverages that may cause symptoms. May be used up to bid.
Norethindrone	MICRONOR, NOR-Q.D.	Oral Contraceptive	**Tab**: 0.35 mg	1 tablet daily po, every day of the year starting on the first day of menstruation.
Norethindrone Acetate	AYGESTIN	Progestin	**Tab**: 5 mg	**Amenorrhea**: 2.5 - 10 mg once daily po, for 5 to 10 days during the second half of the menstrual cycle. **Endometriosis**: 5 mg once daily po for 2 weeks, with increments of 2.5 mg/day q 2 weeks until 15 mg/day is reached.

GENERIC NAME	COMMON TRADE NAMES	THERAPEUTIC CATEGORY	PREPARATIONS	COMMON ADULT DOSAGE
Norfloxacin	NOROXIN	Urinary Tract Anti-Infective	**Tab**: 400 mg	**Urinary Tract Infections -** **Uncomplicated, due to *E. coli, K. pneumonia,* or *P. mirabilis***: 400 mg q 12 h po for 3 days. **Uncomplicated, due to Other Organisms:** 400 mg q 12 h po for 7 - 10 days. **Complicated**: 400 mg q 12 h po for 10 - 21 days. **Gonorrhea (Uncomplicated)**: 800 mg po (as a single dose). **Prostatitis:** 400 mg q 12 h po for 28 days.
	CHIBROXIN	Antibacterial	**Ophth Solution**: 0.3%	1 - 2 drops into the eye(s) qid for up to 7 days.
Norgestrel	OVRETTE	Oral Contraceptive	**Tab**: 0.075 mg	1 tablet daily po, every day of the year starting on the first day of menstruation.
Nortriptyline Hydrochloride	PAMELOR	Antidepressant	**Solution**: 10 mg/5 mL (3.4% alcohol) **Cpsl**: 10, 25, 50, 75 mg	25 mg tid or qid po; or total daily dosage may be given once daily hs po.
Nystatin	MYCOSTATIN	Antifungal	**Susp**: 100,000 Units/mL **Tab**: 500,000 Units **Pastilles**: 200,000 Units **Vaginal Tab**: 100,000 Units **Cream & Oint**: 100,000 Units/g **Powder**: 100,000 Units/g	400,000 - 600,000 Units qid po (1/2 dose in each side of the mouth). 500,000 - 1,000,000 Units tid po. 200,000 - 400,000 Units 4 or 5 times daily po. Allow to dissolve slowly in the mouth. 1 tablet daily intravaginally for 2 weeks. Apply liberally to affected areas bid. Apply to candidal lesions bid or tid.

Ofloxacin	FLOXIN FLOXIN I.V.	Antibacterial	**Tab**: 200, 300, 400 mg **Inj (per mL)**: 4, 10, 20 mg	**Lower Respiratory Tract, Skin & Skin Structure Infections**: 400 mg q 12 h po or by IV infusion (over 60 min.) for 10 days. **Gonorrhea (Uncomplicated)**: 400 mg po or by IV infusion (over 60 min.) as a single dose. **Cervicitis or Urethritis due to *N. gonorrhoeae* and/or *C. trachomatis***: 300 mg q 12 h po or by IV infusion (over 60 min.) for 7 days. **Cystitis due to *E. coli* or *K. pneumoniae***: 200 mg q 12 h po or by IV infusion (over 60 min.) for 3 days. **Cystitis due to other Organisms**: 200 mg q 12 h po or by IV infusion (over 60 min.) for 7 days. **Urinary Tract Infections (Complicated)**: 200 mg q 12 h po or by IV infusion (over 60 min.) for 10 days. **Prostatitis**: 300 mg q 12 h po for 6 weeks or by IV infusion (over 60 min.) for up to 10 days, then switch to oral therapy.
	OCUFLOX	Antibacterial	**Ophth Solution**: 0.3%	**Bacterial Conjunctivitis**: 1 - 2 drops in affected eye(s) q 2 - 4 h for 2 days, then 1 - 2 drops qid for up to 5 more days. **Bacterial Corneal Ulcer**: On Days 1 and 2 instill 1 - 2 drops in affected eye(s) q 30 min. while awake; awaken at approximately 4 and 6 h after retiring and instill 1 or 2 drops. On Days 3 through 7 - 9 instill 1 or 2 drops hourly while awake. On Days 7 - 9 to completion of therapy instill 1 or 2 drops qid.
	FLOXIN OTIC	Antibacterial	**Otic Solution**: 0.3%	**Otitis Externa**: 10 drops (0.5 mL) instilled into the affected ear bid for 10 days. **Chronic Suppurative Otitis Media with Perforated Tympanic Membranes**: 10 drops (0.5 mL) instilled into the affected ear bid for 14 days.

GENERIC NAME	COMMON TRADE NAMES	THERAPEUTIC CATEGORY	PREPARATIONS	COMMON ADULT DOSAGE
Olanzapine	ZYPREXA	Antipsychotic	**Tab**: 2.5, 5, 7.5, 10, 15 mg	Initially 5 - 10 mg once daily po, with a target dose of 10 mg/day within several days. Further dosage adjustments should occur at intervals of not less than 1 week.
Olopatadine Hydrochloride	PATANOL	Antihistamine	**Ophth Solution**: 0.1%	1 - 2 drops in each affected eye bid at an interval of 6 - 8 h.
Olsalazine Sodium	DIPENTUM	Bowel Antiinflam. Agent	**Cpsl**: 250 mg	1000 mg daily po in 2 divided doses.
Omeprazole	PRILOSEC	Gastric Acid Pump Inhibitor, Anti-Ulcer Agent	**Delayed-Rel. Cpsl**: 10, 20, 40 mg	**Acute Duodenal Ulcer, Severe Erosive Esophagitis or Poorly Responsive Gastro-esophageal Reflux Disease (GERD)**: 20 mg once daily po for up to 4 - 8 weeks. **Maintenance of Healing Erosive Esophagitis**: 20 mg daily po. **Active Duodenal Ulcer Associated with *Helicobacter pylori* Infection**: 40 mg po each AM plus clarithromycin 500 mg tid po for days 1 - 14; then 20 mg po each AM for days 15 - 28. **Pathological Hypersecretory Conditions**: 60 mg once daily po, initially; adjust dosage as indicated. Daily dosages over 80 mg po should be given in divided doses.
Ondansetron Hydrochloride	ZOFRAN	Antiemetic	**Tab**: 4, 8, 24 mg **Oral Solution**: 4 mg/5 mL	**Highly Emetogenic Chemotherapy**: 24 mg po as a single dose 30 minutes before the start of single-day chemotherapy. **Moderately Emetogenic Chemotherapy**: 8 mg po q 8 h for 2 doses 30 minutes before chemotherapy, then 8 mg q 12 h for 1 - 2 days after chemotherapy is completed. **Prevention of Postoperative Nausea and Vomiting**: 16 mg po as a single dose 1 hour before induction of anesthesia.

			Inj: 2 mg/mL **Inj (premixed)**: 32 mg/50 mL	**Nausea & Vomiting Associated With Cancer Chemotherapy**: Three 0.15 mg/kg doses IV: The first dose is infused over 15 minutes beginning 30 minutes before the start of emetogenic chemotherapy. Alternatively, 32 mg IV (infused over 15 min) beginning 30 minutes before the start of emetogenic chemotherapy. Subsequent doses are given 4 and 8 h after the first dose. **Prevention of Postoperative Nausea and Vomiting**: Immediately before induction of anesthesia or postoperatively, 4 mg IV (over 2 to 5 min).
Orlistat	XENICAL	Lipase Inhibitor	**Cpsl**: 120 mg	120 mg tid po with each main meal containing fat (during or up to 1 hour pc).
Orphenadrine Citrate	NORFLEX	Skeletal Muscle Relaxant	**Extended-Rel. Tab**: 100 mg **Inj**: 60 mg/2 mL	100 mg bid po, AM and PM. 60 mg q 12 h IM or IV.
Oseltamivir Phosphate	TAMIFLU	Antiviral	**Cpsl**: 75 mg	75 mg bid po for 5 days. Begin treatment within 2 days of symptom onset.
Oxacillin Sodium	BACTOCILL	Antibacterial	**Cpsl**: 250, 500 mg	**Mild to Moderate Infections of the Skin, Soft Tissue or Upper Respiratory Tract**: 500 mg q 4 - 6 h po for a minimum of 5 days. **Serious or Life-Threatening Infections**: After initial parenteral treatment, 1 g q 4 - 6 h po.
			Powd for Inj: 250, 500 mg; 1, 2, 4 g	**Mild to Moderate Upper Respiratory and Local Skin and Soft Tissue Infections**: 250 - 500 mg q 4 - 6 h IM or IV. **Severe Lower Respiratory or Disseminated Infections**: 1 g q 4 - 6 h IM or IV.
Oxamniquine	VANSIL	Anthelmintic	**Cpsl**: 250 mg	12 - 15 mg/kg as a single dose po with food.
Oxandrolone (C-III)	OXANDRIN	Anabolic Steroid	**Tab**: 2.5 mg	2.5 mg bid - qid po. Usually a course of therapy of 2 - 4 weeks is adequate.

GENERIC NAME	COMMON TRADE NAMES	THERAPEUTIC CATEGORY	PREPARATIONS	COMMON ADULT DOSAGE
Oxaprozin	DAYPRO	Antiinflammatory	**Tab**: 600 mg	1200 mg once daily po. For patients of low body weight or mild disease, an initial dose of 600 mg once a day may be appropriate.
Oxazepam (C-IV)	SERAX	Antianxiety Agent	**Cpsl**: 10, 15, 30 mg **Tab**: 15 mg	10 - 30 mg tid or qid po. 15 - 30 mg tid or qid po.
Oxiconazole Nitrate	OXISTAT	Antifungal	**Cream & Lotion**: 1%	***Tinea pedis***: Apply to affected areas once daily or bid for 1 month. ***Tinea corporis*, and *T. cruris***: Apply to affected areas once daily or bid for 2 weeks. ***Tinea versicolor***: Apply to affected areas once daily for 2 weeks.
Oxtriphylline		Bronchodilator	**Tab**: 100, 200 mg	7.8 mg/kg po, followed by 4.7 mg/kg q 8 h po (in nonsmokers) and 4.7 mg/kg q 6 h po (in smokers).
	CHOLEDYL SA		**Sustained-Action Tab**: 400, 600 mg	Therapy should be initiated and daily dosage requirements established using a non-sustained-action form of oxtriphylline. If the total daily dosage of the nonsustained prep. is 1200 mg, then 600 mg of CHOLEDYL SA may be used q 12 h. Similarly, if the total daily dosage is 800 mg, then 400 mg of CHOLEDYL SA may be used q 12 h.
Oxybutynin Chloride	DITROPAN	Urinary Tract Antispasmodic	**Syrup**: 5 mg/5 mL **Tab**: 5 mg	5 mg bid - tid po.
	DITROPAN XL		**Extended-Rel. Tab**: 5, 10, 15 mg	Initially, 5 mg once daily po. May increase weekly in 5 mg increments. Maximum: 30 mg daily po.

Oxycodone Hydrochloride (C-II)	ROXICODONE	Opioid Analgesic	**Solution**: 5 mg/5 mL **Conc Solution**: 20 mg/mL **Tab**: 5 mg	5 mg q 6 h po prn pain.
	OXYCONTIN		**Controlled-Rel. Tab**: 10, 20, 40, 80 mg	Variable po dosages based on patient tolerance to opioids and type of conversion, e.g., from oral morphine, parenteral morphine, or other opioid analgesics. Commonly used q 12 h.
Oxymetazoline Hydrochloride	VISINE L.R.	Ocular Decongestant	**Ophth Solution**: 0.025%	1 - 2 drops in the affected eye(s) q 6 h.
	AFRIN, NTZ	Nasal Decongestant	**Nasal Solution**: 0.05% **Nasal Spray**: 0.05%	2 - 3 drops into each nostril bid, AM and PM. Spray 2 - 3 times into each nostril bid, AM and PM.
	CHERACOL NASAL, DRISTAN 12-HOUR, 4-WAY LONG LASTING, NEO-SYNEPHRINE MAXIMUM STRENGTH, NOSTRILLA LONG ACTING, VICKS SINEX 12-HOUR	Nasal Decongestant	**Nasal Spray**: 0.05%	Same dosage as AFRIN Spray above.
Oxymorphone Hydrochloride (C-II)	NUMORPHAN	Opioid Analgesic	**Inj (per mL)**: 1, 1.5 mg	**IM or SC**: 1 - 1.5 mg q 4 - 6 h, prn pain. **IV**: 0.5 mg q 4 - 6 h, prn pain.
			Rectal Suppos: 5 mg	Insert 1 rectally q 4 - 6 h.
Oxytetracycline	TERRAMYCIN	Antibacterial	**Inj (per mL)**: 50, 125 mg	250 mg q 24 h IM or 300 mg daily in divided doses IM at 8- to 12-hour intervals.
Oxytetracycline Hydrochloride	TERRAMYCIN	Antibacterial	**Cpsl**: 250 mg	**Usual Dosage**: 250 - 500 mg q 6 h po. **Brucellosis**: 500 mg qid po with streptomycin for 3 weeks. **Gonorrhea**: Initially 1.5 g po, followed by 500 mg qid po, for a total of 9.0 g. **Syphilis**: 30 - 40 g po in equally divided doses over a period of 10 - 15 days.

GENERIC NAME	COMMON TRADE NAMES	THERAPEUTIC CATEGORY	PREPARATIONS	COMMON ADULT DOSAGE
Pamidronate Disodium	AREDIA	Bone Stabilizer	**Powd for Inj**: 30, 60, 90 mg	**Hypercalcemia of Malignancy**: **Moderate**: 60 mg - 90 by IV infusion. The 60 mg dose is given over at least 4 hours; the 90 mg dose is given over 24 hours. **Severe**: 90 mg by IV infusion, given over 24 h. **Paget's Disease**: 30 mg daily by IV infusion over 4 hours, on 3 consecutive days, for a total dose of 90 mg. **Osteolytic Bone Lesions of Multiple Myeloma**: 90 mg by IV infusion (over 4 hours) once monthly.
Pancuronium Bromide	PAVULON	Neuromuscular Blocker	**Inj (per mL)**: 1, 2 mg	Initially 0.04 - 0.1 mg/kg IV. Later, use incremental doses starting at 0.01 mg/kg.
Papaverine Hydrochloride	PAVABID	Vasodilator	**Timed-Rel. Cpsl**: 150 mg	150 mg q 12 h po.
Paricalcitol	ZEMPLAR	Vitamin D Analog	**Inj**: 5 μg/mL	Initially 0.04 - 0.1 μg/kg (2.8 - 7 μg) IV (as a bolus injection) no more often than every other day at any time during dialysis. If a satisfactory response is not observed, the dose may be increased by 2 - 4 μg at 2- to 4-week intervals. Doses as high as 0.24 μg/kg (16.8 μg) have been safely given.
Paromomycin Sulfate	HUMATIN	Amebicide	**Cpsl**: 250 mg (of paromomycin base)	**Intestinal Amebiasis**: 25 - 35 mg/kg/day po in 3 divided doses with meals for 5 - 10 days.
Paroxetine Hydrochloride	PAXIL	Antidepressant, Drug for Obsessive-Compulsive Disorder, Drug for Panic Disorder, Drug for Social Anxiety Disorder	**Tab**: 10, 20, 30, 40 mg **Susp**: 10 mg/5 mL	**Depression**: Initially, 20 mg po once daily in the AM. May increase in 10 mg/day increments at intervals ≥ 1 week, up to a maximum of 50 mg/day. **Social Anxiety Disorder**: Initially, 20 mg po once daily in the AM. The usual dosage range is 20 - 60 mg daily po.

				OCD and Panic Disorder: Initially, 20 mg po once daily in the AM. The recommended dose is 40 mg daily po. May increase in 10 mg/day increments at intervals ≥ 1 week, up to a maximum of 60 mg/day.
	PAXIL CR	Antidepressant	**Controlled-Rel. Tab**: 12.5, 25 mg	**Depression**: Initially, 12.5 - 25 mg po once daily in the AM. Doses may be changed at intervals ≥ 1 week, up to a maximum of 62.5 mg/day.
Pegaspargase	ONCASPAR	Antineoplastic	**Inj**: 750 IUnits/mL	2500 IU/m^2 q 14 days by IM (preferred) or IV.
Pemoline (C-IV)	CYLERT	CNS Stimulant	**Chewable Tab**: 37.5 mg **Tab**: 18.75, 37.5, 75 mg	**Attention Deficit Hyperactivity Disorder**: The starting dose is 37.5 mg/day po. Gradually increase daily dose by 18.75 mg at 1 week intervals until the desired response is obtained (Maximum: 112.5 mg).
Penbutolol Sulfate	LEVATOL	Antihypertensive	**Tab**: 20 mg	20 mg once daily po.
Penciclovir	DENAVIR	Antiviral	**Cream**: 10 mg/g	Apply q 2 h while awake for 4 days. Start treatment as early as possible when lesions appear.
Penicillin G Benzathine	BICILLIN L-A	Antibacterial	**Inj (per mL)**: 300,000; 600,000 Units	**Streptococcal Upper Respiratory Infections (e.g., Pharyngitis)**: 1,200,000 Units IM. **Syphilis (Primary, Secondary & Latent)**: 2,400,000 Units IM. **Syphilis (Late)**: 2,400,000 Units IM at 7-day intervals for 3 doses. **Rheumatic Fever and Glomerulonephritis (Prophylaxis)**: 1,200,000 Units IM once a month or 600,000 Units IM q 2 weeks.
Penicillin G Potassium	PFIZERPEN	Antibacterial	**Powd for Inj**: 5,000,000; 20,000,000 Units	5,000,000 to 80,000,000 Units daily IM or by IV drip, depending on the severity of the infection and the susceptibility of the infecting organism.

GENERIC NAME	COMMON TRADE NAMES	THERAPEUTIC CATEGORY	PREPARATIONS	COMMON ADULT DOSAGE
Penicillin G Procaine	PFIZERPEN-AS	Antibacterial	**Inj**: 300,000 Units/mL	**Usual Dosage**: 600,000 - 1,000,000 Units daily IM.
	WYCILLIN		**Inj**: 600,000 Units/mL	**Syphilis**: 600,000 Units daily IM for 8 - 15 days. **Gonorrhea**: 4,800,000 Units IM divided into at least 2 doses and inj. at diff. sites at the same visit, with probenecid (1 g po).
Penicillin V Potassium	PEN-VEE K	Antibacterial	**Tab**: 250, 500 mg **Powd for Solution (per 5 mL)**: 125, 250 mg	**Streptococcal Upper Respiratory Infections**: 125 - 250 mg q 6 - 8 h po for 10 days. **Pneumococcal Infections**: 250 - 500 mg q 6 h po until afebrile for at least 48 hours. **Staphylococcal Infections**: 250 - 500 mg q 6 to 8 h po. **Vincent's Gingivitis and Pharyngitis**: 250 - 500 mg q 6 - 8 h po.
Pentamidine Isethionate	NEBUPENT	Antiprotozoal	**Powd for Solution**: 300 mg	300 mg once q 4 weeks, administered via a Respirgard II nebulizer.
	PENTAM 300		**Powd for Inj**: 300 mg	4 mg/kg once daily IV (over 60 minutes) or IM for 14 days.
Pentazocine Lactate (C-IV)	TALWIN	Opioid Analgesic	**Inj**: 30 mg/mL	**Usual Dosage**: 30 mg q 3 - 4 h IM, SC or IV. **Patients in Labor**: 30 mg IM or 20 mg q 2 - 3 h IV.
Pentobarbital Sodium (C-II)	NEMBUTAL SODIUM	Sedative - Hypnotic	**Cpsl**: 50, 100 mg **Elixir**: 20 mg/5 mL (18% alcohol)	**Sedation**: Reduce hypnotic dose appropriately. **Hypnosis**: 100 mg po hs.
			Rectal Suppos: 30, 60, 120, 200 mg	**Sedation**: Reduce hypnotic dose appropriately. **Hypnosis**: 120 - 200 mg rectally.
		Hypnotic	**Inj**: 50 mg/mL	**IM**: 150 - 200 mg as a single dose. **IV**: Initially, 100 mg/70 kg. May increase in small increment to 200 - 500 mg if needed.
Pentosan Polysulfate Sodium	ELMIRON	Urinary Tract Analgesic	**Cpsl**: 100 mg	100 mg tid po. Take 1 h ac or 2 h pc with water.

Pentostatin	NIPENT	Antineoplastic	**Powd for Inj**: 10 mg	After hydration with 500 - 1000 mL of 5% Dextrose in 0.5 normal saline, give 4 mg/m^2 IV every other week. An additional 500 mL of 5% Dextrose should be given after the drug is administered.
Pentoxifylline	TRENTAL	Hemorheologic Agent	**Tab**: 400 mg	400 mg tid po with meals.
Pergolide Mesylate	PERMAX	Antiparkinsonian	**Tab**: 0.05, 0.25, 1 mg	0.05 mg po for first 2 days; then increase the dosage by 0.1 or 0.15 mg/day every third day for the next 12 days. The dosage may then be increased by 0.25 mg/day every 3rd day until optimal response is reached. Daily dose is usually given in 3 divided doses.
Perindopril Erbumine	ACEON	Antihypertensive	**Tab**: 2, 4, 8 mg	Initially, 4 mg once daily po. The usual maintanence dose range is 4 - 8 mg administered as a single daily dose or in 2 divided doses.
Permethrin	ELIMITE	Scabicide	**Cream**: 5%	Throughly massage into skin from the head to the soles of the feet. Wash off (bath or shower) after 8 - 14 h.
	NIX		**Liquid**: 1%	Shampoo hair, rinse with water and towel dry. Saturate the hair and scalp; allow solution to remain for 10 minutes before rinsing off with water. If live lice are observed 7 days or more after the first application, a second treatment should be given.
Perphenazine	TRILAFON	Antipsychotic, Antiemetic	**Tab**: 2, 4, 8, 16 mg **Liquid Conc**: 16 mg/5 mL **Inj**: 5 mg/mL	**Psychoses**: **Outpatients**: 4 - 8 mg tid po. **Hospitalized Patients**: 8 - 16 mg bid - qid po; or 5 mg q 6 h IM. **Nausea & Vomiting**: 8 - 16 mg daily in divided doses po; or 5 mg IM.
Phenazopyridine Hydrochloride	PYRIDIUM	Urinary Tract Analgesic	**Tab**: 100, 200 mg	200 mg tid po after meals.

GENERIC NAME	COMMON TRADE NAMES	THERAPEUTIC CATEGORY	PREPARATIONS	COMMON ADULT DOSAGE
Phendimetrazine Tartrate (C-III)	BONTRIL PDM, PLEGINE	Anorexiant	**Tab**: 35 mg	35 mg bid - tid po, 1 h ac.
	BONTRIL SLOW RELEASE PRELU-2		**Slow-Rel. Cpsl**: 105 mg **Timed-Rel. Cpsl**: 105 mg	105 mg po, 30 - 60 minutes before the morning meal.
Phenelzine Sulfate	NARDIL	Antidepressant	**Tab**: 15 mg	Initially, 15 mg tid po. Increase dosage to at least 60 mg/day at a rapid pace as patient tolerates drug. After several weeks, dosage may be reduced (over several weeks) to as low as 15 mg daily or every other day.
Phenindamine Tartrate	NOLAHIST	Antihistamine	**Tab**: 25 mg	25 mg q 4 - 6 h po.
Phenobarbital (C-IV)		Sedative - Hypnotic, Anticonvulsant	**Tab**: 15, 30, 60, 100 mg **Elixir**: 20 mg/5 mL (alcohol)	**Sedation**: 30 - 120 mg daily po in 2 - 3 divided doses. **Hypnosis**: 100 - 200 mg hs po. **Convulsions**: 60 - 200 mg daily po.
Phenobarbital Sodium (C-IV)		Sedative - Hypnotic, Anticonvulsant	**Inj (per mL)**: 30, 60, 65, 130 mg	**Sedation**: 30 - 120 mg daily IM or IV in 2 - 3 divided doses. **Preoperative Sedation**: 100 - 200 mg IM, 60 to 90 minutes before surgery. **Hypnosis**: 100 - 320 mg IM or IV. **Acute Convulsions**: 200 - 320 mg IM or IV, repeated in 6 h prn.
Phenoxybenzamine Hydrochloride	DIBENZYLINE	Antihypertensive	**Cpsl**: 10 mg	Initially, 10 bid po; increase dosage every other day, usually to 20 - 40 mg, bid - tid po.
Phentermine Hydrochloride (C-IV)	ADIPEX-P	Anorexiant	**Cpsl & Tab**: 37.5 mg	37.5 mg daily po, before breakfast or 1 - 2 h after breakfast.
	FASTIN		**Cpsl**: 30 mg	30 mg daily po, approximately 2 h after breakfast.

Phentermine Resin (C-IV)	IONAMIN	Anorexiant	**Cpsl**: 15, 30 mg	15 - 30 mg daily po, before breakfast or 10 to 14 hours before retiring.
Phentolamine Mesylate	REGITINE	Antihypertensive	**Powd for Inj**: 5 mg	**Preoperative**: 5 mg IM or IV, 1 - 2 h before surgery, and repeated if necessary. **During Surgery**: 5 mg IV as required.
Phenylephrine Hydrochloride	NEO-SYNEPHRINE	Nasal Decongestant	**Nasal Solution & Spray**: 0.25,	2 - 3 drops or sprays in each nostril q 4 h.
	NŌSTRIL		**Nasal Spray**: 0.25, 0.5%	2 - 3 sprays (of 0.25%) in each nostril q 3 - 4 h; 0.5% may be used in resistant cases.
	NEO-SYNEPHRINE	Sympathomimetic	**Inj**: 10 mg/mL (1%)	**Mild or Moderate Hypotension**: 2 - 5 mg SC; or 0.2 mg by slow IV. Repeat injections no more often than every 10 - 15 minutes. **Severe Hypotension & Shock**: Infuse a dilute solution IV (10 mg in 500 mL of Dextrose Injection) at 100 - 180 μg/min (approx. 100 to 180 drops/min). When blood pressure stabilizes, use maintenance rate of 40 - 60 μg/min (approx. 40 - 60 drops/min).
Phenylpropanolamine Hydrochloride	DEXATRIM	Anorexiant	**Timed-Rel. Cplt & Tab**: 75 mg	75 mg po at mid-morning with a full glass of water.
Phenytoin	DILANTIN-125 DILANTIN INFATAB	Antiepileptic	**Susp**: 125 mg/5 mL **Chewable Tab**: 50 mg	Initially, 125 mg tid po; adjust dosage prn. Initially, 100 mg tid po; adjust dosage prn.
Phentoin Sodium	DILANTIN	Antiepileptic	**Inj**: 50 mg/mL	**Status Epilepticus**: A loading dose of 10 - 15 mg/kg slow IV (at a rate not exceeding 50 mg/min). Follow with maintenance doses of 100 mg po or IV q 6 - 8 h.
			Cpsl: 100 mg	Initially, 100 mg tid po; adjust dosage prn. For patients controlled at 100 mg tid, a single daily dose of 300 mg po may be given.
Phytonadione	AQUA-MEPHYTON	Vitamin K_1	**Inj (per mL)**: 2, 10 mg	2.5 - 25 mg SC or IM. Repeat in 6 - 8 h if necessary.

GENERIC NAME	COMMON TRADE NAMES	THERAPEUTIC CATEGORY	PREPARATIONS	COMMON ADULT DOSAGE
Pilocarpine	OCUSERT PILO-20	Anti-Glaucoma Agent	**Ocular Therapeutic System**: releases 20 μg/h for 1 week	Place in conjunctival cul-de-sac hs; replace every 7 days.
	OCUSERT PILO-40		**Ocular Therapeutic System**: releases 40 μg/h for 1 week	Place in conjunctival cul-de-sac hs; replace every 7 days.
Pilocarpine Hydrochloride	ISOPTO CARPINE	Anti-Glaucoma Agent	**Ophth Solution**: 0.25, 0.5, 1, 2, 3, 4, 5, 6, 8, 10%	1 or 2 drops in eye(s) up to 6 times daily. The usual range is 0.5 to 4%.
	PILOCAR, PILOSTAT		**Ophth Solution**: 0.5, 1, 2, 3, 4, 6%	1 or 2 drops in eye(s) up to 6 times daily. The usual range is 0.5 to 4%.
	PILOPINE HS GEL		**Ophth Gel**: 4%	Apply a 0.5 in. ribbon in the lower conjunctival sac of the affected eye(s) once daily hs.
	SALAGEN	Cholinomimetic	**Tab**: 5 mg	Initially, 5 mg tid po. Dosage may be increased to 10 mg tid, if necessary and tolerated.
Pilocarpine Nitrate	PILAGAN	Anti-Glaucoma Agent	**Ophth Solution**: 1, 2, 4%	1 or 2 drops in the affected eye(s) bid to qid.
Pimozide	ORAP	Antipsychotic	**Tab**: 2 mg	Initially, 1 - 2 mg daily in divided doses po; may increase thereafter every other day. Most are maintained at less than 0.2 mg/kg daily or 10 mg daily, whichever is less.
Pindolol	VISKEN	Antihypertensive	**Tab**: 5, 10 mg	Initially, 5 mg bid po. After 3 - 4 weeks dosage may be increased in increments of 10 mg/day q 2 - 4 weeks, to a maximum of 60 mg/day.
Pioglitazone Hydrochloride	ACTOS	Hypoglycemic Agent	**Tab**: 15, 30, 45 mg	**Monotherapy or Combination Therapy:** Usually 15 or 30 mg po once daily. For patients who do not respond adequately (as determined by fasting serum glucose), the dose may be increased to 45 mg po once daily.

Pipecuronium Bromide	ARDUAN	Neuromuscular Blocker	**Powd for Inj**: 10 mg	**Endotracheal Intubation**: 70 - 85 μg/kg IV. **Maintenance**: 10 - 15 μg/kg IV.
Piperacillin Sodium	PIPRACIL	Antibacterial	**Powd for Inj**: 2, 3, 4 g	**Urinary Tract Infections (Uncomplicated) and Most Community-Acquired Pneumonia**: 100 to 125 mg/kg/day IM or IV in divided doses q 6 - 12 h. **Urinary Tract Infections (Complicated)**: 125 to 200 mg/kg/day IV in divided doses q 6 - 8 h. **Serious Infections**: 200 - 300 mg/kg/day IV in divided doses q 4 - 6 h. **Gonorrhea (Uncomplicated)**: 2 g IM as a single dose with probenecid (1 g po).
Pirbuterol Acetate	MAXAIR	Bronchodilator	**Aerosol**: 200 μg/spray	2 inhalations q 4 - 6 h.
Piroxicam	FELDENE	Antiinflammatory	**Cpsl**: 10, 20 mg	20 mg daily po.
Plicamycin	MITHRACIN	Antineoplastic	**Powd for Inj**: 2.5 mg	**Testicular Tumors**: 25 - 30 μg/kg daily by IV infusion (over 4 - 6 h) for 8 - 10 days. Repeat monthly if necessary. **Hypercalcemia & Hypercalciuria**: 25 μg/kg daily by IV infusion (over 4 - 6 h) for 3 or 4 days.
Polyethylene Glycol 3350	MIRALAX	Saline Laxative	**Powder**: (with measuring cup)	Dissolve 17 g in 8 fl. oz. of water and drink once daily. May need 2 - 4 days to induce bowel movement.
Polythiazide	RENESE	Diuretic, Antihypertensive	**Tab**: 1, 2, 4 mg	**Diuresis**: 1 - 4 mg daily po. **Hypertension**: 2 - 4 mg daily po.

GENERIC NAME	COMMON TRADE NAMES	THERAPEUTIC CATEGORY	PREPARATIONS	COMMON ADULT DOSAGE
Potassium Chloride	K-DUR	Potassium Supplement	**Extended-Rel. Tab**: 10, 20 mEq	Dosage must be adjusted to the individual needs of each patient. Typical dosages are given below. **Prevention of Hypokalemia**: 20 - 30 mEq daily po as a single dose or in divided doses with meals and with water or other liquids. **Treatment of Potassium Depletion**: 40 - 100 mEq daily po in divided doses with meals and with water or other liquids.
	K-TAB		**Extended-Rel. Tab**: 10 mEq	
	KLOTRIX		**Slow-Rel. Tab**: 10 mEq	
	K-NORM		**Extended-Rel. Cpsl**: 10 mEq	
	KLOR-CON		**Extended-Rel. Tab**: 8, 10 mEq	
	MICRO-K EXTENCAPS		**Extended-Rel. Cpsl**: 8, 10 mEq	
	SLOW-K		**Extended-Rel. Tab**: 8 mEq	
	TEN-K		**Extended-Rel. Tab**: 10 mEq	
	KLORVESS 10% LIQUID		**Liquid**: 20 mEq/15 mL (0.75% alcohol)	15 mL (20 mEq) diluted in 3 - 4 oz. of cold water bid - qid po.
	KLOR-CON POWDER		**Powd for Solution**: 20 mEq	Same dosages as shown above. Dissolve each each packet in at least 3 oz. of fluid.
	KLOR-CON/25 POWDER		**Powd for Solution**: 25 mEq	
	MICRO-K LS		**Extended-Rel. Formulation (Powd for Susp)**: 20 mEq	Dissolve each packet in 2 - 6 oz. of cold water. Drink solution 1 - 5 times daily with meals.
	KLORVESS		**Effervescent Powd for Solution**: 20 mEq	Dissolve each packet in 3 - 4 oz. of cold water, fruit juice or other liquid. Drink solution bid to qid.
	K-LYTE/CL		**Effervescent Tab**: 25, 50 mEq	Dissolve 1 tablet completely in cold water (3 to 4 oz. for the 25 mEq tab and 6 to 8 oz. for the 50 mEq tab); drink solution bid - qid.
Potassium Gluconate	KAON	Potassium Supplement	**Elixir**: 20 mEq/15 mL (5% alcohol)	15 mL (20 mEq) diluted in 3 - 4 oz. of cold water bid - qid po.

Pramipexole	MIRAPEX	Antiparkinsonian	**Tab**: 0.125, 0.25, 0.5, 1, 1.5 mg	Increase dosage gradually from a starting dose of 0.125 mg tid po and do not increase more often than q 5 - 7 days. The table below shows a suggested ascending dosage schedule:

Week	Oral Dosage	Total Daily Dose
1	0.125 mg tid	0.375 mg
2	0.25 mg tid	0.75 mg
3	0.5 mg tid	1.5 mg
4	0.75 mg tid	2.25 mg
5	1.0 mg tid	3.0 mg
6	1.25 mg tid	3.75 mg
7	1.5 mg tid	4.5 mg

Pramoxine Hydrochloride	TRONOLANE	Local Anesthetic, Antihemorrhoidal	**Cream**: 1%	**Topical**: Apply to affected areas tid or qid. **Anorectal**: Apply up to 5 times daily, especially morning, night, and after bowel movements. **Intrarectal**: Insert 1 applicatorful into rectum.
Pravastatin Sodium	PRAVACHOL	Hypolipidemic	**Tab**: 10, 20, 40 mg	10 - 20 mg once daily po, hs.
Praziquantel	BILTRICIDE	Anthelmintic	**Tab**: 600 mg	Three 20 mg/kg doses po for 1 day only.
Prazosin Hydrochloride	MINIPRESS	Antihypertensive	**Cpsl**: 1, 2, 5 mg	Initially, 1 mg bid - tid po. Dosage may be slowly increased to 20 mg daily, given in divided doses.
Prednicarbate	DERMATOP	Corticosteroid	**Cream**: 0.1%	Apply a thin film to skin bid.
Prednisolone	PRELONE	Corticosteroid	**Syrup**: 15 mg/5 mL	Initial dosage varies from 5 - 60 mg daily po depending on the disease being treated and the patient's response.

GENERIC NAME	COMMON TRADE NAMES	THERAPEUTIC CATEGORY	PREPARATIONS	COMMON ADULT DOSAGE
Prednisolone Acetate	PRED-MILD PRED FORTE	Corticosteroid	**Ophth Susp**: 0.12% **Ophth Susp**: 1%	1 - 2 drops into affected eye(s) bid - qid. During the initial 24 - 48 h, the dosing frequency may be increased if necessary.
Prednisolone Sodium Phosphate	HYDELTRASOL	Corticosteroid	**Inj**: 20 mg/mL	**For IV and IM Injection**: Dose requirements are variable and must be individualized on the basis of the disease and the response of the patient. The initial dosage varies from 4 to 60 mg a day. Usually the daily parenteral dose of HYDELTRASOL is the same as the oral dose of prednisolone and the dosage interval is q 4 to 8 h. **For Intra-articular, Intralesional and Soft Tissue Injection**: Dose requirements are variable and must be individualized on the basis of the disease, the response of the patient, and the site of injection. The usual dose is from 2 to 30 mg. The frequency usually ranges from once every 3 to 5 days to once every 2 to 3 weeks.
	INFLAMASE MILD 1/8% INFLAMASE FORTE 1%	Corticosteroid	**Ophth Solution**: 0.125% **Ophth Solution**: 1%	1 - 2 drops into affected eye(s) up to q h during the day & q 2 h at night. When a favorable response occurs, reduce dosage to 1 drop q 4 h.
Prednisone	DELTASONE	Corticosteroid	**Tab**: 2.5, 5, 10, 20, 50 mg	Initial dosage may vary from 5 - 60 mg daily po, depending on the disease being treated.
Primaquine Phosphate	PRIMAQUINE PHOSPHATE	Antimalarial	**Tab**: 26.3 mg (equal to 15 mg of primaquine base)	15 mg (of base) daily po for 14 days.
Primidone	MYSOLINE	Antiepileptic	**Susp**: 250 mg/5 mL **Tab**: 50, 250 mg	100 - 125 mg hs po (for 3 days); 100 - 125 mg bid po (for 3 days); 100 - 125 mg tid po (for 3 days); then 250 mg tid po.

Probenecid		Anti-Gout Agent, Penicillin/Cephalosporin Adjunct	**Tab**: 500 mg	**Gout**: 250 mg bid po for 1 week, followed by 500 mg bid thereafter. **Penicillin/Cephalosporin Therapy**: The recommended dosage is 2 g po daily in divided doses. Usually 1 g po with or just before each administration of antibacterial therapy.
Procainamide Hydrochloride	PRONESTYL	Antiarrhythmic	**Cpsl & Tab**: 250, 375, 500 mg **Inj (per mL)**: 100, 500 mg	Up to 50 mg/kg daily in divided doses q 3 h po. **IM**: 50 mg/kg daily in divided doses given q 3 to 6 h until oral therapy is possible. **IV**: 100 mg q 5 minutes (at a rate not to exceed 50 mg/min) until the arrhythmia is suppressed or until 500 mg has been given. **IV Infusion**: Loading dose of 20 mg/mL (1 g diluted in 50 mL of 5% Dextrose Injection) at a rate of 1 mL/min for 25 - 30 min; then a maintenance dose of 2 or 4 mg/mL (1 g diluted in 500 or 250 mL of 5% Dextrose Injection) at a rate of 0.5 - 1.5 mL/min.
	PROCANBID PRONESTYL-SR		**Extended-Rel. Tab**: 500, 1000 mg **Extended-Rel. Tab**: 500 mg	Up to 50 mg/kg daily in divided doses q 6 h po.
Procarbazine Hydrochloride	MATULANE	Antineoplastic	**Cpsl**: 50 mg	2 - 4 mg/kg/day po as a single dose or in divided doses for 1 week; then maintain the dosage at 4 - 6 mg/kg/day until maximum response occurs. Then give 1 - 2 mg/kg/day.
Prochlorperazine	COMPAZINE	Antiemetic	**Rectal Suppos**: 25 mg	**Nausea & Vomiting**: 25 mg bid rectally.

GENERIC NAME	COMMON TRADE NAMES	THERAPEUTIC CATEGORY	PREPARATIONS	COMMON ADULT DOSAGE
Prochlorperazine Edisylate	COMPAZINE	Antiemetic, Antipsychotic	**Syrup**: 5 mg/5 mL	**Nausea & Vomiting**: 5 - 10 mg tid or qid po.
			Inj: 5 mg/mL	**Nausea & Vomiting**: 5 - 10 mg q 3 - 4 h deep IM; or 2.5 - 10 mg by slow IV injection or IV infusion (maximum rate of 5 mg/min). **Psychosis**: Initially, 10 - 20 mg deep IM. May repeat q 2 - 4 h, if necessary, for a few doses; then switch to oral medication.
Prochlorperazine Maleate	COMPAZINE	Antiemetic, Antipsychotic	**Tab**: 5, 10 mg	**Nausea & Vomiting**: 5 - 10 mg tid or qid po. **Non-Psychotic Anxiety**: 5 mg tid or qid po. **Psychosis:** **Mild or in Outpatients**: 5 - 10 mg tid - qid po. **Moderate-to-Severe or in Hospitalized Patients**: Initially, 10 mg tid - qid po; raise the dosage slowly until symptoms are controlled. **More Severe Cases**: Optimum dosage is 100 to 150 mg daily po.
			Sustained-Rel. Cpsl: 10, 15 mg	**Nausea & Vomiting or Non-Psychotic Anxiety**: 15 mg po on arising or 10 mg q 12 h po.
Procyclidine Hydrochloride	KEMADRIN	Antiparkinsonian	**Tab**: 5 mg	Initially, 2.5 mg tid po pc. If well tolerated, gradually increase to 5 mg tid pc.
Progesterone	PROGESTASERT	Intrauterine Contraceptive	**Intrauterine System**: unit containing a reservoir of 38 mg of progesterone	Insert a single unit into the uterine cavity. Replace 1 year after insertion.
Progesterone, Micronized	CRINONE 8%	Progestin	**Vaginal Gel**: 8% (90 mg in prefilled applicators)	**Assisted Reproductive Technology:** **Supplementation**: 1 applicatorful intravaginally once daily (see Note, below). **Replacement**: 1 applicatorful intravaginally bid (see Note, below). Note: if pregnancy occurs, treatment may be continued until placental autonomy is achieved (10 - 12 weeks).

	CRINONE 4%		**Vaginal Gel**: 4% (45 mg in prefilled applicators)	**Secondary Amenorrhea**: 1 applicatorful intravaginally every other day up to a total of 6 doses. For women who fail to respond, a trial of CRINONE 8% (see above) every other day for up to a total of 6 doses may be tried.
Promazine Hydrochloride	SPARINE	Antipsychotic	**Tab**: 25, 50, 100 mg **Inj**: 50 mg	10 - 200 mg q 4 - 6 h po. 10 - 200 mg q 4 - 6 h IM.
Promethazine Hydrochloride	PHENERGAN	Antihistamine, Antiemetic, Sedative	**Tab**: 12.5, 25, 50 mg **Syrup (PLAIN)**: 6.25 mg/5 mL (7% alcohol) **Syrup (FORTIS)**: 25 mg/5 mL (1.5% alcohol) **Inj (per mL)**: 25, 50 mg **Rectal Suppos**: 12.5, 25, 50 mg	**Allergy**: 25 mg po hs, or 12.5 mg po ac & hs. By deep IM injection, 25 mg; may repeat once in 2 h, then switch to oral medication. **Motion Sickness**: 25 mg po, taken 30 - 60 min before travel; repeat once in 8 - 12 h. On succeeding days, 25 mg bid, on arising & hs. **Nausea & Vomiting**: 25 mg po, followed by 12.5 - 25 mg q 4 - 6 h po. When oral medication is not tolerated, dose by injection (deep IM) or by rectal suppositories. **Sedation**: 25 - 50 mg hs po or by deep IM.
Propafenone Hydrochloride	RYTHMOL	Antiarrhythmic	**Tab**: 150, 225, 300 mg	Initiate with 150 mg q 8 h po. Dosage may be increased at a minimum of 3 - 4 day intervals to 225 mg q 8 h po, and if needed to 300 mg q 8 h po.
Propantheline Bromide	PRO-BANTHINE	Anticholinergic	**Tab**: 7.5, 15 mg	15 mg po 30 minutes ac and 30 mg hs. For mild symptoms, 7.5 mg tid po may be used.
Propoxyphene Hydrochloride (C-IV)	DARVON	Opioid Analgesic	**Cpsl**: 65 mg	65 mg q 4 h po, prn pain.
Propoxyphene Napsylate (C-IV)	DARVON-N	Opioid Analgesic	**Tab**: 100 mg	100 mg q 4 h po, prn pain.

GENERIC NAME	COMMON TRADE NAMES	THERAPEUTIC CATEGORY	PREPARATIONS	COMMON ADULT DOSAGE
Propranolol Hydrochloride	INDERAL	Antihypertensive, Antianginal, Antiarrhythmic, Antimigraine Agent, Post-MI Drug	**Tab**: 10, 20, 40, 60, 80 mg	**Hypertension**: Initially, 40 mg bid po; increase dosage gradually. The usual maintenance dosage is 120 - 240 mg daily. **Angina**: 80 - 320 mg daily po in divided doses (bid to qid). **Hypertrophic Subaortic Stenosis**: 20 - 40 mg tid - qid po. ac & hs. **Arrhythmias**: 10 - 30 mg tid - qid po, ac & hs. **Migraine Headaches**: Initially, 80 mg daily po in divided doses; increase dosage gradually. The usual maintenance dosage is 160 - 240 mg daily. **Post-Myocardial Infarction**: 180 - 240 mg daily po in divided doses (bid to tid).
		Antiarrhythmic	**Inj**: 1 mg/mL	**Life-Threatening Arrhythmias**: 1 - 3 mg IV (at a rate not exceeding 1 mg/min). May repeat dose after 2 minutes, if necessary. Then no additional drug should be given for 4 h.
	INDERAL LA	Antihypertensive, Antianginal, Antimigraine Agent	**Long-Acting Cpsl**: 60, 80, 120, 160 mg	**Hypertension**: Initially, 80 mg once daily po; may increase to usual maintenance dosage of 120 - 160 mg daily. **Angina**: Initially, 80 mg once daily po; increase at 3 - 7 day intervals. The average optimal dosage is 160 mg once daily. **Hypertrophic Subaortic Stenosis**: 80 - 160 mg once daily po. **Migraine Headaches**: Initially, 80 mg once daily po; increase gradually. The usual effective dosage range is 160 - 240 mg once daily.
Propylhexedrine	BENZEDREX INHALER	Nasal Decongestant	**Inhalant Tube**: delivers 0.4 to 0.5 mg/800 mL of air	2 inhalations in each nostril not more often than q 2 h.

Propylthiouracil		Antithyroid Agent	**Tab**: 50 mg	**Initial**: 300 mg/day po, usually administered in 3 equal doses at 8 hour intervals. **Maintenance**: Usually, 100 - 150 mg daily po in 3 equal doses at 8 hour intervals.
Protamine Sulfate		Heparin Antagonist	**Inj**: 10 mg/mL	1 mg per 90 - 115 Units of heparin activity by slow IV (over 10 minutes). Maximum dose: 50 mg.
Protriptyline Hydrochloride	VIVACTIL	Antidepressant	**Tab**: 5, 10 mg	15 - 40 mg daily po in 3 - 4 divided doses.
Pseudoephedrine Hydrochloride	SUDAFED CHILDREN'S NASAL DECONGESTANT	Decongestant	**Liquid**: 15 mg/5 mL	20 mL (60 mg) q 4 - 6 h po.
	SUDAFED		**Tab**: 30, 60 mg	60 mg q 4 - 6 h po.
	SUDAFED 12 HOUR		**Extended-Rel. Cplt**: 120 mg	120 mg q 12 h po.
	EFIDAC/24		**Extended-Rel. Tab**: 240 mg	240 mg once daily po.
Pseudoephedrine Sulfate	DRIXORAL NON-DROWSY	Decongestant	**Extended-Rel. Tab**: 120 mg	120 mg q 12 h po.
Psyllium	PERDIEM FIBER	Bulk Laxative	**Granules**: 4.03 g/rounded teaspoonful (6.0 g)	In the evening and/or before breakfast, 1 - 2 rounded teaspoonfuls should be swallowed with at least 8 oz. of a cool beverage.
	SERUTAN		**Granules**: 2.5 g/heaping teaspoonful	1 - 3 heaping teaspoonfuls on cereal or other food 1 - 3 times daily po. Drink at least 8 oz. of liquid with the food.

GENERIC NAME	COMMON TRADE NAMES	THERAPEUTIC CATEGORY	PREPARATIONS	COMMON ADULT DOSAGE
Psyllium Hydrophilic Mucilloid	FIBERALL	Bulk Laxative	**Powder**: 3.4 g/rounded teaspoonful (5.0 - 5.9 g) **Wafer**: 3.4 g	1 rounded teaspoonful in 8 oz. of liquid 1 - 3 times daily po. 1 - 2 wafers with 8 oz. of liquid 1 - 3 times daily po.
	METAMUCIL		**Powder (Regular)**: 3.4 g per rounded teaspoonful **Powder (Flavored)**: 3.4 g per tablespoonful	1 rounded teaspoonful (Regular) or tablespoonful (Flavored) in 8 oz. of liquid 1 - 3 times daily po.
	SYLLACT		**Powder**: 3.3 g/rounded teaspoonful	1 rounded teaspoonful in 8 oz. of liquid 1 - 3 times daily po.
Pyrantel Pamoate	ANTIMINTH	Anthelmintic	**Susp**: 144 mg/mL (equivalent to 50 mg/mL of pyrantel)	5 mg/lb (to a maximum of 1 g) as a single dose po.
	REESE'S PINWORM MEDICINE		**Liquid**: 144 mg/mL (equivalent to 50 mg/mL of pyrantel) **Cpsl**: 180 mg (equivalent to 62.5 mg of pyrantel)	5 mg/lb (to a maximum of 1 g) as a single dose po.
Pyrazinamide		Tuberculostatic	**Tab**: 500 mg	15 - 30 mg/kg once daily po (Maximum: 2 g/day).
Pyridostigmine Bromide	MESTINON	Cholinomimetic	**Syrup**: 60 mg/5 mL (5% alcohol) **Tab**: 60 mg	600 mg (10 tsp. or 10 tab) daily po in divided doses, spaced to provide maximum relief when maximum strength is needed.
	MESTINON TIMESPAN		**Slow-Rel. Tab**: 180 mg	1 - 3 tablets once or twice daily po.
Pyrimethamine	DARAPRIM	Antimalarial	**Tab**: 25 mg	**Chemoprophylaxis**: 25 mg once weekly po.
Quazepam (C-IV)	DORAL	Hypnotic	**Tab**: 7.5, 15 mg	7.5 - 15 mg hs po.

Quetiapine Fumarate	SEROQUEL	Antipsychotic	**Tab**: 25, 100, 200 mg	**Over 18 yrs**: Initially 25 mg bid po. Increase in increments of 25 - 50 mg bid - tid on Days 2 and 3; by Day 4, dose should be in the range of 300 - 400 mg/day in 2 - 3 divided doses. Make further dosage adjustments prn at intervals of at least 2 days in increments or decrements of 25 - 50 mg bid. Usual dose range: 150 - 750 mg/day.
Quinapril Hydrochloride	ACCUPRIL	Antihypertensive, Heart Failure Drug	**Tab**: 5, 10, 20, 40 mg	**Hypertension**: **Initial**: 10 mg once daily po. Adjust dosage at intervals of at least 2 weeks. **Maintenance**: Most patients require 20 - 80 mg daily po as a single dose or in 2 equally divided doses. **Heart Failure**: Used in conjunction with other conventional therapies including diuretics or digoxin. Initially, give 5 mg bid po. Titrate patients at weekly intervals until an effective dose is attained, usually 10 - 20 mg bid.
Quinidine Gluconate	QUINAGLUTE	Antiarrhythmic	**Extended-Rel. Tab**: 324 mg	324 - 648 mg q 8 - 12 h po.
Quinidine Polygalacturonate	CARDIOQUIN	Antiarrhythmic	**Tab**: 275 mg	Initially 275 mg q 6 - 8 h po. If tolerated and the serum level is well within the therapeutic range, the dose may be increased cautiously.
Quinidine Sulfate	QUINIDEX EXTENTABS	Antiarrhythmic	**Extended-Rel. Tab**: 300 mg	Initially 300 mg q 8 - 12 h po. If tolerated and the serum level is well within the therapeutic range, the dose may be increased cautiously.
Quinine Sulfate		Antimalarial	**Cpsl**: 200, 260, 325 mg **Tab**: 260 mg	260 - 650 mg tid po for 6 - 12 days.

GENERIC NAME	COMMON TRADE NAMES	THERAPEUTIC CATEGORY	PREPARATIONS	COMMON ADULT DOSAGE
Rabeprazole Sodium	ACIPHEX	Gastric Acid Pump Inhibitor, Anti-Ulcer Agent	**Delayed-Rel. Tab**: 20 mg	**Healing of Duodenal Ulcers**: 20 mg once daily po after the morning meal for ≤ 4 weeks. **Healing of Erosive or Ulcerative GERD**: 20 mg once daily po for 4 - 8 weeks. **Maintenance of Healing of Erosive or Ulcerative GERD**: 20 mg once daily po. **Treatment of Pathological Hypersecretory Conditions, including Zollinger-Ellison Syndrome**: Initially, 60 mg once daily po. Adjust dosage to patient needs and continue for as long as clinically indicated.
Raloxifene Hydrochloride	EVISTA	Antiosteoporotic	**Tab**: 60 mg	60 mg once daily po.
Ramipril	ALTACE	Antihypertensive, Heart Failure Drug	**Cpsl**: 1.25, 2.5, 5, 10 mg	**Hypertension**: Initially, 2.5 mg once daily po. The usual maintenance dosage range is 2.5 to 20 mg daily administered as a single dose or in two equally divided doses. **Heart Failure Post-M.I.**: Initially 2.5 mg bid po. If hypotension occurs, reduce dosage to 1.25 mg bid po, but all patients should be titrated toward a target dosage of 5 mg bid.
Ranitidine Bismuth Citrate	TRITEC	Anti-Ulcer Agent	**Tab**: 400 mg	**Eradication of *Helicobacter pylori* Infection**: 400 mg bid po for 4 weeks in conjunction with clarithromycin 500 mg tid po for the first 2 weeks.
Ranitidine Hydrochloride	ZANTAC 75	Histamine H_2-Blocker	**Tab**: 84 mg (equivalent to 75 mg of ranitidine)	**Heartburn, Acid Indigestion, Sour Stomach**: 75 mg once or twice daily po.

	ZANTAC	Histamine H_2-Blocker, Anti-Ulcer Agent	**Syrup**: 15 mg/mL (7.5% alcohol) **Cpsl & Tab**: 150, 300 mg **Effervescent Tab**: 150 mg **Effervescent Granules**: 150 mg/packet	**Active Duodenal Ulcer**: 150 mg bid po; or 300 mg once daily po hs. **Maintenance Therapy**: 150 mg daily po hs. **Pathological Hypersecretory Conditions**: 150 mg bid po, or more frequently if needed. **Gastroesophageal Reflux and Benign Gastric Ulcer**: 150 mg bid po. **Erosive Esophagitis**: 150 mg qid po.
			Inj: 25 mg/mL	**IM**: 50 mg q 6 - 8 h. **Intermittent IV**: 50 mg q 6 - 8 h as a bolus (diluted solution) or as an infusion (at a rate not greater than 5 - 7 mL/min). **Continuous IV Infusion**: 6.25 mg/h.
Repaglinide	PRANDIN	Hypoglycemic Agent	**Tab**: 0.5, 1, 2 mg	There is no fixed dosage regimen for the management of type 2 diabetes with this drug. **Starting Dose**: **For patients not previously treated or whose HbA_{1C} is < 8%**: 0.5 mg po ac. **For patients previously treated with blood glucose lowering drugs or whose HbA_{1C} is > 8%**: 1 - 2 mg po ac. Dosage adjustments should be determined by blood glucose response. The recommended dose range is 0.5 - 4 mg po with meals and the drug may be given bid - qid ac.
Reserpine		Antihypertensive	**Tab**: 0.1, 0.25 mg	Initially, 0.5 mg daily po for 1 - 2 weeks; for maintenance, reduce to 0.1 - 0.25 mg daily.
Reteplase, Recombinant	RETAVASE	Thrombolytic	**Powd for Inj**: 18.8 mg (10.8 IUnits)	10 IUnits by bolus IV injection (given over 2 min), followed by a second 10 IU bolus IV injection (over 2 min) 30 minutes after the initiation of the first injection.
Rifabutin	MYCOBUTIN	Tuberculostatic	**Cpsl**: 150 mg	300 mg once daily po.

GENERIC NAME	COMMON TRADE NAMES	THERAPEUTIC CATEGORY	PREPARATIONS	COMMON ADULT DOSAGE
Rifampin	RIFADIN RIFADIN I.V.	Tuberculostatic	**Cpsl**: 150, 300 mg **Powd for Inj**: 600 mg	600 mg daily in a single administration, po (1 hour before or 2 hours after a meal) or IV.
Rifapentine	PRIFTIN	Tuberculostatic	**Tab**: 150 mg	**Intensive Phase**: 600 mg twice weekly po with an interval of ≥ 3 days between doses continued for 2 months. Administer in combination as part of an appropriate drug regimen that includes daily companion drugs. **Continuation Phase**: Continue treatment once weekly for 4 months in combination with isoniazid or an appropriate drug for susceptible organisms.
Riluzole	RILUTEK	Drug for Amyotrophic Lateral Sclerosis	**Tab**: 50 mg	50 mg q 12 h po, taken at least 1 h ac or 2 h pc.
Rimantadine Hydrochloride	FLUMADINE	Antiviral	**Syrup**: 50 mg/5 mL **Tab**: 100 mg	**Prophylaxis:** 100 mg bid po. **Treatment:** 100 mg bid po. Start therapy within 48 h of symptoms; continue for 7 days from initial onset of symptoms.
Rimexolone	VEXOL	Corticosteroid	**Ophth Susp**: 1%	**Post-Operative Inflammation**: 1 - 2 drops into the affected eye(s) qid beginning 24 h after surgery & continuing for 2 weeks. **Anterior Uveitis**: 1 - 2 drops into the affected eye(s) q 1 h during waking hours for the first week, 1 drop q 2 h during waking hours of the second week, and then taper off until the uveitis is resolved.
Risedronate Sodium	ACTONEL	Bone Stabilizer	**Tab**: 30 mg	30 mg once daily po for 2 months. Take ≥ 30 min before the first food or drink of the day other than water. Take while in a upright position with a full glass (6 - 8 oz.) of plain water and avoid lying down for 30 min to minimize the possibility of GI side effects.

Risperidone	RISPERDAL	Antipsychotic	**Tab**: 0.25, 0.5, 1, 2, 3, 4 mg **Oral Solution**: 1 mg/mL	Initially, 1 mg bid po. Increase in increments of 1 mg bid on 2nd & 3rd day, as tolerated, to a target dose of 3 mg bid. Further dosage adjustaments should be made at intervals of ≥ 1 week.
Ritonavir	NORVIR	Antiviral	**Solution**: 80 mg/mL **Cpsl**: 100 mg	600 mg bid po with food. For patients who experience nausea, initiate therapy with 300 mg bid po for 1 day, 400 mg bid for 2 days, 500 mg bid for 1 day, then 600 mg bid po thereafter.
Rizatriptan Benzoate	MAXALT	Antimigraine Agent	**Tab**: 5, 10 mg	5 - 10 mg po. For redosing, doses should be separated by at least 2 h. Maximum: 30 mg within 24 h.
	MAXALT-MLT		**Oral Disintegrating Tab**: 5, 10 mg	5 - 10 mg placed on the tongue where it will dissolve. For redosing, doses should be separated by at least 2 h. Maximum: 30 mg within 24 h.
Rofecoxib	VIOXX	Antiinflammatory, Non-Opioid Analgesic	**Tab**: 12.5, 25 mg **Susp (per 5 mL)**: 12.5, 25 mg	**Osteoarthritis**: Initially 12.5 mg once daily po. Some patients may benefit by an increase to the maximum of 25 mg once daily po. **Acute Pain and Primary Dysmenorrhea**: Initially 50 mg once daily po for up to 5 days.
Ropinirole Hydrochloride	REQUIP	Antiparkinsonian	**Tab**: 0.25, 0.5, 1, 2, 4, 5 mg	The recommended initial dose is 0.25 mg tid po. Based on patient response titrate the dosage in weekly increments as follows: **Week 1**: 0.25 mg tid po. **Week 2**: 0.5 mg tid po. **Week 3**: 0.75 mg tid po. **Week 4**: 1.0 mg tid po. After week 4, if necessary, the dosage may be increased by 1.5 mg/day on a weekly basis up to a dose of 9 mg/day, and then by ≤ 3 mg/day weekly to a total dose of 24 mg/day.

GENERIC NAME	COMMON TRADE NAMES	THERAPEUTIC CATEGORY	PREPARATIONS	COMMON ADULT DOSAGE
Rosiglitazone Maleate	AVANDIA	Hypoglycemic Agent	**Tab**: 2, 4, 8 mg	**Monotherapy or With Metformin**: Usually 4 mg po as a single dose once daily or in divided doses bid. For patients who do not respond adequately after 12 weeks of therapy (as determined by fasting serum glucose), the dose may be increased to 8 mg po as a single daily dose or in divided doses bid.
Salmeterol	SEREVENT	Bronchodilator	**Aerosol**: 25 μg base/spray (as the xinafoate salt)	**Asthma and Bronchospasm**: 2 inhalations bid, approximately q 12 h. **Prevention of Exercise-Induced Bronchospasm**: 2 inhalations at least 30 - 60 min. before exercise.
	SEREVENT DISKUS		**Powder**: 50 μg base (as the xinafolate salt) in a blister strip	**Asthma**: 1 inhalation (50 μg) orally via the inhalation device bid (AM & PM, approximately 12 h apart).
Salsalate	DISALCID	Antiinflammatory	**Cpsl**: 500 mg **Tab**: 500, 750 mg	3000 mg daily po, given in divided doses as 1500 mg bid or 1000 mg tid.
	SALFLEX		**Tab**: 500, 750 mg	Same dosage as for DISALCID above.
Saquinavir	FORTOVASE	Antiviral	**Cpsl**: 200 mg	1200 mg tid po taken within 2 h after a meal in combination with a nucleoside analog.
Scopolamine	TRANSDERM SCŌP	Anticholinergic, Antiemetic	**Transdermal**: 1.5 mg/patch	Apply 1 patch to the area behind one ear at least 4 hours before the antiemetic effect is required. Effective for 3 days.
Scopolamine Hydrobromide	ISOPTO HYOSCINE	Mydriatic - Cycloplegic	**Ophth Solution**: 0.25%	**Refraction**: Instill 1 - 2 drops in the eye(s) 1 hour before refracting. **Uveitis**: Instill 1 - 2 drops in the eye(s) up to qid.
Secobarbital Sodium (C-II)		Sedative - Hypnotic	**Inj**: 50 mg/mL	**Hypnotic**: 100 - 200 mg IM or 50 - 250 mg IV. **Preoperative Sedation**: 1 mg/kg IM, 10 - 15 minutes before the procedure.

Selegiline Hydrochloride	ELDEPRYL	Antiparkinsonian	**Cpsl**: 5 mg	5 mg bid po, at breakfast and lunch.
Selenium Sulfide	EXSEL, SELSUN Rx	Antiseborrheic, Antifungal	**Lotion**: 2.5%	**Seborrheic Dermatitis & Dandruff**: Massage 5 to 10 mL into wet scalp; let stand for 2 - 3 minutes. Rinse & repeat. Apply twice a week for 2 weeks; then may be used once weekly or once every 2 - 4 weeks. **Tinea Versicolor**: Apply to affected areas and lather with water; leave on skin for 10 minutes, then rinse. Repeat once daily for 7 days.
Sennosides	AGORAL	Irritant Laxative	**Liquid**: 25 mg/15 mL	15 - 30 mL once daily or bid po.
	EX-LAX EX-LAX CHOCOLATED	Irritant Laxative	**Tab**: 15 mg **Tab**: 15 mg	2 tabs once daily or bid with water. 2 tabs once daily or bid with water.
	EX-LAX, MAXIMUM RELIEF		**Tab**: 25 mg	2 tabs once daily or bid with water.
	SENOKOT	Irritant Laxative	**Syrup**: 8.8 mg/5 mL	10 - 15 mL daily po, preferably hs. (Maximum: 15 mL bid po).
			Tab: 8.6 mg	2 tablets daily po, preferably hs. (Maximum: 2 bid po).
			Granules: 15 mg/tsp.	1 teaspoonful daily po, preferably hs. (Maximum: 2 teaspoonfuls bid po).
	SENOKOTXTRA		**Tab**: 17 mg	1 tablet daily po, preferably hs. (Maximum: 2 tablets bid po).
Sertraline Hydrochloride	ZOLOFT	Antidepressant, Drug for Obsessive-Compulsive Disorder	**Tab**: 25, 50, 100 mg	Initially, 50 mg once daily po, either in the morning or evening. The dosage may be increased, at intervals of not less than 1 week, up to a maximum of 200 mg daily.
Sibutramine	MERIDIA	Anorexiant	**Cpsl**: 5, 10, 15 mg	Initially, 10 mg once daily po. If there is inadequate weight loss after 4 weeks, the dose may be titrated to a total of 15 mg once daily.

GENERIC NAME	COMMON TRADE NAMES	THERAPEUTIC CATEGORY	PREPARATIONS	COMMON ADULT DOSAGE
Sildenafil Citrate	VIAGRA	Agent for Impotence	**Tab**: 25, 50, 100 mg	50 mg po, taken prn approximately 1 h prior to sexual activity. May be taken between 30 min and 4 h before sexual activity and dose may be decreased to 25 mg or increased to 100 mg. The maximum dosing frequency is once per day.
Silver Sulfadiazine	SSD	Burn Preparation	**Cream**: 1%	Apply to a thickness of 1/16 inch once or twice daily.
Simethicone	MYLICON	Antiflatulant	**Solution (Drops)**: 40 mg/0.6 mL	0.6 mL (40 mg) qid po pc and hs.
	MYLANTA GAS		**Gelcap**: 62.5 mg **Chewable Tab**: 80, 125 mg	62.5 mg qid, po, pc and hs. Chew 80 - 125 mg qid, pc and hs.
	PHAZYME		**Solution (Drops)**: 40 mg/0.6 mL **Tab**: 60 mg	1.2 mL (80 mg) qid po pc and hs. 60 mg qid po, pc and hs.
	PHAZYME-95		**Tab**: 95 mg	95 mg qid po, pc and hs.
	PHAZYME-125		**Softgel**: 125 mg **Liquid**: 62.5 mg/5 mL	125 mg qid po, pc and hs. 10 mL qid po, pc and hs.
	PHAZYME-166		**Softgel & Chewable Tab**: 166 mg	166 mg tid po, pc and hs.
Simvastatin	ZOCOR	Hypolipidemic	**Tab**: 5, 10, 20, 40, 80 mg	Initialy 5 - 10 mg once daily po, in the evening. Dosage range: 5 - 40 mg once daily po, in the evening. Adjust dose at intervals of ≥ 4 weeks.
Sodium Chloride	AFRIN MOISTURIZING SALINE MIST	Nasal Moisturizer	**Nasal Solution**: 0.64%	2 - 6 sprays into each nostril prn.
	AYR SALINE, NASAL	Nasal Moisturizer	**Nasal Solution & Spray**: 0.65%	2 - 4 drops or 2 sprays into each nostril prn.

Sodium Nitroprusside		Antihypertensive, Heart Failure Drug	**Inj**: 50 mg (in 1 L D_5W)	**Acute Hypertension**: The average effective IV infusion rate is about 3 μg/kg/min. At this rate, some patients will become dangerously hypotensive. Begin IV infusion at a very low rate (0.3 μg/kg/min), with gradual upward titration every few minutes until the desired effect is achieved or the maximum infusion rate (10 μg/kg/min) has been reached. **Congestive Heart Failure**: Titrate by increasing the infusion rate until measured cardiac output is no longer increasing, systemic blood pressure cannot be further reduced without compromising the perfusion of vital organs, or the maximum recommended infusion rate (10 μg/kg/min) has been reached, whichever comes first.
Sodium Polystyrene Sulfonate	KAYEXALATE	Potassium-Removing Resin	**Powder**: 10 - 12 g/heaping teaspoonful	Average daily dose is 15 - 60 g po. Usually, 15 g mixed in liquid 1 - 4 times daily po.
	SODIUM POLYSTYRENE SULFONATE SUSP.		**Susp**: 15 g/60 mL (0.1% alcohol)	Same dosage as for KAYEXALATE above.
Sotalol Hydrochloride	BETAPACE	Antiarrhythmic	**Tab**: 80, 120, 160, 240 mg	Initially, 80 mg bid po. Dosage may be increased at 2 - 3 day intervals up to 320 mg/day po given in 2 or 3 divided doses.
Sparfloxacin	ZAGAM	Antibacterial	**Tab**: 200 mg	400 mg po as a loading dose, followed by 200 mg once daily for a total of 10 days (i.e., 11 tablets).
Spectinomycin Hydrochloride	TROBICIN	Antibacterial	**Powd for Inj**: 2, 4 g	2 g as a single deep IM injection.
Spironolactone	ALDACTONE	Antihypertensive, Diuretic	**Tab**: 25, 50, 100 mg	**Diuresis**: Initially, 100 mg po, as a single dose or in divided doses, for at least 5 days. **Hypertension**: Initially 50 - 100 mg po as a single dose or in divided doses.

GENERIC NAME	COMMON TRADE NAMES	THERAPEUTIC CATEGORY	PREPARATIONS	COMMON ADULT DOSAGE
Stanozolol (C-III)	WINSTROL	Anabolic Steroid	**Tab**: 2 mg	Initially, 2 mg tid po. After a favorable response, decrease dosage at intervals of 1 to 3 months to a maintenance dosage of 2 mg once daily.
Stavudine	ZERIT	Antiviral	**Cpsl**: 15, 20, 30, 40 mg **Powd for Solution**: 1 mg/mL	**Initial Dosage**: < **60 kg**: 30 mg twice daily (q 12 h) po. ≥ **60 kg**: 40 mg twice daily (q 12 h) po. **Dosage Adjustment**: Monitor patients for the development of peripheral neuropathy. If symptoms develop, stop the drug. If the symptoms resolve completely, consider resumption of therapy with half of the above mg dosages.
Streptokinase	STREPTASE	Thrombolytic	**Powd for Inj**: 250,000 IUnits, 750,000 IUnits, and 1,500,000 IUnits	250,000 IU IV (over 30 minutes), followed by 100,000 IU/h by IV infusion. Length of therapy determined by condition (see below). **Pulmonary Embolism**: 24 h (72 h if concurrent deep vein thrombosis is suspected). **Deep Vein Thrombosis**: 72 h. **Arterial Thrombosis or Embolism**: 24 - 72 h.
Streptomycin Sulfate		Antibacterial, Tuberculostatic	**Inj**: 1 g/2.5 mL	**Tuberculosis**: either of the following regimens are used. Generally no more than 120 g is given over the course of therapy. 15 mg/kg daily IM (Maximum: 1 g). 25 - 30 mg/kg two or three times weekly IM (Maximum: 1.5 g). **Tularemia**: 1 - 2 g daily IM in divided doses for 7 - 14 days until afebrile for 5 - 7 days. **Plague**: 2 g daily IM in 2 divided doses for a minimum of 10 days.

				Bacterial Endocarditis: **Streptococcal Endocarditis**: 1 g bid IM for the 1st week, followed by 500 mg bid IM for the 2nd week. **Enterococcal Endocarditis**: 1 g bid IM for 2 weeks, followed by 500 mg bid IM for an additional 4 weeks (with penicillin).
Streptozocin	ZANOSAR	Antineoplastic	**Powd for Inj**: 1 g	**Daily Schedule**: 500 mg/m^2 IV for 5 consecutive days q 6 weeks. **Weekly Schedule**: 1000 mg/m^2 IV weekly for the first 2 weeks. Dosage may be increased in selected patients to a maximum of 1500 mg/m^2 IV once a week.
Succinylcholine Chloride	ANECTINE	Neuromuscular Blocker	**Inj**: 20 mg/mL **Powd for IV Infusion**: 500, 1000 mg	**Short Surgical Procedures**: 0.6 mg/kg IV. **Long Surgical Procedures**: 2.5 - 4.3 mg/min by IV infusion; or 0.3 - 1.1 mg/kg initially by IV injection followed, at appropriate intervals, by 0.04 - 0.07 mg/kg.
Sucralfate	CARAFATE	Anti-Ulcer Agent	**Tab**: 1 g **Susp**: 1 g/10 mL	**Active Duodenal Ulcer**: 1 g qid po on an empty stomach. **Maintenance**: 1 g bid po.
Sulconazole Nitrate	EXELDERM	Antifungal	**Cream & Solution**: 1%	Gently massage a small amount into the skin once or twice daily.
Sulfacetamide Sodium	SODIUM SULAMYD	Antibacterial	**Ophth Solution**: 10%	1 - 2 drops into the affected eye(s) q 2 - 3 h during the day, less often at night.
			Ophth Oint: 10%	Apply a small amount to affected eye(s) q 3 - 4 h and hs.
	SODIUM SULAMYD		**Ophth Solution**: 30%	**Conjunctivitis or Corneal Ulcer**: 1 drop into the affected eye(s) q 2 h or less frequently. **Trachoma**: 2 drops into eye(s) q 2 h.

[Continued on the next page]

GENERIC NAME	COMMON TRADE NAMES	THERAPEUTIC CATEGORY	PREPARATIONS	COMMON ADULT DOSAGE
Sulfacetamide Sodium [Continued]	BLEPH-10		**Ophth Solution**: 10%	**Conjunctivitis and other Superficial Ocular Infections**: 1 - 2 drops into the affected eye(s) q 2 - 3 h initially. Dosage may be reduced as the condition responds. The usual duration of therapy is 7 to 10 days. **Trachoma**: 2 drops into eye(s) q 2 h.
			Ophth Oint: 10%	**Conjunctivitis and other Superficial Ocular Infections**: Apply a small amount (approx. 1/2 inch) into the affected eye(s) q 3 - 4 h and hs. Dosage may be reduced as the condition responds. The usual duration of therapy is 7 to 10 days.
	KLARON	Anti-Acne Agent	**Lotion**: 10%	Apply a thin film to affected areas bid.
Sulfamethizole	THIOSULFIL FORTE	Antibacterial	**Tab**: 500 mg	500 - 1000 mg tid or qid po.
Sulfamethoxazole	GANTANOL	Antibacterial	**Tab**: 500 mg	**Mild to Moderate Infections**: Initially, 2 g po; then 1 g bid po thereafter. **Severe Infections**: Initially 2 g po; then 1 g tid po thereafter.
Sulfanilamide	AVC	Antibacterial	**Vaginal Cream**: 15% **Vaginal Suppos**: 1.05 g	1 applicatorful intravaginally once daily or bid. Insert 1 vaginally once daily or bid.
Sulfasalazine	AZULFIDINE-EN	Bowel Antiinflammatory Agent, Antirheumatic	**Enteric-Coated Tab**: 500 mg	**Ulcerative Colitis**: **Initial**: 3 - 4 g daily po in evenly divided doses. **Maintenance**: 2 g daily po. **Rheumatoid Arthritis**: Initially 0.5 - 1 g daily po; then 2 g daily po in evenly divided doses.
Sulfinpyrazone	ANTURANE	Anti-Gout Agent	**Tab**: 100 mg **Cpsl**: 200 mg	**Initial**: 200 - 400 mg daily po in 2 divided doses with meals or milk. **Maintenance**: 400 mg daily po in 2 divided doses with meals or milk.

Sulfisoxazole		Antibacterial	**Tab**: 500 mg	Initially 2 - 4 g po, then 4 - 8 g/day divided in 4 - 6 doses.
Sulfisoxazole Acetyl		Antibacterial	**Syrup**: 500 mg/5 mL (0.9% alcohol)	Initially 2 - 4 g po, then 4 - 8 g/day divided in 4 - 6 doses.
Sulindac	CLINORIL	Antiinflammatory	**Tab**: 150, 200 mg	**Osteoarthritis, Rheumatoid Arthritis, and Ankylosing Spondylitis**: 150 mg bid po with food. **Acute Painful Shoulder**: 200 mg bid po with food for 7 - 14 days. **Acute Gouty Arthritis**: 200 mg bid po with food for 7 days.
Sumatriptan Succinate	IMITREX	Antimigraine Agent	**Inj**: 12 mg/mL	6 mg SC. A second 6 mg dose may be given in patients who failed to respond to the first dose. Maximum: two 6 mg doses in 24 h, separated by ≥ 1 h.
			Tab: 25, 50 mg	25 - 50 mg po taken with fluids as early as possible after the onset of attack. If a suitable response does not occur within 2 h, a second dose of up to 100 mg may be given. If headache returns, additional doses may be taken at 2 h intervals, not to exceed 200 mg per day.
			Nasal Spray (per 0.1 mL): 5, 20 mg	5, 10, or 20 mg administered in one nostril as a single dose. (A 10 mg dose is achieved by administering 5 mg in each nostril).
Suprofen	PROFENAL	Antiinflammatory (Topical)	**Ophth Solution**: 1%	On the day of surgery, instill 2 drops into the conjunctival sac at 3, 2, and 1 hour prior to surgery. Two drops may be instilled into the conjunctival sac q 4 h, while awake, the day preceding surgery.

GENERIC NAME	COMMON TRADE NAMES	THERAPEUTIC CATEGORY	PREPARATIONS	COMMON ADULT DOSAGE
Tacrine Hydrochloride	COGNEX	Drug for Alzheimer's Disease	**Cpsl**: 10, 20, 30, 40 mg	**Initial**: 10 mg qid po. Maintain this dose for ≥ 4 weeks, every other week monitoring transaminase levels beginning at week 4 of therapy. **Titration**: After 4 weeks, increase to 20 mg qid po providing there are no significant transaminase elevations and the patient is tolerating treatment. Titrate to higher doses (30 and 40 mg qid po) at 4 week intervals on the basis of tolerance and transaminase levels during monitoring.
Tacrolimus	PROGRAF	Immunosuppressant	**Cpsl**: 1, 5 mg	0.15 - 0.3 mg/kg/day po in 2 divided doses (q 12 h). Administer initial dose no sooner than 6 h after transplantation. If IV therapy was initiated, begin 8 - 12 h after discontinuing IV therapy.
			Inj: 5 mg/mL	0.05 - 0.1 mg/kg/day as a continuous IV infusion. Administer initial dose no sooner than 6 h after transplantation. Convert to oral therapy as soon as the patient can tolerate oral dosing.
Tamoxifen Citrate	NOLVADEX	Antineoplastic	**Tab**: 10, 20 mg	**Breast Cancer**: 20 - 40 mg daily po. Give doses over 20 mg daily in divided doses (morning and evening). **Reduction in Breast Cancer Incidence in High-Risk Women**: 20 mg daily po for 5 years.
Tamsulosin Hydrochloride	FLOMAX	Benign Prostatic Hyperplasia Drug	**Cpsl**: 0.4 mg	Initially 0.4 mg once daily po; take dose 30 min. after the same meal each day. May increase dose to 0.8 mg once daily po after 2 - 4 weeks if the response is inadequate. If therapy is interrupted, resume at 0.4 mg once daily and re-titrate.

Tazarotene	TAZORAC	Anti-Acne Agent, Anti-Psoriasis Agent	**Gel**: 0.05, 0.1%	After the skin is clean and dry, apply a thin film once daily, in the evening, to the acne or psoriatic lesions. Use enough to cover the entire lesion.
Telmisartan	MICARDIS	Antihypertensive	**Tab**: 40, 80 mg	Initially, 40 mg daily po. The usual dosage range is 20 - 80 mg daily.
Temazepam (C-IV)	RESTORIL	Hypnotic	**Cpsl**: 7.5, 15, 30 mg	7.5 - 30 mg po hs.
Terazosin Hydrochloride	HYTRIN	Antihypertensive, Benign Prostatic Hyperplasia Drug	**Cpsl**: 1, 2, 5, 10 mg	**Hypertension**: Initially, 1 mg po hs. Dosage may be slowly increased to the suggested dosage range of 1 - 5 mg once daily po. **Benign Prostatic Hyperplasia**: Initially, 1 mg po hs. Increase the dose in a stepwise fashion to 2, 5, or 10 mg daily to achieved desired effect. Doses of 10 mg once daily are generally required and may require 4 - 6 weeks of therapy to assess benefits.
Terbinafine Hydrochloride	LAMISIL	Antifungal	**Cream**: 1%	**Interdigital *Tinea pedis***: Apply to affected and surrounding areas bid for at least 1 week. ***Tinea cruris* or *T. corporis***: Apply to affected and surrounding areas once daily or bid for at least 1 week.
			Tab: 250 mg	**Onychomycosis**: **Fingernail**: 250 mg daily po for 6 weeks. **Toenail**: 250 mg daily po for 12 weeks.
Terbutaline Sulfate	BRETHINE, BRICANYL	Bronchodilator	**Tab**: 2.5, 5 mg	**12-15 yrs**: 2.5 mg tid (q 6 h) po. **Over 15 yrs**: 5 mg tid (q 6 h) po.
			Inj: 1 mg/mL	0.25 mg SC; may repeat once in 15 - 30 min.
	BRETHAIRE		**Aerosol**: 0.2 mg/spray	2 inhalations separated by a 60-sec interval q 4 - 6 h.

GENERIC NAME	COMMON TRADE NAMES	THERAPEUTIC CATEGORY	PREPARATIONS	COMMON ADULT DOSAGE
Terconazole	TERAZOL 3	Antifungal	**Vaginal Cream**: 0.8% **Vaginal Suppos**: 80 mg	1 applicatorful intravaginally hs for 3 days. Insert 1 vaginally hs for 3 days.
	TERAZOL 7		**Vaginal Cream**: 0.4%	1 applicatorful intravaginally hs for 7 days.
Testolactone	TESLAC	Antineoplastic	**Tab**: 50 mg	250 mg qid po.
Testosterone		Androgen, Antineoplastic	**Inj (per mL)**: 25, 50, 100 mg (aqueous suspension)	**Replacement Therapy**: 25 - 50 mg 2 - 3 times a week by deep IM injection. **Breast Cancer**: 50 - 100 mg 3 times a week by deep IM injection.
	ANDRODERM	Androgen	**Transdermal**: rate = 2.5 mg/day	**Replacement Therapy**: Apply 2 patches (5 mg) nightly, at approx. 10 PM, for 24 h to intact clean, dry skin of the back, abdomen, thighs, or upper arms. Increase to 3 patches (7.5 mg) or decrease to 1 patch (2.5 mg) as per morning serum testosterone levels.
	TESTODERM	Androgen	**Transdermal**: rate = 4, 6 mg/24 hr	**Replacement Therapy**: Start with a 6 mg/day system applied daily on clean, dry scrotal skin for up to 8 weeks; if scrotal area is inadequate, use a 4 mg/day system.
Testosterone Cypionate	DEPO-TESTOSTERONE	Androgen, Antineoplastic	**Inj (per mL)**: 100, 200 mg (in oil)	**Male Hypogonadism**: 50 - 400 mg q 2 - 4 weeks IM. **Breast Cancer**: 200 - 400 mg q 2 - 4 weeks IM.
Testosterone Enanthate	DELATESTRYL	Androgen, Antineoplastic	**Inj**: 200 mg/mL (in oil)	Same dosages as for DEPO-TESTOSTERONE above.
Tetracaine Hydrochloride	PONTOCAINE	Local Anesthetic	**Cream**: 1%	Apply to the affected area prn.
	PONTOCAINE HCL PONTOCAINE EYE		**Ophth Solution**: 0.5% **Ophth Oint**: 0.5%	1 - 2 drops into eye(s). Apply 0.5 - 1 inch to lower conjunctival fornix.

Tetracycline Hydrochloride	SUMYCIN	Antibacterial	**Cpsl & Tab**: 250, 500 mg **Syrup**: 125 mg/5 mL	**Usual Dosage**: 1 - 2 g po divided into 2 or 4 equal doses. **Brucellosis**: 500 mg qid po for 3 weeks with streptomycin. **Syphilis**: 30 - 40 g po in equally divided doses over a period of 10 - 15 days. **Gonorrhea**: Initially, 1.5 g po followed by 500 mg q 6 h for 4 days (total dose of 9 g). **Uncomplicated Urethral, Endocervical or Rectal Infections due to *Chlamydia trachomatis***: 500 mg qid po for at least 7 days.
	TOPICYCLINE		**Powd for Solution**: 150 mg [with 70 mL of liquid]	Apply generously bid to the entire affected area until the skin is wet.
Tetrahydrozoline Hydrochloride	TYZINE	Nasal Decongestant	**Nasal Solution**: 0.1%	2 - 4 drops in each nostril q 4 - 6 h.
	VISINE	Ocular Decongestant	**Ophth Solution**: 0.05%	1 - 2 drops in affected eye(s) up to qid.
Theophylline, Anhydrous	AEROLATE	Bronchodilator	**Cpsl**: 65, 130, 260 mg	1 cpsl q 12 h po; in severe attacks, 1 cpsl q 8 h po. Usually 260 mg are used in adults.
	ELIXOPHYLLIN		**Elixir**: 80 mg/15 mL (20% alcohol) **Cpsl**: 100, 200 mg	See Oral Theophylline Doses Table, p. 258.
	RESPBID		**Sustained-Rel. Tab**: 250, 500 mg	See Oral Theophylline Doses Table, p. 259.
	SLO-BID		**Extended-Rel. Cpsl**: 50, 75, 100, 125, 200, 300 mg	See Oral Theophylline Doses Table, p. 259.
	SLO-PHYLLIN		**Syrup**: 80 mg/15 mL **Tab**: 100, 200 mg	See Oral Theophylline Doses Table, p. 258.
			Extended-Rel. Cpsl: 60, 125, 250 mg	See Oral Theophylline Doses Table, p. 259.
	THEO-24		**Extended-Rel. Cpsl**: 100, 200, 300, 400 mg	See Oral Theophylline Doses Table, p. 260.

[Continued on the next page]

GENERIC NAME	COMMON TRADE NAMES	THERAPEUTIC CATEGORY	PREPARATIONS	COMMON ADULT DOSAGE
Theophylline, Anhydrous [Continued]	THEO-DUR		**Extended-Rel. Tab**: 100, 200, 300, 450 mg	See Oral Theophylline Doses Table, p. 259.
	THEOLAIR		**Liquid**: 80 mg/15 mL **Tab**: 125, 250 mg	See Oral Theophylline Doses Table, p. 258.
	THEOLAIR-SR		**Sustained-Rel Tab**: 200, 250, 300, 500 mg	See Oral Theophylline Doses Table, p. 259.
	T-PHYL		**Controlled-Rel Tab**: 200 mg	See Oral Theophylline Doses Table, p. 259.
	UNIPHYL		**Controlled-Rel. Tab**: 400, 600 mg	400 - 600 mg po once daily in the morning or in the evening.
Thiabendazole	MINTEZOL	Anthelmintic	**Susp**: 500 mg/5 mL **Chewable Tab**: 500 mg	**Strongyloidiasis, Intestinal Roundworms and Cutaneous Larva Migrans**: 2 doses/day (as below) po for 2 successive days. **Trichinosis**: 2 doses/day (as below) po for 2 - 4 successive days. **Visceral Larva Migrans**: 2 doses/day (as below) po for 7 successive days. Each Dose: 10 mg/lb.
Thiethylperazine Maleate	TORECAN	Antiemetic	**Tab**: 10 mg **Inj**: 10 mg/2 mL	10 mg once daily to tid po. 10 mg once daily to tid IM.
Thioguanine		Antineoplastic	**Tab**: 40 mg	Initially, 2 mg/kg daily po. If no improvement occurs after 4 weeks, the dosage may be increased to 3 mg/kg/day.
Thioridazine	MELLARIL-S	Antipsychotic	**Susp (per 5 mL)**: 25, 100 mg	Initially 50 - 100 mg tid po, with a gradual increment to a maximum of 800 mg daily if necessary. The maintenance dosage varies from 200 - 800 mg daily, divided into 2 or 4 doses.

Thioridazine Hydrochloride	MELLARIL	Antipsychotic	**Liquid Conc (per mL)**: 30, (3% alcohol), 100 mg (4.2% (alcohol) **Tab**: 10, 15, 25, 50, 100, 150, 200 mg	Same dosage as for MELLARIL-S above.
Thiothixene	NAVANE	Antipsychotic	**Cpsl**: 1, 2, 5, 10, 20 mg	**Mild Psychoses**: Initially 2 mg tid po; dosage may be increased to 15 mg/day if needed. **More Severe Psychoses**: Initially 5 mg bid po; the usual optimal dosage is 20 - 30 mg daily. Dosage may be increased to 60 mg/day.
Thiothixene Hydrochloride	NAVANE	Antipsychotic	**Liquid Conc**: 5 mg/mL (7% alcohol) **Inj (per mL)**: 2, 5 mg	Same dosages as for NAVANE Capsules above. 4 mg bid to qid IM.
Thyroid Dessicated	ARMOUR THYROID	Thyroid Hormone	**Tab**: 15, 30, 60, 90, 120, 180, 240, 300 mg	**Initial**: 30 mg daily po, with increments of 15 mg q 2 - 3 weeks. **Maintenance**: Usually 60 - 120 mg daily po.
Tiagabine Hydrochloride	GABITRIL	Antiepileptic	**Tab**: 4, 12, 16, 20 mg	**12-18 yrs**: 4 mg once daily po for 1 week. May increase to 4 mg bid po for 1 week; then may increase by 4 - 8 mg weekly to the clinical response or up to 32 mg/day in 2 - 4 divided doses. Take with food. **Over 18 yrs**: 4 mg once daily po. May increase by 4 - 8 mg weekly to the clinical response or up to 56 mg/day in 2 - 4 divided doses. Take with food.
Ticarcillin Disodium	TICAR	Antibacterial	**Powd for Inj**: 1, 3, 6 g	**Urinary Tract Infections**: **Uncomplicated**: 1 g IM or direct IV q 6 h. **Complicated**: 150 - 200 mg/kg/day by IV infusion in divided doses q 4 or 6 h. **Most Other Infections**: 200 - 300 mg/kg/day by IV infusion in divided doses q 4 or 6 h.
Ticlopidine Hydrochloride	TICLID	Platelet Aggregation Inhibitor	**Tab**: 250 mg	250 mg bid po, taken with food.

GENERIC NAME	COMMON TRADE NAMES	THERAPEUTIC CATEGORY	PREPARATIONS	COMMON ADULT DOSAGE
Tiludronate Sodium	SKELID	Bone Stabilizer	**Tab**: 240 mg (equivalent to 200 mg of tiludronic acid)	400 mg (acid) po daily with 6 - 8 oz. of water for 3 mos. Do not take within 2 h of food.
Timolol Hemihydrate	BETIMOL	Anti-Glaucoma Agent	**Ophth Solution**: 0.25, 0.5%	1 drop (0.25%) into affected eye(s) bid.
Timolol Maleate	BLOCADREN	Antihypertensive, Post-MI Drug, Antimigraine Agent	**Tab**: 5, 10, 20 mg	**Hypertension**: Initially 10 mg bid po. The usual maintenance dosage is 20 - 40 mg daily. **Myocardial Infarction**: 10 mg bid po. **Migraine Headache**: 10 mg bid po. The 20 mg daily dosage may be given as a single dose during maintenance therapy.
	TIMOPTIC TIMOPTIC-XE	Anti-Glaucoma Agent	**Ophth Solution**: 0.25, 0.5% **Ophth Gel**: 0.25, 0.5%	1 drop into affected eye(s) bid. Apply to affected eye(s) once daily.
Tioconazole	VAGISTAT-1	Antifungal	**Vaginal Oint**: 6.5%	Insert 1 applicatorful intravaginally hs.
Tizanidine Hydrochloride	ZANAFLEX	Skeletal Muscle Relaxant	**Tab**: 4 mg	Initially, 4 mg po. May increase by 2 - 4 mg prn q 6 - 8 h to a maximum of 3 doses in 24 h. Maximum: 36 mg per day.
Tobramycin	TOBREX	Antibacterial	**Ophth Oint**: 3 mg/g (0.3%)	**Mild to Moderate Infections**: Apply 1/2 inch ribbon into the affected eye(s) q 4 h. **Severe Infections**: Apply 1/2 inch ribbon into the affected eye(s) q 3 - 4 h until improvement occurs; reduce dosage prior to discontinuation.
			Ophth Solution: 3 mg/mL (0.3%)	**Mild to Moderate Infections**: 1 - 2 drops into the affected eye(s) q 4 h. **Severe Infections**: 2 drops into the affected eye(s) hourly until improvement occurs; reduce dosage prior to discontinuation.

Tobramycin Sulfate	NEBCIN	Antibacterial	**Inj (per mL)**: 10, 40 mg **Powd for Inj**: 30 mg	**Serious Infections**: 3 mg/kg/day IM or IV in 3 equal doses q 8 h. **Life-Threatening Infections**: Up to 5 mg/kg/day may be given IM or IV in 3 or 4 equal doses.
Tocainide Hydrochloride	TONOCARD	Antiarrhythmic	**Tab**: 400, 600 mg	Initially 400 mg q 8 h po. The usual dosage is 1200 - 1800 mg/day in 3 divided doses.
Tolazamide	TOLINASE	Hypoglycemic Agent	**Tab**: 100, 250, 500 mg	**Initial**: 100 - 250 mg daily po, administered with breakfast or the first main meal. Dosage adjustments are made in increments of 100 to 250 mg at weekly intervals. **Maintenance**: Usually 250 - 500 mg daily po.
Tolbutamide	ORINASE	Hypoglycemic Agent	**Tab**: 500 mg	**Initial**: 1 - 2 g daily po, as a single dose in the AM or in divided doses throughout the day. **Maintenance**: Usually 0.25 - 2 g daily po, as a single dose in the AM or in divided doses throughout the day.
Tolcapone	TASMAR	Antiparkinsonian	**Tab**: 100, 200 mg	Initially 100 or 200 mg tid po always as an adjunct to levodopa/carbidopa therapy.
Tolmetin Sodium	TOLECTIN 200 TOLECTIN DS TOLECTIN 600	Antiinflammatory	**Tab**: 200 mg **Cpsl**: 400 mg **Tab**: 600 mg	Initially 400 mg tid po, preferably including a dose on arising and a dose hs; adjust dosage after 1 - 2 weeks. Control is usually achieved at 600 - 1800 mg daily in divided doses (generally tid).
Tolnaftate	AFTATE	Antifungal	**Gel, Powder, Spray Powder & Liquid Spray**: 1%	Apply a thin layer over affected area morning and night for 2 - 3 weeks.
	TINACTIN		**Cream, Solution, Powder, Spray Powder & Spray Liquid**: 1%	Apply to affected areas morning and night for 2 - 4 weeks.
Tolterodine Tartrate	DETROL	Urinary Antispasmodic	**Tab**: 1, 2 mg	Initially 2 mg bid po. The dosage may be reduced to 1 mg bid po based on individual response and tolerability.

GENERIC NAME	COMMON TRADE NAMES	THERAPEUTIC CATEGORY	PREPARATIONS	COMMON ADULT DOSAGE
Topiramate	TOPAMAX	Antiepileptic	**Tab**: 25, 100, 200 mg **Sprinkle Cpsl**: 15, 25 mg	Initiate therapy with 50 mg/day po followed by titration to an effective dose (400 mg/day) as shown in the table below:

Recommended Oral Titration Doses					
Week	**AM Dose**	**PM Dose**	**Week**	**AM Dose**	**PM Dose**
1	None	50 mg	5	100 mg	150 mg
2	50 mg	50 mg	6	150 mg	150 mg
3	50 mg	100 mg	7	150 mg	200 mg
4	100 mg	100 mg	8	200 mg	200 mg

Sprinkle Capsules may be swallowed whole or the contents may be sprinkled onto soft food.

GENERIC NAME	COMMON TRADE NAMES	THERAPEUTIC CATEGORY	PREPARATIONS	COMMON ADULT DOSAGE
Toremifene Citrate	FARESTON	Antineoplastic	**Tab**: 60 mg	60 mg once daily po.
Torsemide	DEMADEX	Diuretic, Antihypertensive	**Tab**: 5, 10, 20, 100 mg **Inj**: 10 mg/mL	**Hypertension**: 5 mg once daily po. After 4 - 6 weeks, the dose may be increased to 10 mg once daily po. **Diuresis in:** **Congestive Heart Failure**: Initially, 10 or 20 mg once daily po or slow IV (over 2 min). If the response is inadequate, titrate dose upward by approximately doubling. Maximum dose: 200 mg. **Chronic Renal Failure**: Initially, 20 mg once daily po or IV (over 2 min). If the response is inadequate, titrate dose upward by approximately doubling. Max.: 200 mg. **Hepatic Cirrhosis**: Initially, 5 or 10 mg once daily po or IV (over 2 min), together with a potassium-spraing diuretic. If the response is inadequate, titrate dose upward by approx. doubling. Maximum dose: 40 mg.

Tramadol Hydrochloride	ULTRAM	Central Analgesic	**Tab**: 50 mg	50 - 100 mg q 4 - 6 h po, not to exceed 400 mg/day.
Trandolapril	MAVIK	Antihypertensive, Heart Failure Drug	**Tab**: 1, 2, 4 mg	**Hypertension**: **African-American Patients**: Initially, 2 mg once daily po. **Other Patients**: Initially, 1 mg once daily po. **Heart Failure Post-MI**: Initially 1 mg daily po, then titrate patient (as tolerated) toward a target dose of 4 mg daily.
Tranexamic Acid	CYKLOKAPRON	Systemic Hemostatic	**Inj**: 100 mg/mL	10 mg/kg IV immediately before dental surgery. After surgery, give 25 mg/kg po tid - qid for 2 to 8 days. In patients unable to take oral medication, give 10 mg/kg tid to qid.
			Tab: 500 mg	25 mg/kg po tid - qid beginning 1 day prior to dental surgery.
Tranylcypromine Sulfate	PARNATE	Antidepressant	**Tab**: 10 mg	30 mg/day po in divided doses. Adjust dosage in approximately 2 weeks in 10 mg increments at intervals of 1 - 3 weeks to a maximum of 60 mg per day.
Trazodone Hydrochloride	DESYREL	Antidepressant	**Tab**: 50, 100, 150, 300 mg	Initially 150 mg/day po in divided doses. The dose may be increased by 50 mg/day q 3 - 4 days to a maximum of 400 mg/day (for outpatients) or 600 mg/day (for more severely-depressed inpatients).
Tretinoin	RETIN-A	Anti-Acne Agent	**Cream**: 0.025, 0.05, 0.1% **Gel**: 0.01, 0.025% **Liquid**: 0.05%	Cover the entire affected area once daily hs.
	AVITA		**Cream**; 0.025%	Cover the entire affected area once daily hs.
	RENOVA		**Cream**: 0.05%	Apply to face once daily hs, using only enough (i.e., "pea-size" amount) to cover the affected area lightly.

GENERIC NAME	COMMON TRADE NAMES	THERAPEUTIC CATEGORY	PREPARATIONS	COMMON ADULT DOSAGE
Triamcinolone	ARISTOCORT	Corticosteroid	**Tab**: 1, 2, 4, 8 mg	Initial dose may vary from 4 to 48 mg po per day. Dose requirements are variable and must be individualized based on the disease and the patient's response.
Triamcinolone Acetonide	KENALOG-10	Corticosteroid	**Inj**: 10 mg/mL	**Intra-articular or Intrabursal Injection and Injection into Tendon Sheaths:** Initially, 2.5 to 5 mg (for smaller joints) and 5 - 15 mg (for larger joints). **Intradermal Injection**: Varies depending on the disease, but should be limited to 1.0 mg per injection site.
	KENALOG-40		**Inj**: 40 mg/mL	**IM (deep)**: Usual initial dose is 60 mg. Dosage is usually adjusted from 40 - 80 mg, depending on the patient response and the duration of relief. **Intra-articular or Intrabursal Injection and Injection into Tendon Sheaths**: Initially, 2.5 to 5 mg (for smaller joints) and 5 - 15 mg (for larger joints).
	ARISTOCORT A		**Cream**: 0.025, 0.1, 0.5% **Oint**: 0.1%	Apply to affected area as a thin film tid - qid depending on the severity of the condition.
	KENALOG		**Oint**: 0.025, 0.1, 0.5%	Apply a thin film to the affected area bid - qid (of the 0.025%) or bid - tid (of the 0.1% or 0.5%). Rub in gently.
			Cream: 0.025, 0.1, 0.5%	Apply to the affected area bid - qid (of the 0.025%) or bid - tid (of the 0.1 or 0.5%). Rub in gently.
			Lotion: 0.025, 0.1%	Apply to the affected area bid - qid (of the 0.025%) or bid - tid (of the 0.1%). Rub in.
			Spray: 0.2%	Spray onto affected area tid - qid.
	AZMACORT		**Aerosol**: 100 μg/spray	2 inhalations tid or qid.

	NASACORT NASACORT AQ		**Aerosol**: 55 μg/spray **Aerosol**: 55 μg/spray	2 sprays in each nostril once a day. If needed, the dose may be doubled, either as a once a day dosage or divided up to 4 times daily.
Triamcinolone Diacetate	ARISTOCORT FORTE	Corticosteroid	**Inj (per mL)**: 25, 40 mg	Initial dosage may vary from 3 - 48 mg daily, depending on the specific disease being treated. The average dose is 40 mg IM once a week or 5 - 40 mg intra-articularly or intrasynovially.
Triamcinolone Hexacetonide	ARISTOSPAN	Corticosteroid	**Inj (per mL)**: 5, 20 mg	Initial dosage may vary from 2 - 48 mg daily, depending on the specific disease being treated. The average dose is 2 - 20 mg intra-articularly (depending on the size of the joint), repeated q 3 - 4 weeks. Up to 0.5 mg/square inch of skin may be given by intralesional or sublesional injection.
Triamterene	DYRENIUM	Diuretic	**Cpsl**: 50, 100 mg	100 mg bid po pc.
Triazolam (C-IV)	HALCION	Hypnotic	**Tab**: 0.125, 0.25 mg	0.25 mg hs po.
Trichlormethiazide	NAQUA	Diuretic, Antihypertensive	**Tab**: 2, 4 mg	**Diuresis**: 1 - 4 mg daily po. **Hypertension**: 2 - 4 mg daily po.
Trifluoperazine Hydrochloride	STELAZINE	Antipsychotic	**Tab**: 1, 2, 5, 10 mg **Conc Liquid**: 10 mg/mL **Inj**: 2 mg/mL	Initially, 2 - 5 mg bid po. Most show optimum response on 15 - 20 mg daily po. 1 - 2 mg by deep IM q 4 - 6 h prn.
Trifluridine	VIROPTIC	Antiviral	**Ophth Solution**: 1%	1 drop into affected eye(s) q 2 h while awake for a maximum of 9 drops daily until the cornea has re-epithelialized. Then use 1 drop q 4 h while awake for 7 days.
Trihexyphenidyl Hydrochloride	ARTANE	Antiparkinsonian	**Elixir**: 2 mg/5 mL **Tab**: 2, 5 mg	Initially 1 mg po on the first day. The dose may be increased by 2 mg increments at intervals of 3 - 5 days to a maximum of 6 - 10 mg daily.

GENERIC NAME	COMMON TRADE NAMES	THERAPEUTIC CATEGORY	PREPARATIONS	COMMON ADULT DOSAGE
Trimethobenzamide Hydrochloride	TIGAN	Antiemetic	**Cpsl**: 100, 250 mg **Rectal Suppos**: 200 mg **Inj**: 100 mg/mL	250 mg tid or qid po. 200 mg tid or qid rectally. 200 mg tid or qid IM.
Trimethoprim	PROLOPRIM	Antibacterial	**Tab**: 100, 200 mg	100 mg q 12 h po for 10 days, or 200 mg q 24 h po for 10 days.
Trimetrexate Glucuronate	NEUTREXIN	Antiparasitic	**Powd for Inj**: 25 mg	**Must be administ. with concurrent leucovorin.** 45 mg/m^2 once daily by IV infusion over 60 to 90 minutes. Leucovorin must be given daily during treatment with NEUTREXIN and for 72 h past the last dose of NEUTREXIN. Leucovorin may be given IV at a dose of 20 mg/m^2 over 5 - 10 minutes q 6 h for a total daily dose of 80 mg/m^2 or orally as 4 doses of 20 mg/m^2 spaced equally during the day. Recommended course of therapy is 21 days of NEUTREXIN and 24 days of leucovorin.
Trimipramine Maleate	SURMONTIL	Antidepressant	**Cpsl**: 25, 50, 100 mg	**Outpatients**: Initially, 75 mg/day po in divided doses. Maintenance doses range from 50 to 150 mg/day po. **Hospitalized Patients**: Initially, 100 mg/day po in divided doses. May gradually increase in a few days to 200 mg/day. If no improvement occurs in 2 - 3 weeks, dose may be raised to a maximum dose of 250 - 300 mg/day.
Tripelennamine Hydrochloride	PBZ PBZ-SR	Antihistamine	**Tab**: 25, 50 mg **Extended-Rel. Tab**: 100 mg	25 - 50 mg q 4 - 6 h po. 100 mg bid po, in the morning and in the evening.
Trolamine Salicylate	MYOFLEX	Analgesic (Topical)	**Cream**: 10%	Apply to affected area not more than tid to qid. Affected areas may be wrapped loosely prn.
Troleandomycin	TAO	Antibacterial	**Cpsl**: 250 mg	250 - 500 mg qid po.

Tropicamide	MYDRIACYL	Mydriatic - Cycloplegic	**Ophth Solution**: 0.5, 1.0%	**Refraction**: Instill 1 - 2 drops of the 1% solution in the eye(s); repeat in 5 minutes if the patient is not seen in 20 - 30 minutes. **Fundus Examination**: Instill 1 - 2 drops of the 0.5% solution 15 - 20 minutes prior to the examination.
Trovafloxacin Mesylate	TROVAN	Antibacterial	**Tab**: 100, 200 mg **Inj**: 5 mg/mL (as alatrofloxacin mesylate)	**Community-Acquired Pneumonia and Skin and Skin Structure Infections (Complicated)**: 200 mg once daily po or by IV infusion, followed by 200 mg once daily po for 7 - 14 days. **Nosocomial Pneumonia**: 300 mg by IV infusion, followed by 200 mg once daily po for 10 - 14 days. **Gynecologic and Pelvic Infections and Intra-Abdominal Infections (Complicated)**: 300 mg by IV infusion, followed by 200 mg once daily po for 7 - 14 days.
Tubocurarine Chloride		Neuromuscular Blocker	**Inj**: 3 mg (20 Units)/mL	**Usual Effective IV Doses (General Reference)**: **Paresis of Limb Muscles**: 0.1 - 0.2 mg/kg. **Abdominal Relaxation**: 0.4 - 0.5 mg/kg. **Endotracheal Intubation**: 0.5 - 0.6 mg/kg. In prolonged procedures, repeat incremental doses in 40 - 60 minutes, as required.
Urea	UREAPHIL	Osmotic Diuretic	**Inj**: 40 g/150 mL	1 - 1.5 g/kg by slow IV infusion, at a rate not to exceed 4 mL/min (Maximum: 120 g/day).
Urokinase	ABBOKINASE	Thrombolytic	**Powd for Inj**: 250,000 IUnits	**Pulmonary Embolism**: A priming dose of 2,000 IUnits/lb IV (at a rate of 90 mL/h over 10 minutes), followed by an IV infusion of 2,000 IU/lb/h (at a rate of 15 mL/h) for 12 h. **Lysis of Coronary Artery Thrombosis**: After an IV bolus of heparin (2,500 - 10,000 units), infuse into occluded artery at a rate of 4 mL/min (6,000 IU/min) for periods up to 2 h.

GENERIC NAME	COMMON TRADE NAMES	THERAPEUTIC CATEGORY	PREPARATIONS	COMMON ADULT DOSAGE
Valacyclovir Hydrochloride	VALTREX	Antiviral	**Tab**: 500 mg	**Herpes zoster**: 1000 mg tid po for 7 days. **Genital Herpes:** **Initial Episodes**: 1000 mg bid po for 10 days. **Recurrent Episodes**: 500 mg bid po for 5 days.
Valproate Sodium	DEPACON	Antiepileptic	**Inj**: 100 mg/mL	Administer as an IV infusion over 60 min. (≤ 20 mg/min) with the same frequency as the oral products (Divalproex sodium (DEPAKOTE) and Valproic acid (DEPAKENE)).
Valproic Acid	DEPAKENE	Antiepileptic	**Syrup**: 250 mg/5 mL **Cpsl**: 250 mg	Initially 15 mg/kg/day po in 2 or 3 divided doses, increasing at 1 week intervals by 5 to 10 mg/kg/day (Maximum: 60 mg/kg/day).
Valsartan	DIOVAN	Antihypertensive	**Cpsl**: 80, 160 mg	Initially, 80 mg daily po. The dosage range is 80 - 320 mg once daily po.
Vancomycin Hydrochloride	VANCOCIN HCL	Antibacterial	**Powd for Solution**: 1, 10 g **Cpsl**: 125, 250 mg	**Pseudomembranous Colitis**: 500 mg - 2 g daily po in 3 or 4 divided doses for 7 - 10 days.
			Powd for Inj: 500 mg; 1, 10 g	2 g daily, divided either as 500 mg q 6 h or 1 g q 12 h, by IV infusion (at a rate no more than 10 mg/min) over at least 60 minutes.
Vasopressin	PITRESSIN	Posterior Pituitary Hormone	**Inj**: 20 pressor Units/mL	**Diabetes Insipidus**: 5 - 10 Units bid - tid IM or SC prn. **Abdominal Distention**: Initially, 5 Units IM; increase to 10 Units at subsequent injections if necessary. Repeat at 3 - 4 hour intervals.
Vecuronium Bromide	NORCURON	Neuromuscular Blocker	**Powd for Inj**: 10, 20 mg	Initially 0.08 - 0.1 mg/kg as an IV bolus. Maintenance doses of 0.010 - 0.015 mg/kg are recommended and are usually required within 25 - 40 minutes.

Venlafaxine	EFFEXOR	Antidepressant	**Tab**: 25, 37.5, 50, 75, 100 mg	Initially, 75 mg/day po, given in 2 or 3 dividec doses, with food. Dose may be increased to 150 mg/day and then to 225 mg/day at intervals of ≥ 4 days.
	EFFEXOR XR		**Extended-Rel. Cpsl**: 37.5, 75, 150 mg	Transferring from EFFEXOR, give total daily dose on a once a day basis. Initially, 75 mg once daily po, with food. May start at 37.5 mg once daily po, with food, for 4 - 7 days. May increase by increments of up to 75 mg daily at intervals of at least 4 days. Usual maximum is 225 mg/day.
Verapamil Hydrochloride	CALAN, ISOPTIN	Antianginal, Antiarrhythmic, Antihypertensive	**Tab**: 40, 80, 120 mg	**Angina**: 80 - 120 mg tid po. **Arrhythmias:** **Digitalized Patients with Chronic Atrial Fibrillation**: 240 - 320 mg/day po in 3 or 4 divided doses. **Prophylaxis of PSVT (Non-Digitalized Patients)**: 240 - 480 mg/day po in 3 or 4 divided doses. **Hypertension**: 80 mg tid po. Adjust dosage up to 360 mg daily.
	COVERA-HS	Antianginal, Antihypertensive	**Extended-Rel. Tab**: 180, 240 mg	**Angina & Hypertension**: Initially, 180 mg once daily po hs. The dose may be increased in the following manner: 240 mg po each evening, 360 mg po each evening (2 x 180 mg), or 480 mg po each evening (2 x 240 mg).
	CALAN SR ISOPTIN SR	Antihypertensive	**Sustained-Rel. Cplt**: 120, 180, 240 mg **Sustained-Rel. Tab**: 120, 180, 240 mg	**Hypertension**: Initially 180 mg po in the AM with food. Adjust doses upward at weekly intervals, until therapeutic goal is reached as follows: (a) 240 mg each AM; (b) 180 mg bid, AM & PM, or 240 mg each AM and 120 mg each PM; (c) 240 mg q 12 h.

[Continued on the next page]

GENERIC NAME	COMMON TRADE NAMES	THERAPEUTIC CATEGORY	PREPARATIONS	COMMON ADULT DOSAGE
Verapamil Hydrochloride [Continued]	VERELAN	Antihypertensive	**Sustained-Rel. Cpsl**: 120, 180, 240, 360 mg	**Hypertension**: Initially 240 mg po in the AM with food. Adjust doses upward until the therapeutic goal is reached as follows: (a) 240 mg each AM; (b) 360 mg each AM; (c) 480 mg each AM.
	ISOPTIN	Antiarrhythmic	**Inj**: 2.5 mg/mL	5 - 10 mg IV (over at least 2 minutes). Repeat with 10 mg after 30 minutes if response is not adequate.
Vidarabine Monohydrate	VIRA-A	Antiviral	**Ophth Oint**: 3%	Apply 1/2 inch into lower conjunctival sac 5 times daily at 3 h intervals.
Vinblastine Sulfate	VELBAN	Antineoplastic	**Powd for Inj**: 10 mg	Dose at weekly intervals as follows: 1st dose- 3.7 mg/m^2 IV; 2nd dose- 5.5 mg/m^2 IV; 3rd dose- 7.4 mg/m^{2}IV; 4th dose- 9.25 mg/m^2 IV; 5th dose- 11.1 mg/m^2 IV. The dose should not be increased after that dose which reduces the WBC to approx. 3,000 cell/mm^2.
Vincristine Sulfate	ONCOVIN	Antineoplastic	**Inj**: 1 mg/mL	1.4 mg/m^2 IV (at weekly intervals).
Vinorelbine Tartrate	NAVELBINE	Antineoplastic	**Inj**: 10 mg/mL	Initially, 30 mg/m^2 weekly by IV injection (over 6 - 10 minutes). If granulocyte counts fall to 1000 - 1499 cells/mm^2, reduce dose to 15 mg/m^2; below 100, do not administer.
Warfarin Sodium	COUMADIN	Anticoagulant	**Tab**: 1, 2, 2.5, 3, 4, 5, 6, 7.5, 10 mg	Must be individualized for each patient based on the prothrombin time. Maintenance dosage for most patients is 2 - 10 mg daily po.
			Powd for Inj: 5 mg	Individualize dosage. Give as an IV bolus dose over 1 - 2 min into a peripheral vein.

Xylometazoline Hydrochloride	OTRIVIN	Nasal Decongestant	**Nasal Solution**: 0.1% **Nasal Spray**: 0.1%	2 -3 drops into each nostril q 8 - 10 h. 2 - 3 sprays into each nostril q 8 - 10 h.
Zafirukast	ACCOLATE	Drug for Asthma	**Tab**: 20 mg	20 mg bid po. Take at least 1 h ac or 2 h pc.
Zalcitabine	HIVID	Antiviral	**Tab**: 0.375, 0.750 mg	**Monotherapy**: 0.750 mg q 8 h po. **Combination Therapy**: 0.750 mg po, given concomitantly with 200 mg of zidovudine, q 8 h.
Zaleplon	SONATA	Hypnotic	**Cpsl**: 5, 10 mg	5 - 10 mg hs po.
Zidovudine	RETROVIR	Antiviral	**Syrup**: 50 mg/5 mL **Cpsl**: 100 mg **Tab**: 300 mg	**Symptomatic HIV Infection**: 100 mg q 4 h po (600 mg total daily dose). **Asymptomatic HIV Infection**: 100 mg q 4 h po while awake (500 mg/day).
	RETROVIR I.V. INFUSION		**Inj**: 10 mg/mL	1 - 2 mg/kg infused IV over 1 hour at a constant rate; administer q 4 h around the clock (6 times daily).
Zileuton	ZYFLO	Drug for Asthma	**Tab**: 600 mg	600 mg qid po.
Zinamivir	RELENZA	Antiviral	**Powd for Inhalation**: 5 mg	2 inhalations (5 mg per inhalation; total dose of 10 mg) bid (at an interval of at least 2 h) on the 1st day; then 2 inhalations (total dose of 10 mg) bid (12 h apart AM and PM) for a total of 5 days.
Zinc Oxide		Skin Protectant	**Oint**: 20%	Apply topically prn.
Zolmitriptan	ZOMIG	Antimigraine Agent	**Tab**: 2.5, 5 mg	Initially, 2.5 mg or lower po. If the headache returns, the dose may be repeated after 2 h. Do not exceed 10 mg within a 24 h period.

GENERIC NAME	COMMON TRADE NAMES	THERAPEUTIC CATEGORY	PREPARATIONS	COMMON ADULT DOSAGE
Zolpidem Tartrate (C-IV)	AMBIEN	Hypnotic	**Tab**: 5, 10 mg	10 mg po hs.

C-II: Controlled Substance, Schedule II
C-III: Controlled Substance, Schedule III
C-IV: Controlled Substance, Schedule IV

SELECTED COMBINATION DRUG PREPARATIONS

TRADE NAME	THERAPEUTIC CATEGORY	DOSAGE FORMS AND COMPOSITION	COMMON ADULT DOSAGE
A-200	Pediculicide	**Shampoo**: pyrethrum extract (0.33%), piperonyl butoxide (4%)	Apply to affected area until all the hair is thoroughly wet. Allow product to remain on the area for 10 minutes but no longer. Add sufficient warm water to form a lather and shampoo as usual. Rinse thoroughly. Remove dead lice and eggs from the hair with a fine-toothed comb. Repeat treatment in 7 - 10 days to kll any newly hatched lice.
ACNOMEL	Anti-Acne Agent	**Cream**: sulfur (8%), resorcinol (2%), alcohol (11%)	Apply a thin coating once or twice daily.
ACTIFED	Decongestant-Antihistamine	**Syrup (per 5 mL)**: pseudoephedrine HCl (30 mg), triprolidine HCl (1.25 mg)	10 mL q 4 - 6 h po.
ACTIFED ALLERGY DAYTIME/NIGHTTIME	Decongestant-Antihistamine	**Daytime Cplt**: pseudoephedrine HCl (30 mg) **Nighttime Cplt**: pseudoephedrine HCl (30 mg), diphenhydramine HCl (25 mg)	2 Daytime cplts q 4 - 6 h po during waking hours. 2 Nighttime cplts hs po, prn. Do not take during waking hours unless confined to bed or resting at home; 2 Nighttime cplts may then be taken q 4 to 6 h po. Do not exceed 8 cplts (Daytime and/or Nighttime) in 24 h.
ACTIFED COLD & ALLERGY	Decongestant-Antihistamine	**Tab**: pseudoephedrine HCl (60 mg), triprolidine HCl (2.5 mg)	1 tab q 4 - 8 h po.
ACTIFED PLUS	Decongestant-Antihistamine-Analgesic	**Tab & Cplt**: pseudoephedrine HCl (30 mg), triprolidine HCl (1.25 mg), acetaminophen (500 mg)	2 tab (or cplt) q 6 h po.

ACTIFED SINUS DAYTIME/NIGHTTIME	Decongestant-Antihistamine-Analgesic	**Daytime Tab & Cplt**: pseudoephedrine HCl (30 mg), acetaminophen (500 mg) **Nighttime Tab & Cplt**: pseudoephedrine HCl (30 mg), diphenhydramine HCl (25 mg), acetaminophen (500 mg)	2 Daytime cplts (or tabs) q 6 h po during waking hours. 2 Nighttime cplts (or tabs) hs po, prn. Do not take during waking hours unless confined to bed or resting at home; 2 Nighttime cplts (or tabs) may then be taken q 6 h po. Do not exceed 8 cplts (or tabs) (Daytime and/or Nighttime) in 24 h.
ADVIL COLD & SINUS	Decongestant-Analgesic	**Cplt**: pseudoephedrine HCl (30 mg), ibuprofen (200 mg)	1 - 2 cplt q 4 - 6 h po.
AGGRENOX	Platelet Aggregation Inhibitor	**Cpsl**: aspirin (25 mg) [immediate-release], dipyridamole (200 mg) [extended-release]	1 cpsl bid po. Swallow whole; do not chew or crush.
ALDACTAZIDE	Diuretic, Antihypertensive	**Tab**: spironolactone (25 mg), hydrochlorothiazide (25 mg) **Tab**: spirololactone (50 mg), hydrochlorothiazide (50 mg)	**Diuresis**: The usual maintenance dose is 100 mg of each component daily po, as a single dose or in divided doses, but may range from 25 to 200 mg of each component daily. **Hypertension**: Usually 50 - 100 mg of each component daily po, as a single dose or in divided doses.
ALDOCLOR-250	Antihypertensive	**Tab**: chlorothiazide (250 mg), methyldopa (250 mg)	1 tab bid or tid po.
ALDORIL-15 ALDORIL-25 ALDORIL D30 ALDORIL D50	Antihypertensive	**Tab**: hydrochlorothiazide (15 mg), methyldopa (250 mg) **Tab**: hydrochlorothiazide (25 mg), methyldopa (250 mg) **Tab**: hydrochlorothiazide (30 mg), methyldopa (500 mg) **Tab**: hydrochlorothiazide (50 mg), methyldopa (500 mg)	1 tab bid or tid po. 1 tab bid or tid po. 1 tab bid or tid po. 1 tab bid or tid po.
ALESSE	Oral Contraceptive	**Tab**: ethinyl estradiol (20 μg), levonorgestrel (0.10 mg) in 21-Day and 28-Day Minipacks (contains 7 inert tabs)	21-Day regimen po or 28-Day regimen po.

TRADE NAME	THERAPEUTIC CATEGORY	DOSAGE FORMS AND COMPOSITION	COMMON ADULT DOSAGE
ALLEGRA-D	Decongestant-Antihistamine	**Extended-Rel. Tab**: pseudoephedrine HCl (120 mg), fexofenadine HCl (60 mg)	1 tab bid po.
ALLEREST MAXIMUM STRENGTH	Decongestant-Antihistamine	**Tab**: pseudoephedrine HCl (30 mg), chlorpheniramine maleate (2 mg)	2 tab q 4 - 6 h po.
ALLEREST, NO DROWSINESS	Decongestant-Analgesic	**Tab**: pseudoephedrine HCl (30 mg), acetaminophen (325 mg)	2 tab q 4 - 6 h po.
AMBENYL (C-V)	Antitussive-Antihistamine	**Syrup (per 5 mL)**: codeine phosphate (10 mg), bromodiphenhydramine HCl (12.5 mg), alcohol (5%)	5 - 10 mL q 4 - 6 h po.
ANALPRAM-HC	Corticosteroid-Local Anesthetic	**Cream**: hydrocortisone acetate (1%), pramoxine HCl (1%) **Cream & Lotion**: hydrocortisone acetate (2.5%), pramoxine HCl (1%)	Apply to the affected area as a thin film tid or qid.
ANEXSIA 5/500 (C-III)	Analgesic	**Tab**: hydrocodone bitartrate (5 mg), acetaminophen (500 mg)	1 - 2 tab q 4 - 6 h po, prn pain.
ANEXSIA 7.5/650 (C-III)	Analgesic	**Tab**: hydrocodone bitartrate (7.5 mg), acetaminophen (650 mg)	1 tab q 4 - 6 h po, prn pain.
ANEXSIA 10/660 (C-III)	Analgesic	**Tab**: hydrocodone bitartrate (10 mg), acetaminophen (660 mg)	1 tab q 4 - 6 h po, prn pain.
ANUSOL	Antihemorrhoidal	**Oint**: pramoxine HCl (1%), mineral oil (46.7%), zinc oxide (12.5%)	Apply externally to the affected area up to 5 times daily.
APRESAZIDE 25/25	Antihypertensive	**Cpsl**: hydralazine HCl (25 mg), hydrochlorothiazide (25 mg)	1 cpsl bid po.
APRESAZIDE 50/50		**Cpsl**: hydralazine HCl (50 mg), hydrochlorothiazide (50 mg)	1 cpsl bid po.
APRESAZIDE 100/50		**Cpsl**: hydralazine HCl (100 mg), hydrochlorothiazide (50 mg)	1 cpsl bid po.
ARTHROTEC 50	Antiinflammatory	**Enteric-Coated Tab**: diclofenac sodium (50 mg), misoprostol (200 μg)	**Osteoarthritis**: 1 tab tid po. **Rheumatoid Arthritis**: 1 tab tid to qid po.
ARTHROTEC 75	Antiinflammatory	**Enteric-Coated Tab**: diclofenac sodium (75 mg), misoprostol (200 μg)	**Osteoarthritis and Rheumatoid Arthritis**: 1 tab bid po.

AUGMENTIN 125	Antibacterial	**Powd for Susp (per 5 mL)**: amoxicillin (125 mg), clavulanic acid (31.25 mg) **Chewable Tab**: amoxicillin (125 mg), clavulanic acid (31.25 mg)	**Usual Dosage**: 1 AUGMENTIN 250 tablet q 8 h po or 1 AUGMENTIN 500 tablet q 12 h po. The 125 mg/5 mL or 250 mg/5 mL suspension may be given in place of the 500 mg tablet. **Severe Infections & Respiratory Infections**: 1 AUGMENTIN 500 tablet q 8 h po or 1 AUGMENTIN 875 tablet q 12 h po. The 200 mg/5 mL or 400 mg/5 mL suspension may be given in place of the 875 mg tablet.
AUGMENTIN 200		**Powd for Susp (per 5 mL)**: amoxicillin (200 mg), clavulanic acid (28.5 mg) **Chewable Tab**: amoxicillin (200 mg), clavulanic acid (28.5 mg)	
AUGMENTIN 250		**Powd for Susp (per 5 mL)**: amoxicillin (250 mg), clavulanic acid (62.5 mg) **Chewable Tab**: amoxicillin (250 mg), clavulanic acid (62.5 mg) **Tab**: amoxicillin (250 mg), clavulanic acid (125 mg)	
AUGMENTIN 400		**Powd for Susp (per 5 mL)**: amoxicillin (400 mg), clavulanic acid (57 mg) **Chewable Tab**: amoxicillin (400 mg), clavulanic acid (57 mg)	
AUGMENTIN 500 AUGMENTIN 875		**Tab**: amoxicillin (500 mg), clavulanic acid (125 mg) **Tab**: amoxicillin (875 mg), clavulanic acid (125 mg)	
AURALGAN OTIC	Analgesic (Topical)	**Otic Solution (per mL)**: benzocaine (14 mg = 1.4%), antipyrine (54 mg = 5.4%), glycerin	Instill in ear canal until filled, then insert a cotton pledget moistened with solution into meatus. Repeat q 1 - 2 h.
AVALIDE 150/12.5 AVALIDE 300/12.5	Antihypertensive	**Tab**: irbesartan (150 mg), hydrochlorothiazide (12.5 mg) **Tab**: irbesartan (300 mg), hydrochlorothiazide (12.5 mg)	1 tab (150/12.5) daily po. [Used to titrate after the above].
BACTRIM	Antibacterial	**Susp (per 5 mL)**: sulfamethoxazole (200 mg), trimethoprim (40 mg) **Tab**: sulfamethoxazole (400 mg), trimethoprim (80 mg)	**Urinary Tract Infections**: 1 BACTRIM DS tab, 2 BACTRIM tab or 20 mL of Suspension q 12 h po for 10 - 14 days. **Shigellosis**: 1 BACTRIM DS tab, 2 BACTRIM tab or 20 mL of Suspension q 12 h for 5 days. **Acute Exacerbations of Chronic Bronchitis**: 1 BACTRIM DS tab, 2 BACTRIM tab or 20 mL of Suspension q 12 h po for 14 days.
BACTRIM DS		**Tab**: sulfamethoxazole (800 mg), trimethoprim (160 mg)	

[Continued on the next page]

TRADE NAME	THERAPEUTIC CATEGORY	DOSAGE FORMS AND COMPOSITION	COMMON ADULT DOSAGE
BACTRIM & BACTRIM DS [Continued]			***P. carinii*** **Pneumonia Treatment:** 20 mg/kg trimethoprim and 100 mg/kg sulfamethoxazole per 24 h in equally divided doses q 6 h for 14 days. ***P. carinii*** **Pneumonia Prophylax.:** 1 BACTRIM DS tab, 2 BACTRIM tab or 20 mL of Suspension q 24 h po. **Travelers' Diarrhea:** 1 BACTRIM DS tab, 2 BACTRIM tab or 20 mL of Suspension q 12 h po for 5 days.
BACTRIM I.V. INFUSION	Antibacterial	**Inj (per 5 mL):** sulfamethoxazole (400 mg), trimethoprim (80 mg)	**Severe Urinary Tract Infections and Shigellosis:** 8 - 10 mg/kg daily (based on trimethoprim) in 2 - 4 equally divided doses q 6, 8 or 12 h by IV infusion for up to 14 days for UTI and 5 days for shigellosis. ***P. carinii*** **Pneumonia:** 15 - 20 mg/kg daily (based on trimethoprim) in 3 - 4 equally divided doses q 6 - 8 h by IV infusion for up to 14 days.
BANCAP HC (C-III)	Analgesic	**Cpsl:** hydrocodone bitartrate (5 mg), acetaminophen (500 mg)	1 cpsl q 6 h po, prn pain. Maximum: 2 cpsl q 6 h po.
BENADRYL ALLERGY / COLD	Decongestant-Antihistamine-Analgesic	**Tab:** pseudoephedrine HCl (30 mg), diphenhydramine HCl (12.5 mg), acetaminophen (500 mg)	2 tab q 6 h po while symptoms persist.
BENADRYL ALLERGY DECONGESTANT	Decongestant-Antihistamine	**Liquid (per 5 mL):** pseudoephedrine HCl (30 mg), diphenhydramine HCl (12.5 mg) **Tab:** pseudoephedrine HCl (60 mg), diphenhydramine HCl (25 mg)	10 mL q 4 - 6 h po. Maximum: 40 mL/day. 1 tab q 4 - 6 h po. Maximum: 4 tabs daily.

BENADRYL ITCH RELIEF MAXIMUM STRENGTH	Antihistamine	**Cream & Spray**: diphenhydramine HCl (2%), zinc acetate (0.1%)	Apply to affected areas not more than tid or qid.
BENADRYL ITCH STOPPING GEL - EXTRA STRENGTH	Antihistamine	**Gel**: diphenhydramine HCl (2%), zinc acetate (0.1%)	Apply to affected areas sparingly not more than tid or qid.
BENYLIN EXPECTORANT	Antitussive-Expectorant	**Liquid (per 5 mL)**: dextromethorphan HBr (5 mg), guaifenesin (100 mg)	10 - 20 mL q 4 h po, not to exceed 120 mL in 24 h.
BENYLIN MULTI-SYMPTOM	Antitussive-Expectorant-Decongestant	**Liquid (per 5 mL)**: dextromethorphan HBr (5 mg), guaifenesin (100 mg), pseudoephedrine HCl (15 mg)	20 mL q 4 h po. Do not exceed 80 mL in 24 h.
BENZAMYCIN	Anti-Acne Agent	**Gel (per g)**: erythromycin (30 mg = 3%), benzoyl peroxide (50 mg = 5%)	Apply topically bid, AM and PM.
BICILLIN C-R	Antibacterial	**Inj (per mL)**: penicillin G benzathine (150,000 Units), penicillin G procaine (150,000 Units) **Inj (per mL)**: penicillin G benzathine (300,000 Units), penicillin G procaine (300,000 Units)	**Streptococcal Infections:** 2,400,000 Units by deep IM injection (multiple sites). **Pneumococcal Infections (except Meningitis):** 1,200,000 Units by deep IM injection, repeated q 2 - 3 days until the temperature is normal for 48 hours.
BICILLIN C-R 900/300		**Inj (per 2 mL)**: penicillin G benzathine (900,000 Units), penicillin G procaine (300,000 units)	**Streptococcal Infections:** A single deep IM injection is usually sufficient. **Pneumococcal Infections (except Meningitis)**: One 2 mL deep IM injection, repeated q 2 - 3 days until the temp. is normal for 48 hours.
BLEPHAMIDE	Antibacterial-Corticosteroid	**Ophth Susp**: sulfacetamide sodium (10%), prednisolone acetate (0.2%) **Ophth Oint**: sulfacetamide sodium (10%), prednisolone acetate (0.2%)	1 drop into affected eye(s) bid to qid. Apply to affected eye(s) tid - qid and once or twice at night.

TRADE NAME	THERAPEUTIC CATEGORY	DOSAGE FORMS AND COMPOSITION	COMMON ADULT DOSAGE
BREVICON	Oral Contraceptive	**Tab**: ethinyl estradiol (35 μg), norethindrone (0.5 mg) in 21-Day and 28-Day Wallettes (contains 7 inert tabs)	21-Day regimen po or 28-Day regimen po.
BRONTEX (C-III) BRONTEX LIQUID (C-V)	Antitussive-Expectorant	**Tab**: codeine phosphate (10 mg), guaifenesin (300 mg) **Liquid (per 20 mL)**: codeine phosphate (10 mg), guaifenesin (300 mg)	1 tab q 4 h po, prn. 20 mL q 4 h po, prn.
CAFERGOT	Antimigraine Agent	**Tab**: ergotamine tartrate (1 mg), caffeine (100 mg)	2 tab stat po, then 1 tab q 0.5 h if needed (maximum of 6 tab per attack).
		Rectal Suppos: ergotamine tartrate (2 mg), caffeine (100 mg)	Insert 1 rectally stat, then 1 suppos. after 1 h if needed.
CAPOZIDE 25/15 CAPOZIDE 25/25 CAPOZIDE 50/15 CAPOZIDE 50/25	Antihypertensive	**Tab**: captopril (25 mg), hydrochlorothiazide (15 mg) **Tab**: captopril (25 mg), hydrochlorothiazide (25 mg) **Tab**: captopril (50 mg), hydrochlorothiazide (15 mg) **Tab**: captopril (50 mg), hydrochlorothiazide (25 mg)	1 CAPOZIDE 25/15 tab bid po, 1 h ac. Increased captopril dosage may be obtained by utilizing CAPOZIDE 50/15 bid, or higher hydrochlorothiazide dosage may be obtained by utilizing CAPOZIDE 25/25 bid. CAPOZIDE 25/15 and 50/15 may also be used tid po.
CEROSE-DM	Decongestant-Antihistamine-Antitussive	**Liquid (per 5 mL)**: phenylephrine HCl (10 mg), chlorpheniramine maleate (4 mg), dextromethorphan HBr (15 mg), alcohol (2.4%)	5 mL q 4 h po prn.
CHERACOL (C-V)	Antitussive-Expectorant	**Syrup (per 5 mL)**: codeine phosphate (10 mg), guaifenesin (100 mg), alcohol (4.75%)	10 mL q 4 - 6 h po.
CHERACOL D	Antitussive-Expectorant	**Liquid (per 5 mL)**: dextromethorphan HBr (10 mg), guaifenesin (100 mg), alcohol (4.75%)	10 mL q 4 h po.
CHERACOL PLUS	Decongestant-Antihistamine-Antitussive	**Liquid (per 5 mL)**: phenylpropanolamine HCl (8.3 mg), chlorpheniramine maleate (1.3 mg), dextromethorphan HBr (6.7 mg), alcohol (8%)	15 mL q 4 h po.

CHLOROMYCETIN HYDROCORTISONE	Antibacterial-Corticosteroid	**Powd for Ophth Susp**: chloramphenicol (12.5 mg), hydrocortisone acetate (25 mg) in vials with diluent	2 drops in the affected eye(s) q 3 h. Continue dosing day & night for the first 48 h, after which the interval between applications may be increased. Treatment should continue for 48 h after the eye appears normal.
CHLOR-TRIMETON 4 HOUR RELIEF	Decongestant-Antihistamine	**Tab**: pseudoephedrine sulfate (60 mg), chlorpheniramine maleate (4 mg)	1 tab q 4 - 6 h po, up to 4 tabs per day.
CHLOR-TRIMETON 12 HOUR RELIEF	Decongestant-Antihistamine	**Sustained-Rel. Tab**: pseudoephedrine sulfate (120 mg), chlorpheniramine maleate (8 mg)	1 tab q 12 h po.
CIPRO HC OTIC	Antibacterial-Corticosteroid	**Otic Susp (per mL)**: ciprofloxacin HCl (equivalent to 2 mg of base), hydrocortisone (10 mg)	Instill 3 drops into the affected ear(s) bid for 7 days.
CLARITIN-D 12-HOUR	Decongestant-Antihistamine	**Extended-Rel. Tab**: pseudoephedrine sulfate (120 mg), loratidine (5 mg)	1 tab q 12 h po.
CLARITIN-D 24-HOUR	Decongestant-Antihistamine	**Extended-Rel. Tab**: pseudoephedrine sulfate (240 mg), loratidine (10 mg)	1 tab q 24 h po.
COLY-MYCIN S OTIC	Antibacterial-Corticosteroid	**Otic Susp (per mL)**: neomycin sulfate (4.71 mg, equivalent to 3.3 mg neomycin base), colistin sulfate (3 mg), hydrocortisone acetate (10 mg = 1%)	5 instilled drops into the affected ear(s) tid - qid.
COMBIPRES 0.1 COMBIPRES 0.2 COMBIPRES 0.3	Antihypertensive	**Tab**: clonidine HCl (0.1 mg), chlorthalidone (15 mg) **Tab**: clonidine HCl (0.2 mg), chlorthalidone (15 mg) **Tab**: clonidine HCl (0.3 mg), chlorthalidone (15 mg)	1 tab once daily or bid po. 1 tab once daily or bid po. 1 tab once daily or bid po.
COMBIVENT	Drug for COPD	**Aerosol**: ipratropium bromide (18 μg), albuterol sulfate (103 μg) per spray	2 inhalations qid.
COMBIVIR	Antiviral	**Tab**: lamivudine (150 mg), zidovudine (300 mg)	1 tab bid po.
COMHIST LA	Decongestant-Antihistamine	**Cpsl**: phenylephrine HCl (20 mg), chlorpheniramine maleate (4 mg), phenyltoloxamine citrate (50 mg)	1 cpsl q 8 - 12 h po.

TRADE NAME	THERAPEUTIC CATEGORY	DOSAGE FORMS AND COMPOSITION	COMMON ADULT DOSAGE
COMTREX	Antitussive-Decongestant-Antihistamine-Analgesic	**Cplt & Tab**: dextromethorphan HBr (15 mg), pseudoephedrine HCl (30 mg), chlorpheniramine maleate (2 mg), acetaminophen (500 mg)	2 cplt (or tab) q 6 h po, not to exceed 8 cplt (or tab) in 24 h.
		Liqui-Gel Cpsl: dextromethorphan HBr (15 mg), phenylpropanolamine HCl (12.5 mg), chlorpheniramine maleate (2 mg), acetaminophen (500 mg)	2 cpsl q 6 h po, not to exceed 8 cpsl in 24 h.
		Liquid (per 30 mL): dextromethorphan HBr (30 mg), pseudoephedrine HCl (60 mg), chlorpheniramine maleate (4 mg), acetaminophen (1000 mg), alcohol (10%)	30 mL q 6 h po, not to exceed 4 doses in 24 h.
COMTREX, ALLERGY-SINUS	Decongestant-Antihistamine-Analgesic	**Cplt & Tab**: pseudoephedrine HCl (30 mg), chlorpheniramine maleate (2 mg), acetaminophen (500 mg)	2 cplt (or tab) q 6 h po.
COMTREX, NON-DROWSY	Antitussive-Decongestant-Analgesic	**Cplt**: dextromethorphan HBr (15 mg), pseudoephedrine HCl (30 mg), acetaminophen (500 mg)	2 cplt q 6 h po, not to exceed 4 doses in 24 h.
CORICIDIN HB	Antihistamine-Analgesic	**Tab**: chlorpheniramine maleate (2 mg), acetaminophen (325 mg)	2 tab q 4 - 6 h po.
CORICIDIN "D"	Decongestant-Antihistamine-Analgesic	**Tab**: phenylpropanolamine HCl (12.5 mg), chlorpheniramine maleate (2 mg), acetaminophen (325 mg)	2 tab q 4 h po.
CORICIDIN MAXIMUM STRENGTH SINUS HEADACHE	Decongestant-Antihistamine-Analgesic	**Cplt**: phenylpropanolamine HCl (12.5 mg), chlorpheniramine maleate (2 mg), acetaminophen (500 mg)	2 cplt q 6 h po.
CORTISPORIN	Antibacterial-Corticosteroid	**Ophth Susp (per mL)**: polymyxin B sulfate (10,000 Units), neomycin sulfate (equal to 3.5 mg of neomycin base), hydrocortisone (10 mg = 1%)	1 - 2 drops into the affected eye(s) q 3 - 4 h, depending on the severity of the condition.
		Ophth Oint (per g): polymyxin B sulfate (10,000 Units), neomycin sulfate (equal to 3.5 mg of neomycin base), bacitracin zinc (400 Units), hydrocortisone (10 mg = 1%)	Apply to the affected eye(s) q 3 - 4 h, depending on the severity of the condition.
		Cream (per g): polymyxin B sulfate (10,000 Units), neomycin sulfate (equal to 3.5 mg of neomycin base), hydrocortisone acetate (5 mg = 0.5%)	Apply topically bid - qid. If the conditions permit, gently rub into the affected areas.
		Oint (per g): polymyxin B sulfate (5,000 Units), neomycin sulfate (equal to 3.5 mg of neomycin base), bacitracin zinc (400 Units), hydrocortisone (10 mg = 1%)	Apply topically as a thin film bid to qid prn.

CORTISPORIN OTIC	Antibacterial-Corticosteroid	**Otic Solution & Susp (per mL)**: polymyxin B sulfate (10,000 Units), neomycin sulfate (equal to 3.5 mg of neomycin base), hydrocortisone (10 mg = 1%)	4 drops instilled in the affected ear(s) tid to qid.
CORZIDE 40/5	Antihypertensive	**Tab**: nadolol (40 mg), bendroflumethiazide (5 mg)	1 tab daily po.
CORZIDE 80/5		**Tab**: nadolol (80 mg), bendroflumethiazide (5 mg)	1 tab daily po.
COSOPT	Anti-Glaucoma Agent	**Ophth Solution**: dorzolamide HCl (2%), timolol maleate (0.5%)	1 drop in the affected eye(s) bid.
DARVOCET-N 50 (C-IV)	Analgesic	**Tab**: propoxyphene napsylate (50 mg), acetaminophen (325 mg)	2 tab q 4 h prn pain po.
DARVOCET-N 100 (C-IV)		**Tab**: propoxyphene napsylate (100 mg), acetaminophen (650 mg)	1 tab q 4 h prn pain po.
DARVON COMPOUND-65 (C-IV)	Analgesic	**Cpsl**: propoxyphene HCl (65 mg), aspirin (389 mg), caffeine (32.4 mg)	1 cpsl q 4 h po, prn pain.
DECADRON W/XYLOCAINE	Corticosteroid-Local Anesthetic	**Inj (per mL)**: dexamethasone sodium phosphate (4 mg), lidocaine HCl (10 mg)	Initial dose ranges from 0.1 to 0.75 mL by injection. Some patients respond to a single injection; in others, additional doses may be needed, usually at 4 - 7 day intervals.
DECONAMINE	Decongestant-Antihistamine	**Syrup (per 5 mL)**: pseudoephedrine HCl (30 mg), chlorpheniramine maleate (2 mg)	5 - 10 mL tid - qid po.
		Tab: pseudoephedrine HCl (60 mg), chlorpheniramine maleate (4 mg)	1 tab tid - qid po.
DECONAMINE CX (C-III)	Decongestant-Expectorant-Antitussive	**Liquid (per 5 mL)**: pseudoephedrine HCl (60 mg), hydrocodone bitartrate (5 mg), guiafenesin (200 mg)	5 mL qid po.
DECONAMINE SR	Decongestant-Antihistamine	**Sustained-Rel. Cpsl**: pseudoephedrine HCl (120 mg), chlorpheniramine maleate (8 mg)	1 cpsl q 12 h po.
DEMULEN 1/35	Oral Contraceptive	**Tab**: ethinyl estradiol (35 μg), ethynodiol diacetate (1 mg) in 21-Day and 28-Day Compaks (contains 7 inert tabs)	21-Day regimen po or 28-Day regimen po.
DEMULEN 1/50		**Tab**: ethinyl estradiol (50 μg), ethynodiol diacetate (1 mg) in 21-Day and 28-Day Compaks (contains 7 inert tabs)	21-Day regimen po or 28-Day regimen po.

TRADE NAME	THERAPEUTIC CATEGORY	DOSAGE FORMS AND COMPOSITION	COMMON ADULT DOSAGE
DESENEX (Original)	Antifungal	**Oint, Cream, & Powder**: total undecylenate = 25% as undecylenic acid and zinc undecylenate	Cleanse the skin with soap and water and dry thoroughly. Apply to the affected skin areas morning and night.
DESOGEN	Oral Contraceptive	**Tab**: ethinyl estradiol (30 μg), desogestrel (0.15 mg) in 28-Day packs (contains 7 inert tabs)	28-Day regimen po.
DEXACIDIN	Antibacterial-Corticosteroid	**Ophth Oint (per g)**: neomycin sulfate (equal to 3.5 mg of neomycin base), polymyxin B sulfate (10,000 Units), dexamethasone (1 mg)	Apply a small amount (about 0.5 in.) into the conjunctival sac tid - qid.
DIMETANE DECONGESTANT	Decongestant-Antihistamine	**Elixir (per 5 mL)**: phenylephrine HCl (5 mg), brompheniramine maleate (2 mg), alcohol (2.3%)	10 mL q 4 h po.
		Cplt: phenylephrine HCl (10 mg), brompheniramine maleate (4 mg)	1 cplt q 4 h po.
DIMETANE-DC (C-V)	Antitussive-Decongestant-Antihistamine	**Syrup (per 5 mL)**: codeine phosphate (10 mg), phenylpropanolamine HCl (12.5 mg), brompheniramine maleate (2 mg), alcohol (0.95%)	10 mL q 4 h po.
DIMETANE-DX	Antitussive-Decongestant-Antihistamine	**Syrup (per 5 mL)**: dextromethorphan HBr (10 mg), pseudoephedrine HCl (30 mg), brompheniramine maleate (2 mg), alcohol (0.95%)	10 mL q 4 h po.
DIMETAPP	Decongestant-Antihistamine	**Elixir (per 5 mL)**: phenylpropanolamine HCl (12.5 mg), brompheniramine maleate (2 mg)	10 mL q 4 h po.
		Tab & Liqui-Gel Cpsl: phenylpropanolamine HCl (25 mg), brompheniramine maleate (4 mg)	1 tab (or Softgel) q 4 h po.
DIMETAPP EXTENTAB		**Sustained-Rel. Tab**: phenylpropanolamine HCl (75 mg), brompheniramine maleate (12 mg)	1 tab q 12 h po.
DIMETAPP COLD & FLU	Decongestant-Antihistamine-Analgesic	**Cplt**: phenylpropanolamine HCl (12.5 mg), brompheniramine maleate (2 mg), acetaminophen (500 mg)	2 cplt q 6 h po.
DIMETAPP DM	Decongestant-Antihistamine-Antitussive	**Elixir (per 5 mL)**: phenylpropanolamine HCl (12.5 mg), brompheniramine maleate (2 mg), dextromethorphan HBr (10 mg)	10 mL q 4 h po.

DIOVAN HCT 80/12.5	Antihypertensive	**Tab**: valsartan (80 mg), hydrochlorothiazide (12.5 mg)	1 tab daily po.
DIOVAN HCT 160/12.5	Antihypertensive	**Tab**: valsartan (160 mg), hydrochlorothiazide (12.5 mg)	1 tab daily po.
DOMEBORO	Astringent	**Powder (per packet)**: aluminum sulfate (1191 mg), calcium acetate (938 mg) **Effervescent Tab**: aluminum sulfate (878 mg), calcium acetate (604 mg)	**As a Compress**: Dissolve 1 or 2 packets (or tabs) in 16 fl. oz. of warm water. Saturate a clean dressing in the sol'n, gently squeeze and apply loosely to the affected area. Remove, remoisten and reapply q 15 - 30 minutes prn. **As a Soak**: Dissolve 1 or 2 packets (or tablets) in 16 fl. oz. of warm water. Soak the affected area for 15 - 30 minutes. Repeat tid.
DONNATAL	Antispasmodic, Anticholinergic	**Cpsl & Tab**: atropine sulfate (0.0194 mg), scopolamine HBr (0.0065 mg), hyoscyamine sulfate (0.1037 mg), phenobarbital (16.2 mg)	1 - 2 cpsl (or tab) tid or qid po.
		Elixir (per 5 mL): atropine sulfate (0.0194 mg), scopolamine HBr (0.0065 mg), hyoscyamine sulfate (0.1037 mg), phenobarbital (16.2 mg), alcohol (23%)	5 - 10 mL tid or qid po.
DONNATAL EXTENTABS	Antispasmodic, Anticholinergic	**Extended-Rel. Tab**: atropine sulfate (0.0582 mg), scopolamine HBr (0.0195 mg), hyoscyamine sulfate (0.3111 mg), phenobarbital (48.6 mg)	1 tab q 8 - 12 h po.
DOXIDAN	Irritant Laxative-Stool Softener	**Cpsl**: casanthranol (30 mg), docusate sodium (100 mg)	1 - 3 cpsl daily po.
DRIXORAL COLD & ALLERGY	Decongestant-Antihistamine	**Sustained-Rel. Tab**: pseudoephedrine sulfate (120 mg), dexbrompheniramine maleate (6 mg)	1 tab q 12 h po.
DRIXORAL COLD & FLU	Decongestant-Antihistamine-Analgesic	**Sustained-Rel. Tab**: pseudoephedrine sulfate (60 mg), dexbrompheniramine maleate (3 mg), acetaminophen (500 mg)	2 tab q 12 h po.
DURATUSS	Decongestant-Expectorant	**Sustained-Rel. Tab**: pseudoephedrine HCl (120 mg), guaifenesin (600 mg)	1 tab q 12 h po.

TRADE NAME	THERAPEUTIC CATEGORY	DOSAGE FORMS AND COMPOSITION	COMMON ADULT DOSAGE
DURATUSS HD (C-III)	Antitussive-Decongestant-Expectorant	**Elixir (per 5 mL)**: hydrocodone bitartrate (2.5 mg), pseudoephedrine HCl (30 mg), guaifenesin (100 mg), alcohol (5%)	10 mL q 4 - 6 h po.
DYAZIDE	Diuretic, Antihypertensive	**Cpsl**: triamterene (37.5 mg), hydrochlorothiazide (25 mg)	1 - 2 cpsl once daily po.
ELIXOPHYLLIN-GG	Drug for COPD	**Liquid (per 15 mL)**: theophylline anhydrous (100 mg), guaifenesin (100 mg)	Dose based on theophylline; see Oral Theophylline Doses Table, p. 252. **Initial**: 6 mg/kg po; then reduce to 3 mg/kg q 6 h for 2 doses. **Maintenance**: 3 mg/kg q 8 h po.
ELIXOPHYLLIN-KI	Drug for COPD	**Elixir (per 15 mL)**: theophylline anhydrous (80 mg), potassium iodide (130 mg), alcohol (10%)	Dose based on theophylline; see Oral Theophylline Doses Table, p. 252. **Initial**: 6 mg/kg po; then reduce to 3 mg/kg q 6 h for 2 doses. **Maintenance**: 3 mg/kg q 8 h po.
EMETROL	Antiemetic	**Solution (per 5 mL)**: dextrose (1.87 g), levulose (1.87 g), phosphoric acid (21.5 mg)	15 - 30 mL po. Repeat q 15 min. until distress subsides.
EMLA	Local Anesthetic	**Cream**: lidocaine (2.5%), prilocaine (2.5%)	**Minor Dermal Procedures**: Apply 2.5 g over 20 - 25 cm^2 of the skin surface, cover with an occlusive dressing, and allow to remain for at least 1 h. **Major Dermal Procedures**: Apply 2 g per 10 cm^2 of the skin surface, cover with an occlusive dressing, and allow to remain for at least 2 h.
EMPIRIN W/CODEINE	Analgesic		
#3 (C-III)		**Tab**: aspirin (325 mg), codeine phosphate (30 mg)	1 - 2 tab q 4 h po, prn.
#4 (C-III)		**Tab**: aspirin (325 mg), codeine phosphate (60 mg)	1 tab q 4 h po, prn.

ENLON-PLUS	Cholinomimetic-Anticholinergic	**Inj (per mL)**: edrophonium chloride (10 mg), atropine sulfate (0.14 mg)	Dosages range from 0.05 - 1 mL/kg IV given slowly over 45 to 60 seconds at a point of at least 5% recovery of twitch response to neuromuscular stimulation (95% block). The dosage delivered is 0.5 to 1 mg/kg edrophonium and 7 to 14 μg/kg atropine. A total dosage of 1 mg/kg of edrophonium should rarely be exceeded.
ENTEX	Decongestant-Expectorant	**Cpsl**: phenylpropanolamine HCl (45 mg), phenylephrine HCl (5 mg), guaifenesin (200 mg)	1 cpsl qid (q 6 h) po with food or fluid.
		Liquid (per 5 mL): phenylpropanolamine HCl (20 mg), phenylephrine HCl (5 mg), guaifenesin (100 mg), alcohol (5%)	10 mL qid (q 6 h) po.
ENTEX LA	Decongestant-Expectorant	**Long-Acting Tab**: phenylpropanolamine HCl (75 mg), guaifenesin (400 mg)	1 tab bid (q 12 h) po.
ENTEX PSE	Decongestant-Expectorant	**Long-Acting Tab**: pseudoephedrine HCl (120 mg), guaifenesin (600 mg)	1 tab bid (q 12 h) po.
EPIFOAM	Corticosteroid-Local Anesthetic	**Aerosolized Foam**: hydrocortisone acetate (1%), pramoxine HCl (1%)	Apply to affected area tid to qid.
E-PILO-1	Anti-Glaucoma Agent	**Ophth Solution**: epinephrine bitartrate (1%), pilocarpine HCl (1%)	1 - 2 drops into affected eye(s) up to qid.
E-PILO-2		**Ophth Solution**: epinephrine bitartrate (1%), pilocarpine HCl (2%)	1 - 2 drops into affected eye(s) up to qid.
E-PILO-4		**Ophth Solution**: epinephrine bitartrate (1%), pilocarpine HCl (4%)	1 - 2 drops into affected eye(s) up to qid.
E-PILO-6		**Ophth Solution**: epinephrine bitartrate (1%), pilocarpine HCl (6%)	1 - 2 drops into affected eye(s) up to qid.
EQUAGESIC (C-IV)	Analgesic-Antianxiety Agent	**Tab**: aspirin (325 mg), meprobamate (200 mg)	1 - 2 tab tid po, prn pain.

TRADE NAME	THERAPEUTIC CATEGORY	DOSAGE FORMS AND COMPOSITION	COMMON ADULT DOSAGE
ESGIC	Analgesic	**Cpsl & Tab**: acetaminophen (325 mg), butalbital (50 mg), caffeine (40 mg)	1 - 2 cpsl (or tab) q 4 h po, prn pain.
ESGIC-PLUS	Analgesic	**Cpsl & Tab**: acetaminophen (500 mg), butalbital (50 mg), caffeine (40 mg)	1 cpsl (or tab) q 4 h po, prn pain.
ESIMIL	Antihypertensive	**Tab**: guanethidine monosulfate (10 mg), hydrochlorothiazide (25 mg)	2 tab daily po. Dosage may be increased at weekly intervals.
ESTRATEST	Estrogen-Androgen	**Tab**: esterified estrogens (1.25 mg), methyltestosterone (2.5 mg)	1 tab daily po. Administration should be cyclic: 3 weeks on and 1 week off.
ESTRATEST H.S.	Estrogen-Androgen	**Tab**: esterified estrogens (0.625 mg), methyltestosterone (1.25 mg)	1 -2 tab daily po. Administration should be cyclic: 3 weeks on and 1 week off.
ESTROSTEP 21	Oral Contraceptive	**Tab**: 5 triangular tabs: ethinyl estradiol (20 μg), norethindrone acetate (1 mg); 7 square tabs: ethinyl estradiol (30 μg), norethindrone acetate (1 mg); 9 round tabs: ethinyl estradiol (35 μg), norethindrone acetate (1 mg)	21-Day regimen po.
ESTROSTEP FE	Oral Contraceptive	**Tab**: 5 triangular tabs: ethinyl estradiol (20 μg), norethindrone acetate (1 mg); 7 square tabs: ethinyl estradiol (30 μg), norethindrone acetate (1 mg); 9 round tabs: ethinyl estradiol (35 μg), norethindrone acetate (1 mg); 7 (brown) tabs: ferrous fumarate (75 mg)	28-Day regimen po.
ETRAFON	Antipsychotic-Antidepressant	**Tab**: perphenazine (2 mg), amitriptyline HCl (25 mg)	1 tab tid or qid po.
ETRAFON 2-10		**Tab**: perphenazine (2 mg), amitriptyline HCl (10 mg)	1 tab tid or qid po.
ETRAFON-FORTE		**Tab**: perphenazine (4 mg), amitriptyline HCl (25 mg)	1 tab tid or qid po.
EXCEDRIN, ASPIRIN FREE	Analgesic	**Cplt & Geltab**: acetaminophen (500 mg), caffeine (65 mg)	2 cplt (or geltabs) q 6 h po while symptoms persist.
EXCEDRIN EXTRA-STRENGTH	Analgesic	**Tab, Cplt & Geltab**: acetaminophen (250 mg), aspirin (250 mg), caffeine (65 mg)	2 tabs (cplt or geltabs) q 6 h po while symptoms persist.
EXCEDRIN MIGRAINE	Analgesic	**Tab & Cplt**: acetaminophen (250 mg), aspirin (250 mg), caffeine (65 mg)	2 tabs (or cplts) q 6 h po while symptoms persist.

EXCEDRIN PM	Analgesic-Sedative	**Tab, Cplt & Geltab**: acetaminophen (500 mg), diphenhydramine citrate (38 mg)	2 tabs (cplts or geltabs) hs po.
EXTENDRYL	Decongestant-Antihistamine-Anticholinergic	**Syrup (per 5 mL)**: phenylephrine HCl (10 mg), chlorpheniramine maleate (2 mg), methscopolamine nitrate (1.25 mg)	10 mL q 4 h po.
		Tab: phenylephrine HCl (10 mg), chlorpheniramine maleate (2 mg), methscopolamine nitrate (1.25 mg)	2 tab q 4 h po.
EXTENDRYL SR		**Sustained-Rel. Cpsl**: phenylephrine HCl (20 mg), chlorpheniramine maleate (8 mg), methscopolamine nitrate (2.5 mg)	1 cpsl q 12 h po.
FANSIDAR	Antimalarial	**Tab**: sulfadoxine (500 mg), pyrimethamine (25 mg)	**Acute Malarial Attack**: 2 - 3 tab po alone or with quinine. **Malaria Prophylaxis**: 1 tab po once weekly or 2 tab po q 2 weeks 1 to 2 days before departure to an endemic area; continue during stay and for 4 to 6 weeks after return.
FEDAHIST EXPECTORANT	Decongestant-Expectorant	**Syrup (per 5 mL)**: pseudoephedrine HCl (20 mg), guaifenesin (200 mg)	10 mL q 4 - 6 h po, up to 40 mL per day.
FEDAHIST GYROCAPS	Decongestant-Antihistamine	**Timed-Rel. Cpsl**: pseudoephedrine HCl (65 mg), chlorpheniramine maleate (10 mg)	1 cpsl q 12 h po.
FEDAHIST TIMECAPS	Decongestant-Antihistamine	**Timed-Rel. Cpsl**: pseudoephedrine HCl (120), chlorpheniramine maleate (8 mg)	1 cpsl q 12 h po.
FERO-FOLIC-500	Hematinic	**Controlled-Rel. Tab**: ferrous sulfate (525 mg), folic acid (800 μg), sodium ascorbate (500 mg)	1 tab daily po.
FERO-GRAD-500	Hematinic	**Controlled-Rel. Tab**: ferrous sulfate (525 mg), sodium ascorbate (500 mg)	1 tab daily po.
FIORICET	Analgesic	**Tab**: acetaminophen (325 mg), butalbital (50 mg), caffeine (40 mg)	1 - 2 tab q 4 h po. Maximum of 6 tabs daily.
FIORICET W/CODEINE (C-III)	Analgesic	**Cpsl**: acetaminophen (325 mg), butalbital (50 mg), caffeine (40 mg), codeine phosphate (30 mg)	1 - 2 cpsl q 4 h po. Maximum of 6 cpsls daily.

TRADE NAME	THERAPEUTIC CATEGORY	DOSAGE FORMS AND COMPOSITION	COMMON ADULT DOSAGE
FIORINAL (C-III)	Analgesic	**Cpsl & Tab**: aspirin (325 mg), caffeine (40 mg), butalbital (50 mg)	1 - 2 cpsl (or tab) q 4 h po. Maximum of 6 daily.
FIORINAL W/CODEINE (C-III)	Analgesic	**Cpsl**: aspirin (325 mg), caffeine (40 mg), butalbital (50 mg), codeine phosphate (30 mg)	1 - 2 cpsl q 4 h po. Maximum of 6 caps daily.
FML-S	Antibacterial-Corticosteroid	**Ophth Susp**: sulfacetamide sodium (10%), fluorometholone (0.1%)	1 drop in affected eye(s) qid.
HALEY'S M-O	Emollient Laxative-Saline Laxative	**Liquid (per 5 mL)**: mineral oil (1.25 mL), magnesium hydroxide (304 mg)	15 - 30 mL po in the morning and hs.
HUMIBID DM	Antitussive-Expectorant	**Sustained-Rel. Tab**: dextromethorphan HBr (30 mg), guaifenesin (600 mg)	1 or 2 tablets q 12 h po.
HUMIBID DM SPRINKLE	Antitussive-Expectorant	**Sustained-Rel. Cpsl**: dextromethorphan HBr (15 mg), guaifenesin (300 mg)	2 or 4 capsules q 12 h po.
HYCODAN (C-III)	Antitussive-Anticholinergic	**Syrup (per 5 mL)**: hydrocodone bitartrate (5 mg), homatropine methylbromide (1.5 mg)	5 mL q 4 - 6 h po.
		Tab: hydrocodone bitartrate (5 mg), homatropine methylbromide (1.5 mg)	1 tab q 4 - 6 h po.
HYCOMINE (C-III)	Antitussive-Decongestant	**Syrup (per 5 mL)**: hydrocodone bitartrate (5 mg), phenylpropanolamine HCl (25 mg)	5 mL q 4 h po.
HYCOMINE COMPOUND (C-III)	Antitussive-Decongestant-Antihistamine-Analgesic	**Tab**: hydrocodone bitartrate (5 mg), phenylephrine HCl (10 mg), chlorpheniramine maleate (2 mg), acetaminophen (250 mg), caffeine (30 mg)	1 tab qid po.
HYCOTUSS EXPECTORANT (C-III)	Antitussive-Expectorant	**Syrup (per 5 mL)**: hydrocodone bitartrate (5 mg), guaifenesin (100 mg), alcohol (10%)	5 mL q 4 h po, pc & hs.
HYDROCET (C-III)	Analgesic	**Cpsl**: hydrocodone bitartrate (5 mg), acetaminophen (500 mg)	1 - 2 cpsl q 4 - 6 h po, prn pain.
HYDROPRES-50	Antihypertensive	**Tab**: hydrochlorothiazide (50 mg), reserpine (0.125 mg)	1 tab daily po.

HYZAAR 50-12.5	Antihypertensive	**Tab**: losartan potassium (50 mg), hydrochlorothiazide (12.5 mg)	1 tab daily po.
HYZAAR 100-25		**Tab**: losartan potassium (100 mg), hydrochlorothiazide (25 mg)	1 tab daily po.
INDERIDE-40/25	Antihypertensive	**Tab**: propranolol HCl (40 mg), hydrochlorothiazide (25 mg)	1 tab bid po.
INDERIDE-80/25		**Tab**: propranolol HCl (80 mg), hydrochlorothiazide (25 mg)	1 tab bid po.
INDERIDE LA 80/50	Antihypertensive	**Cpsl**: propranolol HCl (80 mg), hydrochlorothiazide (50 mg)	1 cpsl daily po.
INDERIDE LA 120/50		**Cpsl**: propranolol HCl (120 mg), hydrochlorothiazide (50 mg)	1 cpsl daily po.
INDERIDE LA 160/50		**Cpsl**: propranolol HCl (160 mg), hydrochlorothiazide (50 mg)	1 cpsl daily po.
JENEST-28	Oral Contraceptive	**Tab**: 7 tabs: norethindrone (0.5 mg), ethinyl estradiol (35 μg); 14 tabs: norethindrone (1 mg), ethinyl estradiol (35 μg); + 7 placebos in 28-Day Compaks	28-Day regimen po.
LEVLEN	Oral Contraceptive	**Tab**: ethinyl estradiol (30 μg), levonorgestrel (0.15 mg) in 21-Day and 28-Day Slidecases (contains 7 inert tabs)	21-Day regimen po or 28-Day regimen po.
LEVLITE	Oral Contraceptive	**Tab**: ethinyl estradiol (20 μg), levonorgestrel (0.10 mg) in 21-Day and 28-Day Slidecases (contains 7 inert tabs)	21-Day regimen po or 28-Day regimen po.
LEVORA 0.15/30	Oral Contraceptive	**Tab**: levonorgestrel (0.15 mg), ethinyl estradiol (30 μg) in 21-Day and 28-Day Dispensers (contains 7 inert tabs)	21-Day regimen po or 28-Day regimen po.
LEXXEL	Antihypertensive	**Extended-Rel. Tab**: enalapril maleate (5 mg), felodipine (2.5 mg)	1 tab once daily po.
		Extended-Rel. Tab: enalapril maleate (5 mg), felodipine (5 mg)	1 tab once daily po.
LIBRAX	Anticholinergic-Antianxiety	**Cpsl**: clidinium bromide (2.5 mg), chlordiazepoxide HCl (5 mg)	1 - 2 cpsl qid po, ac & hs.
LIMBITROL DS (C-IV)	Antianxiety Agent-Antidepressant	**Tab**: chlordiazepoxide (10 mg), amitriptyline HCl (25 mg)	1 tab tid or qid po.
LOESTRIN 21 1/20	Oral Contraceptive	**Tab**: ethinyl estradiol (20 μg), norethindrone acetate (1 mg) in 21-Day Petipacs	21-Day regimen po.
LOESTRIN 21 1.5/30		**Tab**: ethinyl estradiol (30 μg), norethindrone acetate (1.5 mg) in 21-Day Petipacs	21-Day regimen po.

TRADE NAME	THERAPEUTIC CATEGORY	DOSAGE FORMS AND COMPOSITION	COMMON ADULT DOSAGE
LOESTRIN FE 1/20	Oral Contraceptive	**Tab**: 21 tabs: ethinyl estradiol (20 μg), norethindrone acetate (1 mg) + 7 tabs: ferrous fumarate (75 mg) in 28-Day Petipacs	28-Day regimen po.
LOESTRIN FE 1.5/30		**Tab**: 21 tabs: ethinyl estradiol (30 μg), norethindrone acetate (1.5 mg) + 7 tabs: ferrous fumarate (75 mg) in 28-Day Petipacs	28-Day regimen po.
LOMOTIL (C-V)	Antidiarrheal	**Liquid (per 5 mL)**: diphenoxylate HCl (2.5 mg), atropine sulfate (0.025 mg), alcohol (15%)	10 mL qid po until control of diarrhea is achieved.
		Tab: diphenoxylate HCl (2.5 mg), atropine sulfate (0.025 mg)	2 tab qid po until control of diarrhea is achieved.
LO/OVRAL	Oral Contraceptive	**Tab**: ethinyl estradiol (30 μg), norgestrel (0.3 mg) in 21-Day Pilpaks	28-Day regimen po.
LOPRESSOR HCT 50/25	Antihypertensive	**Tab**: metoprolol tartrate (50 mg), hydrochlorothiazide (25 mg)	2 tab daily po as a single dose or in divided doses.
LOPRESSOR HCT 100/25		**Tab**: metoprolol tartrate (100 mg), hydrochlorothiazide (25 mg)	1 - 2 tab daily po as a single dose or in divided doses.
LOPRESSOR HCT 100/50		**Tab**: metoprolol tartrate (100 mg), hydrochlorothiazide (50 mg)	1 tab daily po as a single dose or in divided doses.
LORTAB (C-III)	Analgesic	**Elixir (per 5 mL)**: hydrocodone bitartrate (2.5 mg), acetaminophen (120 mg), alcohol (7%)	15 mL q 4 h po, prn pain.
LORTAB 2.5/500 (C-III)		**Tab**: hydrocodone bitartrate (2.5 mg), acetaminophen (500 mg)	1 - 2 tab q 4 - 6 h po, prn pain.
LORTAB 5/500 (C-III)		**Tab**: hydrocodone bitartrate (5 mg), acetaminophen (500 mg)	1 - 2 tab q 4 - 6 h po, prn pain.
LORTAB 7.5/500 (C-III)		**Tab**: hydrocodone bitartrate (7.5 mg), acetaminophen (500 mg)	1 tab q 4 - 6 h po, prn pain.
LORTAB 10/500 (C-III)		**Tab**: hydrocodone bitartrate (10 mg), acetaminophen (500 mg)	1 tab q 4 - 6 h po, prn pain.
LORTAB ASA (C-III)	Analgesic	**Tab**: hydrocodone bitartrate (5 mg), aspirin (500 mg)	1 - 2 tab q 4 - 6 h po, prn pain.
LOTENSIN HCT 5/6.25	Antihypertensive	**Tab**: benazepril HCl (5 mg), hydrochlorothiazide (6.25 mg)	1 tab daily po.
LOTENSIN HCT 10/12.5		**Tab**: benazepril HCl (10 mg), hydrochlorothiazide (12.5 mg)	1 tab daily po.
LOTENSIN HCT 20/12.5		**Tab**: benazepril HCl (20 mg), hydrochlorothiazide (12.5 mg)	1 tab daily po.
LOTENSIN HCT 20/25		**Tab**: benazepril HCl (20 mg), hydrochlorothiazide (25 mg)	1 tab daily po.

LOTREL	Antihypertensive	**Cpsl**: amlodipine besylate (2.5 mg), benazepril HCl (10 mg) **Cpsl**: amlodipine besylate (5 mg), benazepril HCl (10 mg) **Cpsl**: amlodipine besylate (5 mg), benazepril HCl (20 mg)	1 cpsl daily po. 1 cpsl daily po. 1 cpsl daily po.
LOTRISONE	Antifungal-Corticosteroid	**Cream**: clotrimazole (1%), betamethasone dipropionate (0.05%)	Massage into affected skin areas bid for up to 4 weeks.
LUFYLLIN-EPG	Drug for COPD	**Elixir (per 10 mL)**: dyphylline (100 mg), guaifenesin (200 mg), ephedrine HCl (16 mg), phenobarbital (16 mg), alcohol (5.5%)	10 - 20 mL q 6 h po.
		Tab: dyphylline (100 mg), guaifenesin (200 mg), ephedrine HCl (16 mg), phenobarbital (16 mg)	1 - 2 tab q 6 h po.
LUFYLLIN-GG	Drug for COPD	**Elixir (per 15 mL)**: dyphylline (100 mg), guiafenesin (100 mg), alcohol (17%)	30 mL qid po.
		Tab: dyphylline (200 mg), guaifenesin (200 mg)	1 tab qid po.
MARAX	Drug for COPD	**Tab**: theophylline (130 mg), ephedrine sulfate (25 mg), hydroxyzine HCl (10 mg)	1 tab bid - qid po. Some patients are adequately controlled with 1/2 - 1 tab hs.
MAXITROL	Antibacterial-Corticosteroid	**Ophth Suspension (per mL)**: polymyxin B sulfate (10,000 Units), neomycin sulfate (equal to 3.5 mg of neomycin base), dexamethasone (0.1%)	1 or 2 drops into the affected eye(s) q 1 h in severe disease; in mild cases, 1 - 2 drops 4 to 6 times daily.
		Ophth Oint (per g): polymyxin B sulfate (10,000 Units), neomycin sulfate (equal to 3.5 mg of neomycin base), dexamethasone (0.1%)	Apply a small amount into the conjunctival sac tid to qid.
MAXZIDE MAXZIDE-25 MG	Antihypertensive, Diuretic	**Tab**: triamterene (75 mg), hydrochlorothiazide (50 mg) **Tab**: triamterene (37.5 mg), hydrochlorothiazide (25 mg)	1 tab daily po. 1 - 2 tab daily po.
METIMYD	Antibacterial-Corticosteroid	**Ophth Susp**: sulfacetamide sodium (10%), prednisolone acetate (0.5%)	2 - 3 drops into the affected eye(s) q 1 - 2 h during the day and hs.
		Ophth Oint: sulfacetamide sodium (10%), prednisolone acetate (0.5%)	Apply to affected eye(s) tid or qid and hs.

TRADE NAME	THERAPEUTIC CATEGORY	DOSAGE FORMS AND COMPOSITION	COMMON ADULT DOSAGE
MIDRIN	Analgesic, Antimigraine Agent	**Cpsl**: isometheptene mucate (65 mg), dichloralphenazone (100 mg), acetaminophen (325 mg)	**Tension Headache**: 1 - 2 cpsl q 4 h po, up to 8 cpsl daily. **Migraine Headache**: 2 cpsl stat, then 1 cpsl q h po until relieved, up to 5 cpsl within a 12-hour period.
MINIZIDE 1 MINIZIDE 2 MINIZIDE 5	Antihypertensive	**Cpsl**: prazosin HCl (1 mg), polythiazide (0.5 mg) **Cpsl**: prazosin HCl (2 mg), polythiazide (0.5 mg) **Cpsl**: prazosin HCl (5 mg), polythiazide (0.5 mg)	1 cpsl bid - tid po, the strength depending upon individual requirement after titration.
MIRCETTE	Oral Contraceptive	**Tab**: 21 white tabs: ethinyl estradiol (20 μg), desogestrel (0.15 mg); 2 green inert tabs; 5 yellow tabs: ethinyl estradiol (10 μg) in 28-Day Dispensers	28-Day regimen po.
MODICON	Oral Contraceptive	**Tab**: ethinyl estradiol (35 μg), norethindrone (0.5 mg) in 21-Day and 28-Day Dialpaks (contains 7 inert tabs)	21-Day regimen po or 28-Day regimen po.
MODURETIC	Diuretic	**Tab**: amiloride HCl (5 mg), hydrochlorothiazide (50 mg)	Initially 1 tab daily po. Dosage may be raised to 2 tab daily as a single dose or in divided doses.
MOTOFEN (C-IV)	Antidiarrheal	**Tab**: difenoxin HCl (1 mg), atropine sulfate (0.025 mg)	2 tab po (1st dose), then 1 tab after each loose stool or 1 tab q 3 - 4 h prn. Maximum: 8 tab per 24 hours.
MOTRIN IB SINUS	Decongestant-Analgesic	**Cplt**: pseudoephedrine HCl (30 mg), ibuprofen (200 mg)	1 - 2 cplt q 4 - 6 h po.
MYCITRACIN PLUS PAIN RELIEVER	Antibacterial-Local Anesthetic	**Oint (per g)**: polymyxin B sulfate (5,000 Units), neomycin sulfate (equal to 3.5 mg of neomycin), bacitracin (500 Units), lidocaine (40 mg)	Apply a small amount to the affected area 1 - 3 times daily.
MYCOLOG-II	Corticosteroid-Antifungal	**Cream & Oint (per g)**: triamcinolone acetonide (1.0 mg), nystatin (100,000 Units)	Apply to the affected areas bid in the morning and evening.

NALDECON	Decongestant-Antihistamine	**Syrup (per 5 mL)**: phenylpropanolamine HCl (20 mg), phenylephrine HCl (5 mg), chlorpheniramine maleate (2.5 mg), phenyltoloxamine citrate (7.5 mg)	5 mL q 3 - 4 h po, not to exceed 4 doses in 24 h.
		Sustained-Action Tab: phenylpropanolamine HCl (40 mg), phenylephrine HCl (10 mg), chlorpheniramine maleate (5 mg), phenyltoloxamine citrate (15 mg)	1 tab tid on arising, in mid-afternoon, and at bedtime po.
NALDECON-CX ADULT (C-V)	Antitussive-Decongestant-Expectorant	**Liquid (per 5 mL)**: codeine phosphate (10 mg), phenylpropanolamine HCl (12.5 mg), guaifenesin (200 mg)	10 mL q 4 h po.
NALDECON-DX ADULT	Antitussive-Decongestant-Expectorant	**Liquid (per 5 mL)**: dextromethorphan HBr (10 mg), phenylpropanolamine HCl (12.5 mg), guaifenesin (200 mg), alcohol (0.06%)	10 mL q 4 h po.
NALDECON SENIOR DX	Antitussive-Expectorant	**Liquid (per 5 mL)**: dextromethorphan HBr (10 mg), guaifenesin (200 mg)	10 mL q 4 h po.
NAPHCON-A	Ocular Decongestant-Antihistamine	**Ophth Solution**: naphazoline HCl (0.025%), pheniramine maleate (0.3%)	1 - 2 drops in the affected eye(s) up to qid.
NECON 0.5/35	Oral Contraceptive	**Tab**: norethindrone (0.5 mg), ethinyl estradiol (35 μg) in 21-Day and 28-Day Dispensers (contains 7 inert tabs)	21-Day regimen po or 28-Day regimen po.
NECON 1/35	Oral Contraceptive	**Tab**: norethindrone (1 mg), ethinyl estradiol (35 μg) in 21-Day and 28-Day Dispensers (contains 7 inert tabs)	21-Day regimen po or 28-Day regimen po.
NECON 1/50	Oral Contraceptive	**Tab**: norethindrone (1 mg), mestranol (50 μg) in 21-Day and 28-Day Dispensers (contains 7 inert tabs)	21-Day regimen po or 28-Day regimen po.
NECON 10/11	Oral Contraceptive	**Tab**: 10 tabs: norethindrone (0.5 mg), ethinyl estradiol (35 μg); 11 tabs: norethindrone (1 mg), ethinyl estradiol (35 μg) in 21-Day and 28-Day Dispensers (contains 7 inert tabs)	21-Day regimen po or 28-Day regimen po.
NELOVA 0.5/35E	Oral Contraceptive	**Tab**: norethindrone (0.5 mg), ethinyl estradiol (35 μg) in 21-Day and 28-Day Compaks (contains 7 inert tabs)	21-Day regimen po or 28-Day regimen po.
NELOVA 1/35E		**Tab**: norethindrone (1.0 mg), ethinyl estradiol (35 μg) in 21-Day and 28-Day Compaks (contains 7 inert tabs)	21-Day regimen po or 28-Day regimen po.
NELOVA 1/50M	Oral Contraceptive	**Tab**: norethindrone (1.0 mg), mestranol (50 μg) in 21-Day and 28-Day Compaks (contains 7 inert tabs)	21-Day regimen po or 28-Day regimen po.

TRADE NAME	THERAPEUTIC CATEGORY	DOSAGE FORMS AND COMPOSITION	COMMON ADULT DOSAGE
NELOVA 10/11	Oral Contraceptive	**Tab**: 10 tabs: norethindrone (0.5 mg), ethinyl estradiol (35 μg); 11 tabs: norethindrone (1 mg), ethinyl estradiol (35 μg); + 7 placebos in 28-Day Compaks	28-Day regimen po.
NEODECADRON	Antibacterial-Corticosteroid	**Ophth Solution**: neomycin sulfate (equal to 0.35% of neomycin base), dexamethasone sodium phosphate (0.1%)	1 - 2 drops into eye(s) every h during the day and q 2 h at night. When a favorable response occurs, reduce the dosage to 1 drop q 4 h.
		Ophth Oint: neomycin sulfate (equal to 0.35% of neomycin base), dexamethasone sodium phosphate (0.05%)	Apply a thin coating to eye(s) tid - qid. When a favorable response occurs, reduce the dosage to bid.
		Topical Cream: neomycin sulfate (equal to 0.35% of base), dexamethasone sodium phosphate (0.1%)	Apply topically to the affected area as a thin film tid - qid.
NEOSPORIN	Antibacterial	**Ophth Solution (per mL)**: polymyxin B sulfate (10,000 Units), neomycin sulfate (equal to 1.75 mg of neomycin base), gramicidin (0.025 mg)	1 - 2 drops in the affected eye(s) bid - qid for 7 - 10 days.
		Ophth Oint (per g): polymyxin B sulfate (10,000 Units), neomycin sulfate (equal to 3.5 mg of neomycin base), bacitracin zinc (400 Units)	Apply to eye(s) q 3 - 4 h for 7 - 10 days.
		Oint (per g): polymyxin B sulfate (5,000 Units), neomycin sulfate (equal to 3.5 mg of neomycin base), bacitracin zinc (400 Units)	Apply topically 1 - 3 times daily.
NEOSPORIN PLUS MAXIMUM STRENGTH	Antibacterial-Local Anesthetic	**Cream (per g)**: polymyxin B sulfate (10,000 Units), neomycin sulfate (equal to 3.5 mg of neomycin base), lidocaine (40 mg)	Apply topically 1 - 3 times daily.
		Oint (per g): polymyxin B sulfate (10,000 Units), neomycin sulfate (equal to 3.5 mg of neomycin base), bacitracin zinc (500 Units), lidocaine (40 mg)	Apply topically 1 - 3 times daily.
NOLAMINE	Decongestant-Antihistamine	**Timed-Rel. Tab**: phenylpropanolamine HCl (50 mg), chlorpheniramine maleate (4 mg), phenindamine tartrate (24 mg)	1 tab q 8 h po. In mild cases, 1 tab q 10 - 12 h po.
NORDETTE	Oral Contraceptive	**Tab**: ethinyl estradiol (30 μg), levonorgestrel (0.15 mg) in 21-Day and 28-Day Pilpaks (contains 7 inert tabs)	21-Day regimen po or 28-Day regimen po.

NORGESIC	Skeletal Muscle Relaxant-Analgesic	**Tab**: orphenadrine citrate (25 mg), aspirin (385 mg), caffeine (30 mg)	1 - 2 tab tid or qid po.
NORGESIC FORTE		**Tab**: orphenadrine citrate (50 mg), aspirin (770 mg), caffeine (60 mg)	1 tab tid or qid po.
NORINYL 1 + 35	Oral Contraceptive	**Tab**: ethinyl estradiol (35 μg), norethindrone (1 mg) in 21-Day and 28-Day Wallettes (contains 7 inert tabs)	21-Day regimen po or 28-Day regimen po.
NORINYL 1 + 50	Oral Contraceptive	**Tab**: mestranol (50 μg), norethindrone (1 mg) in 21-Day and 28-Day Wallettes (contains 7 inert tabs)	21-Day regimen po or 28-Day regimen po.
NOVACET LOTION	Anti-Acne Agent	**Lotion**: sodium sulfacetamide (10%), sulfur (5%)	Apply a thin film to affected areas 1 to 3 times daily.
NOVAFED A	Decongestant-Antihistamine	**Controlled-Rel. Cpsl**: pseudoephedrine HCl (120 mg), chlorpheniramine maleate (8 mg)	1 cpsl q 12 h po.
NUCOFED (C-III)	Decongestant-Antitussive	**Syrup (per 5 mL)**: pseudoephedrine HCl (60 mg), codeine phosphate (20 mg)	5 mL q 6 h po.
		Cpsl: pseudoephedrine HCl (60 mg), codeine phosphate (20 mg)	1 cpsl q 6 h po.
NUCOFED EXPECTORANT (C-III)	Decongestant-Expectorant-Antitussive	**Syrup (per 5 mL)**: pseudoephedrine HCl (60 mg), guiafenesin (200 mg), codeine phosphate (20 mg), alcohol (12.5%)	5 mL q 6 h po.
NUCOFED PEDIATRIC EXPECTORANT (C-III)	Decongestant-Expectorant-Antitussive	**Syrup (per 5 mL)**: pseudoephedrine HCl (30 mg), guiafenesin (100 mg), codeine phosphate (10 mg), alcohol (6%)	10 mL q 6 h po.
ORNADE	Decongestant-Antihistamine	**Controlled-Rel. Cpsl**: phenylpropanolamine HCl (75 mg), chlorpheniramine maleate (12 mg)	1 cpsl q 12 h po.
ORNEX	Decongestant-Analgesic	**Cplt**: pseudoephedrine HCl (30 mg), acetaminophen (325 mg)	2 cplt q 4 h po, not to exceed 8 cplt in 24 h.
ORNEX, MAXIMUM STRENGTH	Decongestant-Analgesic	**Cplt**: pseudoephedrine HCl (30 mg), acetaminophen (500 mg)	2 cplt q 6 h po, not to exceed 8 cplt in 24 h.
ORTHO-CEPT	Oral Contraceptive	**Tab**: ethinyl estradiol (30 μg), desogestrel (0.15 mg) in 21-Day and 28-Day Dialpaks (contains 7 inert tabs)	21-Day regimen po or 28-Day regimen po.

TRADE NAME	THERAPEUTIC CATEGORY	DOSAGE FORMS AND COMPOSITION	COMMON ADULT DOSAGE
ORTHO-CYCLEN	Oral Contraceptive	**Tab**: ethinyl estradiol (35 μg), norgestimate (0.25 mg) in 21-Day and 28-Day Dialpaks (contains 7 inert tabs)	21-Day regimen po or 28-Day regimen po.
ORTHO-NOVUM 1/35	Oral Contraceptive	**Tab**: ethinyl estradiol (35 μg), norethindrone (1 mg) in 21-Day and 28-Day Dialpaks (contains 7 inert tabs)	21-Day regimen po or 28-Day regimen po.
ORTHO-NOVUM 1/50	Oral Contraceptive	**Tab**: mestranol (50 μg), norethindrone (1 mg) in 21-Day and 28-Day Dialpaks (contains 7 inert tabs)	21-Day regimen po or 28-Day regimen po.
ORTHO-NOVUM 7/7/7	Oral Contraceptive	**Tab**: 7 tabs: ethinyl estradiol (35 μg), norethindrone (0.5 mg); 7 tabs: ethinyl estradiol (35 μg), norethindrone (0.75 mg); 7 tabs: ethinyl estradiol (35 μg), norethindrone (1 mg) in 21-Day and 28-Day Dialpaks (contains 7 inert tabs)	21-Day regimen po or 28-Day regimen po.
ORTHO-NOVUM 10/11	Oral Contraceptive	**Tab**: 10 tabs: ethinyl estradiol (35 μg), norethindrone (0.5 mg); 11 tabs: ethinyl estradiol (35 μg), norethindrone (1 mg) in 21-Day and 28-Day Dialpaks (with 7 inert tabs)	21-Day regimen po or 28-Day regimen po.
ORTHO-PREFEST	Estrogen-Progestin	**30 Tab Pkg**: estradiol (1 mg) tabs; estradiol (1 mg) + norgestimate (90 μg) tabs: in an alternating sequence of 3 tablets each	One tablet daily. Take in the correct sequence; repeat without interruption.
ORTHO TRI-CYCLEN	Oral Contraceptive	**Tab**: 7 tabs: ethinyl estradiol (35 μg), norgestimate (0.18 mg); 7 tabs: ethinyl estradiol (35 μg), norgestimate (0.215 mg); 7 tabs: ethinyl estradiol (35 μg), norgestimate (0.25 mg) in 21-Day and 28-Day Dialpaks (contains 7 inert tabs)	21-Day regimen po or 28-Day regimen po.
OTOBIOTIC	Antibacterial-Corticosteroid	**Otic Solution (per mL)**: polymyxin B sulfate (10,000 Units), hydrocortisone (0.5%)	4 drops into ear(s) tid or qid.
OVCON-35	Oral Contraceptive	**Tab**: ethinyl estradiol (35 μg), norethindrone (0.4 mg) in 28-Day dispensers (contains 7 inert tabs)	28-Day regimen po.
OVCON-50		**Tab**: ethinyl estradiol (50 μg), norethindrone (1 mg) in 28-Day dispensers (contains 7 inert tabs)	28-Day regimen po.
OVRAL-28	Oral Contraceptive	**Tab**: ethinyl estradiol (50 μg), norgestrel (0.5 mg) in 28-Day Pilpaks (contains 7 inert tabs)	28-Day regimen po.

P_1E_1	Anti-Glaucoma Agent	**Ophth Solution**: pilocarpine HCl (1%), epinephrine bitartrate (1%)	1 - 2 drops into affected eye(s) up to qid.
P_2E_1		**Ophth Solution**: pilocarpine HCl (2%), epinephrine bitartrate (1%)	1 - 2 drops into affected eye(s) up to qid.
P_4E_1		**Ophth Solution**: pilocarpine HCl (4%), epinephrine bitartrate (1%)	1 - 2 drops into affected eye(s) up to qid.
P_6E_1		**Ophth Solution**: pilocarpine HCl (6%), epinephrine bitartrate (1%)	1 - 2 drops into affected eye(s) up to qid.
PAZO	Antihemorrhoidal	**Oint**: camphor (2%), ephedrine sulfate (0.2%), zinc oxide (5%) **Rectal Suppos**: ephedrine sulfate (3.86 mg), zinc oxide (96.5 mg)	Apply to affected areas up to qid. Insert 1 rectally up to qid.
PEDIOTIC	Antibacterial-Corticosteroid	**Otic Susp (per mL)**: polymyxin B sulfate (10,000 Units), neomycin sulfate (equal to 3.5 mg of neomycin base), hydrocortisone (10 mg = 1%)	4 drops into the affected ear(s) tid to qid.
PERCOCET (C-II)	Analgesic	**Tab**: oxycodone HCl (5 mg), acetaminophen (325 mg)	1 tab q 6 h po, prn pain.
PERCODAN (C-II)	Analgesic	**Tab**: oxycodone HCl (4.5 mg), oxycodone terephthalate (0.38 mg), aspirin (325 mg)	1 tab q 6 h po, prn pain.
PERCODAN-DEMI (C-II)	Analgesic	**Tab**: oxycodone HCl (2.25 mg), oxycodone terephthalate (0.19 mg), aspirin (325 mg)	1 - 2 tab q 6 h po, prn pain.
PERCOGESIC	Antihistamine-Analgesic	**Tab**: phenyltoloxamine citrate (30 mg), acetaminophen (325 mg)	1 - 2 tab q 4 h po, up to 8 tab per day.
PERDIEM OVERNIGHT RELIEF	Bulk Laxative-Irritant Laxative	**Granules (per rounded teaspoonful)**: psyllium (3.25 g), senna (0.74 g)	In the evening and/or before breakfast, 1 - 2 rounded teaspoonfuls in at least 8 oz. of cool beverage po.
PERI-COLACE	Irritant Laxative-Stool Softener	**Cpsl**: casanthranol (30 mg), docusate sodium (100 mg) **Syrup (per 15 mL)**: casanthranol (30 mg), docusate sodium (60 mg), alcohol (10%)	1 - 2 cpsl hs po. 15 - 30 mL hs po.
PHENERGAN VC	Antihistamine-Decongestant	**Syrup (per 5 mL)**: promethazine HCl (6.25 mg), phenylephrine HCl (5 mg), alcohol (7%)	5 mL q 4 - 6 h po.

TRADE NAME	THERAPEUTIC CATEGORY	DOSAGE FORMS AND COMPOSITION	COMMON ADULT DOSAGE
PHENERGAN VC W/ CODEINE (C-V)	Antihistamine-Decongestant-Antitussive	**Syrup (per 5 mL)**: promethazine HCl (6.25 mg), phenylephrine HCl (5 mg), codeine phosphate (10 mg), alcohol (7%)	5 mL q 4 - 6 h po, not to exceed 30 mL in 24 h.
PHENERGAN W/CODEINE (C-V)	Antihistamine-Antitussive	**Syrup (per 5 mL)**: promethazine HCl (6.25 mg), codeine phosphate (10 mg), alcohol (7%)	5 mL q 4 - 6 h po, not to exceed 30 mL in 24 h.
PHENERGAN W/ DEXTROMETHORPHAN	Antihistamine-Antitussive	**Syrup (per 5 mL)**: promethazine HCl (6.25 mg), dextromethorphan HBr (15 mg), alcohol (7%)	5 mL q 4 - 6 h po, not to exceed 30 mL in 24 h.
PHRENILIN PHRENILIN FORTE	Analgesic	**Tab**: acetaminophen (325 mg), butalbital (50 mg) **Cpsl**: acetaminophen (650 mg), butalbital (50 mg)	1 - 2 tab q 4 h po, prn. 1 cpsl q 4 h po, prn.
POLY-PRED	Antibacterial-Corticosteroid	**Ophth Suspension (per mL)**: neomycin sulfate (equal to 3.5 mg of neomycin base), polymyxin B sulfate (10,000 Units), prednisolone acetate (0.5%)	1 or 2 drops q 3 - 4 h into affected eye(s). Acute infections may require dosing q 30 minutes, initially.
POLYSPORIN	Antibacterial	**Ophth Oint (per g)**: polymyxin B sulfate (10,000 Units), bacitracin zinc (500 Units)	Apply to eye(s) q 3 - 4 h.
		Powder & Oint (per g): polymyxin B sulfate (10,000 Units), bacitracin zinc (500 units)	Apply topically 1 - 3 times daily.
POLYTRIM	Antibacterial	**Ophth Solution (per mL)**: trimethoprim sulfate (equal to 1 mg of trimethoprim base), polymyxin B sulfate (10,000 Units)	1 drop into affected eye(s) q 3 h (maximum of 6 doses per day) for 7 - 10 days.
PRED-G	Antibacterial-Corticosteroid	**Ophth Suspension**: gentamicin sulfate (0.3%), prednisolone acetate (1.0%)	1 drop into affected eye(s) bid to qid. During the initial 24 to 48 h, dosage may be raised up to 1 drop every hour.
		Ophth Oint: gentamicin sulfate (0.3%), prednisolone acetate (0.6%)	Apply a small amount (1/2 in.) to the conjunctival sac 1 - 3 times daily.
PREMPHASE	Estrogen-Progestin	**Tab** (PREMARIN [maroon]): conjugated estrogens (0.625 mg); **Tab** (CYCRIN [light-purple]): medroxyprogesterone acetate (5 mg)	1 maroon tab daily po for 28 days; 1 light-purple tab daily po on Days 15 through 28.

PREMPRO	Estrogen-Progestin	**Tab** (PREMARIN [maroon]): conjugated estrogens (0.625 mg); **Tab** (CYCRIN [white]): medroxyprogesterone acetate (2.5 mg)	1 maroon tab daily po; 1 light-purple tab daily po.
PREPARATION H	Antihemorrhoidal	**Ointment**: petrolatum (71.9%), mineral oil (14%), shark liver oil (3%), phenylephrine HCl (0.25%)	Apply to the affected area up to qid, especially at night, in the morning, or after each bowel movement.
		Cream: petrolatum (18%), glycerin (12%), shark liver oil oil (3%), phenylephrine HCl (0.25%)	Apply externally to the affected area up to qid, especially at night, in the morning, or after each bowel movement.
		Rectal Suppositories: cocoa butter (79%), shark liver oil (3%)	Insert 1 into the rectum up to 6 times daily, especially at night, in the morning, or after each bowel movement.
PRIMATENE	Drug for COPD	**Tab**: theophylline anhydrous (130 mg), ephedrine HCl (24 mg)	1 tab initially po, then 1 tab q 4 h po prn.
PRIMATENE DUAL ACTION FORMULA	Drug for COPD	**Tab**: theophylline anhydrous (60 mg), ephedrine HCl (12.5 mg), guaifenesin (100 mg)	2 tab initially po, then 2 tab q 4 h po prn.
PRIMAXIN I.M.	Antibacterial	**Powd for Inj**: imipenem (500 mg), cilastatin sodium (500 mg) **Powd for Inj**: imipenem (750 mg), cilastatin sodium (750 mg)	**Lower Respiratory Tract, Skin & Skin Structure, and Gynecologic Infections**: 500 or 750 mg (of imipenem) q 12 h IM. **Intra-Abdominal Infections**: 750 mg q 12 h IM.

TRADE NAME	THERAPEUTIC CATEGORY	DOSAGE FORMS AND COMPOSITION	COMMON ADULT DOSAGE
PRIMAXIN I.V.	Antibacterial	**Powd for Inj**: imipenem (250 mg), cilastatin sodium (250 mg) **Powd for Inj**: imipenem (500 mg), cilastatin sodium (500 mg)	Administer by IV infusion. Each 250 or 500 mg dose (of imipenem) should be given over 20 - 30 min. Each 1000 mg dose should be infused over 40 - 60 min. **Infections:** **Mild**: 250 - 500 mg q 6 h. **Moderate**: 500 - 1000 mg q 6 to 8 h. **Severe, Life-Threatening**: 500 mg q 6 h to 1000 mg q 6 to 8 h. **Urinary Tract (Uncomplicated)**: 250 mg q 6 h. **Urinary Tract (Complicated)**: 500 mg q 6 h.
PRINZIDE 10-12.5 PRINZIDE 20-12.5 PRINZIDE 20-25	Antihypertensive	**Tab**: lisinopril (10 mg), hydrochlorothiazide (12.5 mg) **Tab**: lisinopril (20 mg), hydrochlorothiazide (12.5 mg) **Tab**: lisinopril (20 mg), hydrochlorothiazide (25 mg)	1 - 2 tab once daily po. 1 - 2 tab once daily po. 1 - 2 tab once daily po.
PROCTOCREAM-HC	Local Anesthetic-Corticosteroid	**Cream**: pramoxine HCl (1%), hydrocortisone acetate (1%)	Apply to the affected area as a thin film tid - qid.
PROCTOFOAM-HC	Local Anesthetic-Corticosteroid	**Aerosol**: pramoxine HCl (1%), hydrocortisone acetate (1%)	Apply to the affected area tid to qid.
QUADRINAL	Drug for COPD	**Tab**: theophylline calcium salicylate (130 mg; equivalent to 65 mg of theophylline base), ephedrine HCl (24 mg), potassium iodide (320 mg), phenobarbital (24 mg)	1 tab tid - qid po; if needed, an additional tab hs for nighttime relief.
QUELIDRINE	Decongestant-Expectorant-Antitussive-Antihistamine	**Syrup (per 5 mL)**: ephedrine HCl (5 mg), phenylephrine HCl (5 mg), ammonium chloride (40 mg), ipecac fluidextract (0.005 mL), dextromethorphan HBr (10 mg), chlorpheniramine maleate (2 mg), alcohol (2%)	5 mL 1 to 4 times daily po.

QUIBRON QUIBRON-300	Drug for COPD	**Cpsl**: theophylline (150 mg), guaifenesin (90 mg) **Cpsl**: theophylline (300 mg), guaifenesin (180 mg)	Dose based on theophylline; see Oral Theophylline Doses Table, p. 252.
R & C	Pediculicide	**Shampoo**: pyrethrins (0.30%), piperonyl butoxide technical (3%)	Apply to dry hair and scalp or other affected areas. Use enough to completely wet area being treated; massage in. Allow the product to remain for 10 min. Rinse and towel dry. Repeat in 7 - 10 days if reinfestation occurs.
RID	Pediculicide	**Shampoo**: pyrethrum extract (0.33%), piperonyl butoxide technical (4%), related compounds (0.8%)	Same dosage and directions as for R & C Shampoo above.
RIFAMATE	Tuberculostatic	**Cpsl**: rifampin (300 mg), isoniazid (150 mg)	2 cpsl daily po, 1 hour before or 2 hours after a meal.
RIFATER	Tuberculostatic	**Tab**: rifampin (120 mg), isoniazid (50 mg), pyrazinamide (300 mg)	**Over 15 yrs and:** **≤ 44 kg**: 4 tab po once daily. **44-54 kg**: 5 tab po once daily. **≥ 55 kg**: 6 tab po once daily. Give on an empty stomach with a full glass of water.
ROBAXISAL	Skeletal Muscle Relaxant-Analgesic	**Tab**: methocarbamol (400 mg), aspirin (325 mg)	2 tab qid po. 3 tab qid po may be used in severe conditions for 1 - 3 days in patients who are able to tolerate salicylates.
ROBITUSSIN A-C (C-V)	Antitussive-Expectorant	**Syrup (per 5 mL)**: codeine phosphate (10 mg), guaifenesin (100 mg), alcohol (3.5%)	10 mL q 4 h po.
ROBITUSSIN-CF	Antitussive-Decongestant-Expectorant	**Syrup (per 5 mL)**: dextromethorphan HBr (10 mg), phenylpropanolamine HCl (12.5 mg), guaifenesin (100 mg)	10 mL q 4 h po.
ROBITUSSIN-DAC (C-V)	Antitussive-Decongestant-Expectorant	**Syrup (per 5 mL)**: codeine phosphate (10 mg), pseudoephedrine HCl (30 mg), guaifenesin (100 mg), alcohol (1.9%)	10 mL q 4 h po.

TRADE NAME	THERAPEUTIC CATEGORY	DOSAGE FORMS AND COMPOSITION	COMMON ADULT DOSAGE
ROBITUSSIN-DM	Antitussive-Expectorant	**Syrup (per 5 mL)**: dextromethorphan HBr (10 mg), guaifenesin (100 mg)	10 mL q 4 h po.
ROBITUSSIN MAXIMUM STRENGTH COUGH & COLD LIQUID	Antitussive-Decongestant	**Syrup (per 5 mL)**: dextromethorphan HBr (15 mg), pseudoephedrine HCl (30 mg)	10 mL q 6 h po.
ROBITUSSIN NIGHT RELIEF	Decongestant-Antihistamine-Antitussive-Analgesic	**Liquid (per 5 mL)**: pseudoephedrine HCl (10 mg), pyrilamine maleate (8.3 mg), dextromethorphan HBr (5 mg), acetaminophen (108.3 mg)	30 mL hs po or 30 mL q 6 h po.
ROBITUSSIN-PE	Decongestant-Expectorant	**Syrup (per 5 mL)**: pseudoephedrine HCl (30 mg), guaifenesin (100 mg)	10 mL q 4 h po. doses/day.
ROBITUSSIN SEVERE CONGESTION LIQUI-GELS	Decongestant-Expectorant	**Softgel**: pseudoephedrine HCl (30 mg), guaifenesin (200 mg)	2 Softgels q 4 h po.
RONDEC	Decongestant-Antihistamine	**Syrup (per 5 mL)**: pseudoephedrine HCl (60 mg), carbinoxamine maleate (4 mg)	5 mL qid po.
		Tab: pseudoephedrine HCl (60 mg), carbinoxamine maleate (4 mg)	1 tab qid po.
RONDEC-DM	Decongestant-Antihistamine-Antitussive	**Syrup (per 5 mL)**: pseudoephedrine HCl (60 mg), carbinoxamine maleate (4 mg), dextromethorphan HBr (15 mg)	5 mL qid po.
RONDEC-TR		**Timed-Rel. Tab**: pseudoephedrine HCl (120 mg), carbinoxamine maleate (8 mg)	1 tab bid po.
ROXICET	Analgesic	**Tab**: oxycodone HCl (5 mg), acetaminophen (325 mg)	1 tab q 6 h po, prn pain.
		Solution (per 5 mL): oxycodone HCl (5 mg), acetaminophen (325 mg), alcohol (0.4%)	5 mL q 6 h po, prn pain.
ROXICET 5/500	Analgesic	**Cplt**: oxycodone HCl (5 mg), acetaminophen (500 mg)	1 cplt q 6 h po, prn pain.
ROXILOX	Analgesic	**Cpsl**: oxycodone HCl (5 mg), acetaminophen (500 mg)	1 cpsl q 6 h po, prn pain.

ROXIPRIN	Analgesic	**Tab**: oxycodone HCl (4.5 mg), oxycodone terephthalate (0.38 mg), aspirin (325 mg)	1 tab q 6 h po, prn pain.
RYNA	Decongestant-Antihistamine	**Liquid (per 5 mL)**: pseudoephedrine HCl (30 mg), chlorpheniramine maleate (2 mg)	10 mL q 6 h po.
RYNA-C (C-V)	Antitussive-Decongestant-Antihistamine	**Liquid (per 5 mL)**: codeine phosphate (10 mg), pseudoephedrine HCl (30 mg), chlorpheniramine maleate (2 mg)	10 mL q 6 h po.
RYNA-CX (C-V)	Antitussive-Decongestant-Expectorant	**Liquid (per 5 mL)**: codeine phosphate (10 mg), pseudoephedrine HCl (30 mg), guaifenesin (100 mg)	10 mL q 6 h po.
RYNATAN	Decongestant-Antihistamine	**Tab**: pseudoephedrine sulfate (120 mg), azatadine maleate (1 mg)	1 tab q 12 h po.
RYNATUSS	Decongestant-Antihistamine-Antitussive	**Tab**: phenylephrine tannate (10 mg), ephedrine tannate (10 mg), chlorpheniramine tannate (5 mg), carbetapentane tannate (60 mg)	1 - 2 tab q 12 h po.
SEMPREX-D	Decongestant-Antihistamine	**Cpsl**: pseudoephedrine HCl (60 mg), acrivastine (8 mg)	1 cpsl qid po.
SEPTRA	Antibacterial	**Susp (per 5 mL)**: sulfamethoxazole (200 mg), trimethoprim (40 mg) **Tab**: sulfamethoxazole (400 mg), trimethoprim (80 mg)	**Urinary Tract Infections**: 1 SEPTRA DS tab, 2 SEPTRA tab or 20 mL of Suspension q 12 h po for 10 - 14 days. **Shigellosis**: 1 SEPTRA DS tab, 2 SEPTRA tab or 20 mL of Suspension for 5 days. **Acute Exacerbations of Chronic Bronchitis**: 1 SEPTRA DS tab, 2 SEPTRA tab or 20 mL of Susp. q 12 h po for 14 days. ***P. carinii* Pneumonia Treatment**: 20 mg/kg trimethoprim and 100 mg/kg sulfamethoxazole per 24 h in equally divided doses q 6 h for 14 days.
SEPTRA DS		**Tab**: sulfamethoxazole (800 mg), trimethoprim (160 mg)	

[Continued on the next page]

TRADE NAME	THERAPEUTIC CATEGORY	DOSAGE FORMS AND COMPOSITION	COMMON ADULT DOSAGE
SEPTRA & SEPTRA DS [Continued]			***P. carinii* Pneumonia Prophylax.**: 1 SEPTRA DS tab, 2 SEPTRA tab or 20 mL of Suspension q 24 h po. **Travelers' Diarrhea**: 1 SEPTRA DS tab, 2 SEPTRA tab or 20 mL of Suspension q 12 h po for 5 days.
SEPTRA I.V. INFUSION	Antibacterial	**Inj (per 5 mL)**: sulfamethoxazole (400 mg), trimethoprim (80 mg)	**Severe Urinary Tract Infections and Shigellosis**: 8 - 10 mg/kg daily (based on trimethoprim) in 2 - 4 equally divided doses q 6, 8 or 12 h by IV infusion for up to 14 days for UTI and 5 days for shigellosis. ***P. carinii* Pneumonia**: 15 - 20 mg/kg daily (based on trimethoprim) in 3 - 4 equally divided doses q 6 - 8 h by IV infusion for up to 14 days.
SER-AP-ES	Antihypertensive	**Tab**: reserpine (0.1 mg), hydralazine HCl (25 mg), hydrochlorothiazide (15 mg)	1 -2 tab tid po.
SINE-AID, MAXIMUM STRENGTH	Decongestant-Analgesic	**Tab, Cplt & Gelcap**: pseudoephedrine HCl (30 mg), acetaminophen (500 mg)	2 tab (cplt or Gelcap) q 4 - 6 h po.
SINE-AID IB	Decongestant-Analgesic	**Cplt**: pseudoephedrine HCl (30 mg), ibuprofen (200 mg)	1 - 2 cplt q 4 - 6 h po.

SINEMET 10-100 SINEMET 25-100	Antiparkinsonian	**Tab**: carbidopa (10 mg), levodopa (100 mg) **Tab**: carbidopa (25 mg), levodopa (100 mg)	The optimum daily dosage of SINEMET must be determined by careful titration in each patient. **Usual Initial Dosage**: 1 tab of SINEMET 25-100 tid po. If SINEMET 10-100 is used, the initial dosage may be 1 tab tid or qid po. The dosage of either preparation may be increased by 1 tab every day or every other day, prn, until 8 tab/day is reached. **Maintenance**: At least 70 to 100 mg of carbidopa/day should be provided. When a greater proportion of carbidopa is required, 1 tab of SINEMET 25-100 may be substituted for each SINEMET 10-100.
SINEMET 25-250	Antiparkinsonian	**Tab**: carbidopa (25 mg), levodopa (250 mg)	**Maintenance Only**: At least 70 to 100 mg of carbidopa/day should be provided. When a larger proportion of levodopa is required, SINEMET 25-250 may be substituted for either of the above two products.
SINE-OFF NO DROWSINESS FORMULA	Decongestant-Analgesic	**Cplt**: pseudoephedrine HCl (30 mg), acetaminophen (500 mg)	2 cplt q 6 h po.
SINE-OFF SINUS MEDICINE	Decongestant-Antihistamine-Analgesic	**Tab**: pseudoephedrine HCl (30 mg), chlorpheniramine maleate (2 mg), acetaminophen (500 mg)	2 tab q 6 h po, up to 8 tab per day.
SINUTAB SINUS ALLERGY MEDICATION, MAXIMUM STRENGTH	Decongestant-Antihistamine-Analgesic	**Cplt & Tab**: pseudoephedrine HCl (30 mg), chlorpheniramine maleate (2 mg), acetaminophen (500 mg)	2 cplt (or tab) q 6 h po.

TRADE NAME	THERAPEUTIC CATEGORY	DOSAGE FORMS AND COMPOSITION	COMMON ADULT DOSAGE
SINUTAB SINUS MEDICAT., MAXIMUM STRENGTH WITHOUT DROWSINESS	Decongestant-Analgesic	**Cplt & Tab**: pseudoephedrine HCl (30 mg), acetaminophen (500 mg)	2 cplt (or tab) q 6 h po.
SLO-PHYLLIN GG	Drug for COPD	**Syrup (per 15 mL)**: theophylline anhydrous (150 mg), guaifenesin (90 mg) **Cpsl**: theophylline anhydrous (150 mg), guaifenesin (90 mg)	Dose based on theophylline; see Oral Theophylline Doses Table, p. 252. Initially 16 mg/kg/day po, up to 400 mg/day in 3 - 4 divided doses q 6 - 8 h. At 3 day intervals, incr. if needed in 25% increments as tolerated.
SLOW FE WITH FOLIC ACID	Hematinic	**Slow-Rel. Tab**: dried ferrous sulfate (160 mg), folic acid (400 μg)	1 or 2 tab once daily po.
SOMA COMPOUND	Skeletal Muscle Relaxant-Analgesic	**Tab**: carisoprodol (200 mg), aspirin (325 mg)	1 - 2 tab qid po.
SOMA COMPOUND W/ CODEINE (C-III)	Skeletal Muscle Relaxant-Analgesic	**Tab**: carisoprodol (200 mg), aspirin (325 mg), codeine phosphate (16 mg)	1 - 2 tab qid po.
SUDAFED COLD & COUGH	Decongestant-Antitussive-Expectorant	**Liquid Cpsl**: pseudoephedrine HCl (60 mg), dextromethorphan HBr (10 mg), guiafenesin (100 mg)	2 cpsl q 4 h po.
SULFACET-R MVL	Anti-Acne Agent	**Lotion**: sulfacetamide sodium (10%), sulfur (5%)	Apply a thin film to affected areas 1 to 3 times daily.
SULTRIN	Antibacterial	**Vaginal Tab**: sulfathiazole (172.5 mg), sulfacetamide (143.75 mg), sulfabenzamide (184 mg) with urea **Vaginal Cream**: sulfathiazole (3.42%), sulfacetamide (2.86%), sulfabenzamide (3.7%), urea (0.64%)	1 tab intravaginally hs and in the morning for 10 days. 1 applicatorful intravaginally bid for 4 - 6 days.
SYNALGOS-DC (C-III)	Analgesic	**Cpsl**: dihydrocodeine bitartrate (16 mg), aspirin (356.4 mg), caffeine (30 mg)	2 cpsl q 4 h po, prn pain.

SYNERCID	Antibacterial	**Powd for Inj**: quinupristin (150 mg), dalfopristin (350 mg)	**Vancomycin-resistant *E. faecium* Bacteremia**: 7.5 mg/kg q 8 h by IV infusion (over 60 min.). Duration of therapy dependent on site of infection and severity. **Complicated Skin and Skin-Structure Infections**: 7.5 mg/kg q 12 h by IV infusion (over 60 min.) for at least 7 days.
TALACEN (C-IV)	Analgesic	**Tab**: pentazocine HCl (equal to 25 mg pentazocine base), acetaminophen (650 mg)	1 tab q 4 h po, prn pain.
TALWIN COMPOUND (C-IV)	Analgesic	**Cplt**: pentazocine HCl (equal to 12.5 mg pentazocine base), aspirin (325 mg)	2 cplt tid or qid po, prn pain.
TALWIN NX	Analgesic	**Tab**: pentazocine HCl (equal to 50 mg pentazocine base), naloxone HCl (0.5 mg)	1 tab q 3 - 4 h po.
TARKA 2/180 TARKA 1/240 TARKA 2/240 TARKA 4/240	Antihypertensive	**Tab**: trandolapril (2 mg), verapamil HCl ER (180 mg) **Tab**: trandolapril (1 mg), verapamil HCl ER (240 mg) **Tab**: trandolapril (2 mg), verapamil HCl ER (240 mg) **Tab**: trandolapril (4 mg), verapamil HCl ER (240 mg) (ER = Extended-Release formulation)	1 tab daily po. 1 tab daily po. 1 tab daily po. 1 tab daily po.
TAVIST-D	Decongestant-Antihistamine	**Tab**: phenylpropanolamine HCl (75 mg), clemastine fumarate (1.34 mg)	1 tab q 12 h po.
TECZEM	Antihypertensive	**Extended-Rel. Tab**: enalapril maleate (5 mg), diltiazem malate (180 mg)	1 tab daily po.
TENORETIC 50 TENORETIC 100	Antihypertensive	**Tab**: atenolol (50 mg), chlorthalidone (25 mg) **Tab**: atenolol (100 mg), chlorthalidone(25 mg)	1 tab daily po. 1 tab daily po.
TERRA-CORTRIL	Antibacterial-Corticosteroid	**Ophth Suspension (per mL)**: oxytetracycline (5 mg), hydrocortisone acetate (15 mg)	1 or 2 drops into the affected eye(s) tid.

TRADE NAME	THERAPEUTIC CATEGORY	DOSAGE FORMS AND COMPOSITION	COMMON ADULT DOSAGE
THYROLAR 1/4	Thyroid Hormone	**Tab**: levothyroxine sodium (12.5 μg), liothyronine sodium (3.1 μg)	**Initial**: Usually 50 μg of levothyroxine po or its isocaloric
THYROLAR 1/2		**Tab**: levothyroxine sodium (25 μg), liothyronine sodium (6.25 μg)	**Initial**: Usually 50 μg of levothyroxine po or its isocaloric equivalent (THYROLAR 1/2), with increments of 25 μg q 2 to 3 weeks.
THYROLAR 1		**Tab**: levothyroxine sodium (50 μg), liothyronine sodium (12.5 μg)	**Maintenance**: Usually 100 - 200 μg/day po (THYROLAR 1 or THYROLAR 2).
THYROLAR 2		**Tab**: levothyroxine sodium (100 μg), liothyronine sodium (25 μg)	
THYROLAR 3		**Tab**: levothyroxine sodium (150 μg), liothyronine sodium (37.5 μg)	
TIMENTIN	Antibacterial	**Powd for Inj**: 3.1 g (3 g ticarcillin, 0.1 g clavulanic acid) **Powd for Inj**: 3.2 g (3 g ticarcillin, 0.2 g clavulanic acid)	**Systemic and Urinary Tract Infections and ≥ 60 kg**: 3.1 g q 4 - 6 h by IV infusion. **Gynecologic Infections:** **Moderate and ≥ 60 kg**: 200 mg/kg/day in divided doses q 6 h by IV infusion. **Severe and ≥ 60 kg**: 300 mg/kg/day in divided doses q 4 h by IV infusion. **Adults < 60 kg**: 200 - 300 mg/kg/day in divided doses q 4 - 6 h by IV infusion.
TIMOLIDE 10-25	Antihypertensive	**Tab**: timolol maleate (10 mg), hydrochlorothiazide (25 mg)	1 tab bid po or 2 tab once daily.
TOBRADEX	Antibacterial-Corticosteroid	**Ophth Suspension**: tobramycin (0.3%), dexamethasone (0.1%)	1 or 2 drops into affected eye(s) q 4 - 6 h. During the initial 24 to 48 h, the dosage may be increased to 1 or 2 drops q 2 h.
		Ophth Oint: tobramycin (0.3%), dexamethasone (0.1%)	Apply a small amount (1/2 in.) to the conjunctival sac tid or qid.

TRIAMINIC AM COUGH AND DECONGESTANT	Decongestant-Antitussive	**Liquid (per 5 mL)**: pseudoephedrine HCl (15 mg), dextromethorphan HBr (7.5 mg)	20 mL q 6 h po.
TRIAMINIC-DM	Decongestant-Antitussive	**Liquid (per 5 mL)**: phenylpropanolamine HCl (6.25 mg), dextromethorphan HBr (5 mg)	20 mL q 4 h po.
TRIAMINIC EXPECTORANT	Decongestant-Expectorant	**Liquid (per 5 mL)**: phenylpropanolamine HCl (6.25 mg), guaifenesin (50 mg)	20 mL q 4 h po.
TRIAMINIC EXPECTORANT DH (C-III)	Decongestant-Expectorant-Antitussive-Antihistamine	**Liquid (per 5 mL)**: phenylpropanolamine HCl (12.5 mg), guaifenesin (100 mg), hydrocodone bitartrate (1.67 mg), pyrilamine maleate (6.25 mg), pheniramine maleate (6.25 mg), alcohol (5%)	10 mL q 4 h po.
TRIAMINIC EXPECTORANT W/CODEINE (C-V)	Decongestant-Expectorant-Antitussive	**Liquid (per 5 mL)**: phenylpropanolamine HCl (12.5 mg), guaifenesin (100 mg), codeine phosphate (10 mg), alcohol (5%)	10 mL q 4 h po.
TRIAMINIC NIGHT TIME	Decongestant-Antihistamine-Antitussive	**Liquid (per 5 mL)**: pseudoephedrine HCl (15 mg), chlorpheniramine maleate (1 mg), dextromethorphan HBr (7.5 mg)	20 mL q 6 h po.
TRIAMINIC SORE THROAT FORMULA	Decongestant-Antitussive-Analgesic	**Liquid (per 5 mL)**: pseudoephedrine HCl (15 mg), dextromethorphan HBr (7.5 mg), acetaminophen (160 mg)	20 mL q 6 h po.
TRIAMINIC SYRUP	Decongestant-Antihistamine	**Liquid (per 5 mL)**: phenylpropanolamine HCl (6.25 mg), chlorpheniramine maleate (1 mg)	20 mL q 4 - 6 h po.
TRIAMINICIN	Decongestant-Antihistamine-Analgesic	**Tab**: phenylpropanolamine HCl (25 mg), chlorpheniramine maleate (4 mg), acetaminophen (650 mg)	1 tab q 4 h po.
TRIAMINICOL MULTI-SYMPTOM COLD TABLETS	Decongestant-Antihistamine-Expectorant	**Tab**: phenylpropanolamine HCl (12.5 mg), chlorpheniramine maleate (2 mg), dextromethorphan HBr (10 mg)	2 tab q 4 h po.
TRIAMINICOL MULTI-SYMPTOM RELIEF	Decongestant-Antihistamine-Expectorant	**Syrup (per 5 mL)**: phenylpropanolamine HCl (6.25 mg), chlorpheniramine maleate (1 mg), dextromethorphan HBr (5 mg)	20 mL q 4 h po.

TRADE NAME	THERAPEUTIC CATEGORY	DOSAGE FORMS AND COMPOSITION	COMMON ADULT DOSAGE
TRIAVIL 2-10 TRIAVIL 2-25 TRIAVIL 4-10 TRIAVIL 4-25 TRIAVIL 4-50	Antipsychotic-Antidepressant	**Tab**: perphenazine (2 mg), amitriptyline HCl (10 mg) **Tab**: perphenazine (2 mg), amitriptyline HCl (25 mg) **Tab**: perphenazine (4 mg), amitriptyline HCl (10 mg) **Tab**: perphenazine (4 mg), amitriptyline HCl (25 mg) **Tab**: perphenazine (4 mg), amitriptyline HCl (50 mg)	**Psychoneuroses**: 1 tab TRIAVIL 2-25 or TRIAVIL 4-25 tid - qid po or 1 tab of TRIAVIL 4-50 bid po. **Schizophrenia**: 2 tab of TRIAVIL 4-25 tid po and, if needed, hs.
TRI-LEVLEN	Oral Contraceptive	**Tab**: 6 tabs: ethinyl estradiol (30 μg), levonorgestrel (0.05 mg); 5 tabs: ethinyl estradiol (40 μg), levonorgestrel (0.075 mg); 10 tabs: ethinyl estradiol (30 μg), levonorgestrel (0.125 mg) in 21-Day and 28-Day Compacts (contains 7 inert tabs)	21-Day regimen po or 28-Day regimen po.
TRILISATE	Non-Opioid Analgesic, Antipyretic, Antiinflammatory	**Tab**: choline magnesium salicylate (500 mg as: choline salicylate (293 mg) and magnesium salicylate (362 mg)) **Tab**: choline magnesium salicylate (750 mg as: choline salicylate (440 mg) and magnesium salicylate (544 mg)) **Tab**: choline magnesium salicylate (1000 mg as: choline salicylate (587 mg) and magnesium salicylate (725 mg)) **Liquid (per 5 mL)**: choline magnesium salicylate (500 mg as: choline salicylate (293 mg) and magnesium salicylate (362 mg))	**Pain & Fever**: 1000 - 1500 mg bid po. **Inflammation**: 1500 mg bid po or 3000 mg once daily hs po.
TRINALIN REPETABS	Decongestant-Antihistamine	**Long-Acting Tab**: pseudoephedrine sulfate (120 mg), azatadine maleate (1 mg)	1 tab bid po.
TRI-NORINYL	Oral Contraceptive	**Tab**: 7 tabs: ethinyl estradiol (35 μg), norethindrone (0.5 mg); 9 tabs: ethinyl estradiol (35 μg), norethindrone (1 mg); 5 tabs: ethinyl estradiol (35 μg), norethindrone (0.5 mg) in 21-Day and 28-Day Wallettes (contains 7 inert tabs)	21-Day regimen po or 28-Day regimen po.
TRIPHASIL	Oral Contraceptive	**Tab**: 6 tabs: ethinyl estradiol (30 μg), levonorgestrel (0.05 mg); 5 tabs: ethinyl estradiol (40 μg), levonorgestrel (0.075 mg); 10 tabs: ethinyl estradiol (30 μg), levonorgestrel (0.125 mg) in 21-Day and 28-Day Pilpaks (contains 7 inert tabs)	21-Day regimen po or 28-Day regimen po.

TUINAL 100 MG (C-II)	Hypnotic	**Cpsl**: amobarbital sodium (50 mg), secobarbital sodium (50 mg)	1 cpsl po hs.
TUINAL 200 MG (C-II)		**Cpsl**: amobarbital sodium (100 mg), secobarbital sodium (100 mg)	1 cpsl po hs.
TUSSAR-2 (C-V)	Decongestant-Expectorant-Antitussive	**Liquid (per 5 mL)**: pseudoephedrine HCl (30 mg), guaifenesin (100 mg), codeine phosphate (10 mg), alcohol (2.5%)	10 mL q 4 h po. Maximum: 40 mL/day.
TUSSAR DM	Decongestant-Antihistamine-Antitussive	**Liquid (per 5 mL)**: pseudoephedrine HCl (30 mg), chlorpheniramine maleate (2 mg), dextromethorphan HBr (15 mg)	10 mL q 6 h po.
TUSSAR SF (C-V)	Decongestant-Expectorant-Antitussive	**Liquid (per 5 mL)**: pseudoephedrine HCl (30 mg), guaifenesin (100 mg), codeine phosphate (10 mg), alcohol (2.5%)	10 mL q 4 h po. Maximum: 40 mL/day.
TUSSEND (C-III)	Decongestant-Antihistamine-Antitussive	**Syrup (per 5 mL)**: pseudoephedrine HCl (30 mg), chlorpheniramine maleate (2 mg), hydrocodone bitartrate (2.5 mg), alcohol (5%)	10 mL q 4 - 6 h po.
TUSSEND EXPECTORANT (C-III)	Decongestant-Expectorant-Antitussive	**Syrup (per 5 mL)**: pseudoephedrine HCl (30 mg), guaifenesin (100 mg), hydrocodone bitartrate (2.5 mg), alcohol (5%)	10 mL q 4 - 6 h po.
TUSSIONEX (C-III)	Antihistamine-Antitussive	**Extended-Rel. Susp (per 5 mL)**: chlorpheniramine polistirex (8 mg), hydrocodone polistirex (10 mg)	5 mL q 12 h po.
TUSSI-ORGANIDIN NR (C-V)	Antitussive-Expectorant	**Liquid (per 5 mL)**: codeine phosphate (10 mg), guaifenesin (100 mg)	10 mL q 4 h po.
TUSSI-ORGANIDIN DM NR	Antitussive-Expectorant	**Liquid (per 5 mL)**: dextromethorphan HBr (10 mg), guaifenesin (100 mg)	10 mL q 4 h po.
TYLENOL W/CODEINE (C-V)	Analgesic	**Elixir (per 5 mL)**: acetaminophen (120 mg), codeine phosphate (12 mg), alcohol (7%)	15 mL q 4 h po, prn pain.
TYLENOL W/CODEINE	Analgesic		
#2 (C-III)		**Tab**: acetaminophen (300 mg), codeine phosphate (15 mg)	2 - 3 tab q 4 h po, prn pain.
#3 (C-III)		**Tab**: acetaminophen (300 mg), codeine phosphate (30 mg)	1 - 2 tab q 4 h po, prn pain.
#4 (C-III)		**Tab**: acetaminophen (300 mg), codeine phosphate (60 mg)	1 tab q 4 h po, prn pain.

TRADE NAME	THERAPEUTIC CATEGORY	DOSAGE FORMS AND COMPOSITION	COMMON ADULT DOSAGE
TYLOX (C-II)	Analgesic	**Cpsl**: oxycodone HCl (5 mg), acetaminophen (500 mg)	1 cpsl q 6 h po, prn pain.
TYMPAGESIC	Analgesic (Topical)-Otic Decongestant	**Otic Solution (per mL)**: benzocaine (5%), antipyrine (5%), phenylephrine HCl (0.25%)	Instill in ear canal until filled, then insert a cotton pledget moistened with solution into meatus. Repeat q 2 - 4 h.
UNASYN	Antibacterial	**Powd for Inj**: 1.5 g (1 g ampicillin sodium, 0.5 g sulbactam sodium) **Powd for Inj**: 3.0 g (2 g ampicillin sodium, 1 g sulbactam sodium)	1.5 - 3.0 g q 6 h by deep IM inj, by slow IV injection (over at least 10 - 15 min), or by IV infusion (diluted with 50 - 100 mL of a compatible diluent and given over 15 - 30 mins).
UNIRETIC 7.5/12.5	Antihypertensive	**Tab**: moexipril HCl (7.5 mg), hydrochiorothiazide (12.5 mg)	1 tab once daily po at least 1 h before a meal.
UNIRETIC 15/25		**Tab**: moexipril HCl (15 mg), hydrochlorothiazide (25 mg)	1 tab once daily po at least 1 h before a meal.
UNISOM WITH PAIN RELIEF	Analgesic-Sedative	**Tab**: acetaminophen (650 mg), diphenhydramine HCl (50 mg)	1 tab po, 30 minutes before retiring.
URISED	Urinary Analgesic	**Tab**: methenamine (40.8 mg), phenyl salicylate (18.1 mg), methylene blue (5.4 mg), benzoic acid (4.5 mg), atropine sulfate (0.03 mg), hyoscyamine (0.03 mg)	2 tab qid po.
VANOXIDE-HC	Anti-Acne Agent	**Lotion (per g)**: benzoyl peroxide (50 mg), hydrocortisone acetate (5 mg)	Gently massage a thin film into affected skin areas 1 to 3 times daily.
VASERETIC 5-12.5 VASERETIC 10-25	Antihypertensive	**Tab**: enalapril maleate (5 mg), hydrochlorothiazide (12.5 mg) **Tab**: enalapril maleate (10 mg), hydrochlorothiazide (25 mg)	1 - 2 tab once daily po. 1 - 2 tab once daily po.

VASOCIDIN	Antibacterial-Corticosteroid	**Ophth Solution**: sulfacetamide sodium (10%), prednisolone acetate (0.25%)	2 drops into affected eye(s) q 4 h. Prolong dosing interval as the condition improves.
		Ophth Oint: sulfacetamide sodium (10%), prednisolone acetate (0.5%)	Apply to affected eye(s) tid or qid during the day and 1 - 2 times at night.
VICODIN (C-III)	Analgesic	**Tab**: hydrocodone bitartrate (5 mg), acetaminophen (500 mg)	1 - 2 tab q 4 - 6 h po, prn pain.
VICODIN ES (C-III)		**Tab**: hydrocodone bitartrate (7.5 mg), acetaminophen (750 mg)	1 tab q 4 - 6 h po, prn pain.
VICODIN HP	Analgesic	**Tab**: hydrocodone bitartrate (10 mg), acetaminophen (660 mg)	1 tab q 4 - 6 h po, prn pain.
VICODIN TUSS (C-III)	Antitussive-Expectorant	**Syrup (per 5 mL)**: hydrocodone bitartrate (5 mg), guaifenesin (100 mg)	5 mL po after meals and hs (not less than 4 hours apart).
VICOPROFEN	Analgesic	**Tab**: hydrocodone bitartrate (7.5 mg), ibuprofen (200 mg)	1 tab q 4 - 6 h po, prn pain.
VOSOL HC	Antibacterial-Corticosteroid	**Otic Solution**: acetic acid (2%), hydrocortisone (1%)	Carefully remove all cerumen & debris. Insert a wick saturated with the solution into the ear canal. Keep in for at least 24 h and keep moist by adding 3 to 5 drops of solution q 4 - 6 h.
WIGRAINE	Antimigraine Agent	**Rectal Suppos**: ergotamine tartrate (2 mg), caffeine (100 mg)	Insert 1 rectally at the first sign of a migraine attack. Maximum: 2 suppositories for an individual attack.
		Tab: ergotamine tartrate (1 mg), caffeine (100 mg)	2 tab po at the first sign of a migraine attack; followed by 1 tab q 30 minutes, prn, up to 6 tabs per attack. Maximum of 10 tabs per week.
WYGESIC (C-IV)	Analgesic	**Tab**: propoxyphene HCl (65 mg), acetaminophen (650 mg)	1 tab q 4 h po, prn pain.
ZESTORETIC 10-12.5	Antihypertensive	**Tab**: lisinopril (10 mg), hydrochlorothiazide (12.5 mg)	1 - 2 tab once daily po.
ZESTORETIC 20-12.5		**Tab**: lisinopril (20 mg), hydrochlorothiazide (12.5 mg)	1 - 2 tab once daily po.
ZESTORETIC 20-25		**Tab**: lisinopril (20 mg), hydrochlorothiazide (25 mg)	1 - 2 tab once daily po.

TRADE NAME	THERAPEUTIC CATEGORY	DOSAGE FORMS AND COMPOSITION	COMMON ADULT DOSAGE
ZIAC	Antihypertensive	**Tab**: bisoprolol fumarate (2.5 mg), hydrochlorothiazide (6.25 mg) **Tab**: bisoprolol fumarate (5 mg), hydrochlorothiazide (6.25 mg) **Tab**: bisoprolol fumarate (10 mg), hydrochlorothiazide (6.25 mg)	Initially, one 2.5/6.25 mg tab once daily po. Adjust dosage at 14 day intervals. Maximum: two 10/ 6.25 mg tabs once daily po.
ZOSYN	Antibacterial	**Powd for Inj**: 2.25 g (2 g piperacillin, 0.25 g tazobactam) **Powd for Inj**: 3.375 g (3 g piperacillin, 0.375 g tazobactam) **Powd for Inj**: 4.5 g (4 g piperacillin, 0.5 g tazobactam)	**Usual Dosage**: 12 g/1.5 g daily by IV infusion (over 30 min), given as 3.375 g q 6 h. **Nosocomial Pneumonia**: 3.375 g q 4 h by IV infusion (over 30 min) plus an aminoglycoside.
ZOVIA 1/35E	Oral Contraceptive	**Tab**: ethynodiol diacetate (1 mg), ethinyl estradiol (35 μg) in 21-Day and 28-Day Dispensers (contains 7 inert tabs)	21-Day regimen po or 28-Day regimen po.
ZOVIA 1/50E		**Tab**: ethynodiol diacetate (1 mg), ethinyl estradiol (50 μg) in 21-Day and 28-Day Dispensers (contains 7 inert tabs)	21-Day regimen po or 28-Day regimen po.
ZYDONE (C-III)	Analgesic	**Cpsl**: hydrocodone bitartrate (5 mg), acetaminophen (500 mg)	1 - 2 cpsl q 4 - 6 h po, prn pain.

C-II: Controlled Substance, Schedule II
C-III: Controlled Substance, Schedule III
C-IV: Controlled Substance, Schedule IV
C-V: Controlled Substance, Schedule V

SPECIAL DOSAGE TABLES

DIGOXIN DOSES

I. RAPID DIGITALIZATION WITH A LOADING DOSE -

In most patients with heart failure and normal sinus rhythm, a therapeutic effect with minimum risk of toxicity should occur with peak body digoxin stores of 8 to 12 μg/kg. For adequate control of ventricular rate in patients with atrial flutter or fibrillation, larger digoxin body stores (10 to 15 μg/kg) are often required. In patients with renal insufficiency, the projected peak body stores of digoxin should be conservative (6 to 10 μg/kg) due to altered distribution and elimination.

The loading dose should be based on the projected peak body stores and administered in several portions; approximately half the total is usually given as the first dose.

FOR ORAL DOSING -

Preparation	In previously undigitalized patients, a single initial oral dose of the following produces a detectable effect in 0.5 to 2 hours that becomes maximal in 2 to 6 hours	The following additional doses may be given cautiously at 6 to 8 hour intervals until clinical evidence of an adequate effect is noted	The usual amount of each preparation that a 70 kg patient requires to achieve 8 to 15 μg/kg peak body stores is
LANOXIN Tablets	0.5 - 0.75 mg po	0.125 - 0.375 mg po	0.75 - 1.25 mg po
LANOXIN ELIXIR PEDIATRIC	0.5 - 0.75 mg po	0.125 - 0.375 mg po	0.75 - 1.25 mg po
LANOXICAPS Capsules	0.4 - 0.6 mg po	0.1 - 0.3 mg po	0.6 - 1.0 mg po

FOR INTRAVENOUS DOSING -

Preparation	In previously undigitalized patients, a single initial intravenous dose of the following produces a detectable effect in 5 to 30 minutes that becomes maximal in 1 to 4 hours	The following additional doses may be given cautiously at 4 to 8 hour intervals until clinical evidence of an adequate effect is noted	The usual amount of LANOXIN Injection that a 70 kg patient requires to achieve 8 to 15 μg/kg peak body stores is
LANOXIN Injection	0.4 - 0.6 mg IV	0.1 - 0.3 mg IV	0.6 - 1.0 mg IV

The maintenance dose should be based upon the percentage of the peak body stores lost each day through elimination. The following formula has wide clinical use:

Maintenance Dose = Peak Body Stores (i.e., Loading Dose) x % Daily Loss/100

where: % Daily Loss = 14 + Creatinine Clearance (corrected to 70 kg body weight or 1.73 m^2 surface area)/5

A common practice involves the use of LANOXIN Injection to achieve rapid digitalization, with conversion to LANOXIN Tablets, LANOXIN ELIXIR PEDIATRIC, or LANOXICAPS Capsules for maintenance therapy. If patients are switched from an IV to an oral digoxin preparation, allowances must be made for difference in bioavailability when calculating maintenance doses (see Inset Table below).

PRODUCT	ABSOLUTE BIOAVAILABILITY	EQUIVALENT DOSES (IN MG)		
LANOXIN Tablets	60 to 80%	0.125	0.25	0.5
LANOXIN ELIXIR PEDIATRIC	70 to 85%	0.125	0.25	0.5
LANOXIN Injection / IM	70 to 85%	0.125	0.25	0.5
LANOXIN Injection / IV	100%	0.1	0.2	0.4
LANOXICAPS Capsules	90 to 100%	0.1	0.2	0.4

II. **GRADUAL DIGITALIZATION WITH A MAINTENANCE DOSE -**

The following Table provides average **LANOXIN Tablet** daily maintenance dose requirements for patients with heart failure based upon lean body weight and renal function:

USUAL LANOXIN DAILY MAINTENANCE DOSE REQUIREMENTS (in mg) FOR ESTIMATED PEAK BODY STORES OF 10 μg/kg

		Lean Body Weight (kg / lbs)							
		50 / 110	60 / 132	70 / 154	80 / 176	90 / 198	100 / 220		
Corrected Creatinine Clearance (mL/min per 70 kg)	0	0.063	0.125	0.125	0.125	0.188	0.188	22	Number of Days Before Steady-State is Achieved
	10	0.125	0.125	0.125	0.188	0.188	0.188	19	
	20	0.125	0.125	0.188	0.188	0.188	0.250	16	
	30	0.125	0.188	0.188	0.188	0.250	0.250	14	
	40	0.125	0.188	0.188	0.250	0.250	0.250	13	
	50	0.188	0.188	0.250	0.250	0.250	0.250	12	
	60	0.188	0.188	0.250	0.250	0.250	0.375	11	
	70	0.188	0.250	0.250	0.250	0.250	0.375	10	
	80	0.188	0.250	0.250	0.250	0.375	0.375	9	
	90	0.188	0.250	0.250	0.250	0.375	0.500	8	
	100	0.250	0.250	0.250	0.375	0.375	0.500	7	

The following Table provides average **LANOXICAP Capsule** daily maintenance dose requirements for patients with heart failure based upon lean body weight and renal function:

USUAL LANOXICAP DAILY MAINTENANCE DOSE REQUIREMENTS (in mg) FOR ESTIMATED PEAK BODY STORES OF 10 μg/kg

		Lean Body Weight (kg / lbs)							
		50 / 110	**60 / 132**	**70 / 154**	**80 / 176**	**90 / 198**	**100 / 220**		
Corrected Creatinine Clearance (mL/min per 70 kg)	0	0.050	0.100	0.100	0.100	0.150	0.150	22	Number of Days Before Steady-State is Achieved
	10	0.100	0.100	0.100	0.150	0.150	0.150	19	
	20	0.100	0.100	0.150	0.150	0.150	0.200	16	
	30	0.100	0.150	0.150	0.150	0.200	0.200	14	
	40	0.100	0.150	0.150	0.200	0.200	0.250	13	
	50	0.150	0.150	0.200	0.200	0.250	0.250	12	
	60	0.150	0.150	0.200	0.200	0.250	0.300	11	
	70	0.150	0.200	0.200	0.250	0.250	0.300	10	
	80	0.150	0.200	0.200	0.250	0.300	0.300	9	
	90	0.150	0.200	0.250	0.250	0.300	0.350	8	
	100	0.200	0.200	0.250	0.300	0.300	0.350	7	

ORAL THEOPHYLLINE DOSES

I. IMMEDIATE-RELEASE PREPARATIONS (e.g., ELIXOPHYLLIN Elixir and Capsules, ELIXOPHYLLIN-GG Liquid, ELIXOPHYLLIN-KI Elixir, QUIBRON and QUIBRON-300 Capsules, SLO-PHYLLIN Syrup and Tablets, SLO-PHYLLIN GG Capsules and Syrup, and THEOLAIR Liquid and Tablets) -

Acute Symptoms of Bronchospasm Requiring Rapid Attainment of Theophylline Serum Levels for Bronchodilation -

Otherwise healthy nonsmoking adults: 5 mg/kg po (oral loading dose); then, 3 mg/kg q 8 h po (maintenance doses).

Older patients and those with cor pulmonale: 5 mg/kg po (oral loading dose); then, 2 mg/kg q 8 h po (maintenance doses).

Patients with congestive heart failure: 5 mg/kg po (oral loading dose); then, 1 - 2 mg/kg q 12 h po (maintenance doses).

Chronic Therapy -

Initial Dose: 16 mg/kg/24 h or 400 mg/24 h (whichever is less) in divided doses q 6 - 8 h po.

Increasing Dose: The initial dosage may be increased in approximately 25% increments at 3 day intervals, as long as the drug is tolerated, until the clinical response is satisfactory, or the maximum dose is reached.

Maximum Dose: 13 mg/kg/day po or 900 mg/day, whichever is less

CHECK SERUM CONCENTRATION BETWEEN 1 AND 2 HOURS AFTER A DOSE WHEN NONE HAVE BEEN MISSED OR ADDED FOR AT LEAST 3 DAYS. If serum theophylline concentration is between 10 and 20 μg/mL, maintain dose, if tolerated. RECHECK THEOPHYLLINE CONCENTRATION AT 6- TO 12-MONTH INTERVALS.

II. SUSTAINED-RELEASE PREPARATIONS -

A. RESPBID Sustained-Release Tablets, SLO-BID Extended-Release Capsules, SLO-PHYLLIN Extended-Release Capsules, THEOLAIR-SR Sustained-Release Tablets and T-PHYL Controlled-Release Tablets -

Initial Therapy: 16 mg/kg/24 h or 400 mg/24 h (whichever is less) in 2 or 3 divided doses at 8 or 12 h intervals po.

Maintenance Therapy: The initial dosage may be increased in approximately 25% increments at 3-day intervals, as long as the drug is tolerated, until the clinical response is satisfactory, or the maximum dose is reached.

Maximum Dose: 13 mg/kg/day po or 900 mg/day, whichever is less

CHECK SERUM CONCENTRATION BETWEEN 5 AND 10 HOURS AFTER A DOSE WHEN NONE HAVE BEEN MISSED OR ADDED FOR AT LEAST 3 DAYS. If serum theophylline concentration is between 10 and 20 µg/mL, maintain dose, if tolerated. RECHECK THEOPHYLLINE CONCENTRATION AT 6- TO 12-MONTH INTERVALS.

B. THEO-DUR Extended-Release Tablets -

Initial Therapy: 200 mg q 12 h po

Maintenance Therapy: The dose may be increased in approximately 25% increments at 3 day intervals, as long as the drug is tolerated, until the clinical response is satisfactory, or the maximum dose is reached.

Maximum Doses: 35 - 70 kg: 300 mg q 12 h po. Over 70 kg: 450 mg q 12 h po.

CHECK SERUM CONCENTRATION AT APPROXIMATELY 8 HOURS AFTER A DOSE WHEN NONE HAVE BEEN MISSED OR ADDED FOR AT LEAST 3 DAYS. If serum theophylline concentration is between 10 and 20 µg/mL, maintain dose, if tolerated. RECHECK THEOPHYLLINE CONCENTRATION AT 6- TO 12-MONTH INTERVALS.

C. THEO-24 Extended-Release Capsules -

Initial Therapy: 200 mg q 12 h po

Maintenance Therapy: If serum levels cannot be measured and the response is unsatisfactory, after 3 days the dose may be increased by 100 mg increments. Reevaluated after 3 days.

Maximum Dose: 13 mg/kg/day po or 900 mg/day, whichever is less

CHECK PEAK SERUM CONCENTRATION (12 HOURS AFTER THE MORNING DOSE) AND TROUGH LEVEL (24 HOURS AFTER THE MORNING DOSE) WHEN NO DOSES HAVE BEEN MISSED OR ADDED FOR AT LEAST 3 DAYS. If serum theophylline concentration is between 10 and 20 μg/mL, maintain dose, if tolerated. RECHECK THEOPHYLLINE CONCENTRATION AT 6- TO 12-MONTH INTERVALS.

ORAL AMINOPHYLLINE DOSES

1.2 mg of aminophylline anhydrous = 1.0 mg of theophylline anhydrous

Acute Symptoms of Bronchospasm Requiring Rapid Attainment of Theophylline Serum Levels for Bronchodilation -

Otherwise healthy nonsmoking adults: 5.8 mg/kg po (oral loading dose); then, 3.5 mg/kg q 8 h po (maintenance doses).

Older patients and those with cor pulmonale: 5.8 mg/kg po (oral loading dose); then, 2.3 mg/kg q 8 h po (maintenance doses).

Patients with congestive heart failure: 5.8 mg/kg po (oral loading dose); then, 1.2 - 2.3 mg/kg q 12 h po (maintenance doses).

Chronic Therapy (Slow Clinical Titration is Generally Preferred) -

Initial Dose: 19 mg/kg/24 h or 480 mg/24 h (whichever is less) in divided doses q 6 - 8 h po.

Increasing Dose: The doses may be increased in approximately 25% increments at 3 day intervals, as long as the drug is tolerated, until the clinical response is satisfactory, or the maximum dose is reached.

Maximum Doses: 15.2 mg/kg/day po or 1000 mg/day, whichever is less

IV AMINOPHYLLINE DOSES[a]

PATIENT GROUP	IV LOADING DOSE:[b]	DOSE FOR NEXT 12 HOURS:	DOSE BEYOND 12 HOURS:	MAXIMUM DAILY DOSE:
Otherwise Healthy Nonsmoking Adults	6 mg/kg (5 mg/kg)	0.7 mg/kg/hr (0.58 mg/kg/hr)	0.5 mg/kg/hr (0.42 mg/kg/hr)	Variable; monitor blood levels and maintain below 20 μg/mL
Older Patients and Those with Cor Pulmonale	6 mg/kg (5 mg/kg)	0.6 mg/kg/hr (0.5 mg/kg/hr)	0.3 mg/kg/hr (0.25 mg/kg/hr)	Variable; monitor blood levels and maintain below 20 μg/mL
Patients with CHF or Liver Disease	6 mg/kg (5 mg/kg)	0.5 mg/kg/hr (0.42 mg/kg/hr)	0.1 - 0.2 mg/kg/hr (0.08 - 0.16 mg/kg/hr)	Variable; monitor blood levels and maintain below 20 μg/mL

[a] Anhydrous theophylline equivalent in parentheses

[b] Administer slowly, no faster than 25 mg/minute

MISCELLANEOUS TABLES

COMPARISON OF VARIOUS TYPES OF INSULIN

GENERIC NAME	TRADE NAME	SOURCE OF INSULIN (SPECIES)	ONSET OF ACTION (HOURS)	PEAK ACTIVITY (HOURS)	DURATION OF ACTION (HOURS)	HOW SUPPLIED
Insulin Injection (Regular)			0.5 - 1	2.5 - 4	6 - 8	
	REGULAR ILETIN II	Purified Pork				**Inj**: 100 units/mL
	REGULAR PURIFIED PORK INSULIN INJECTION	Purified Pork				**Inj**: 100 units/mL
	HUMULIN R	Human[a]				**Inj**: 100 units/mL
	NOVOLIN R	Human[b]				**Inj**: 100 units/mL
	VELOSULIN BR	Human[b]				**Inj**: 100 units/mL
	NOVOLIN R PENFILL	Human[b]				**Inj**: 100 units/mL
	NOVOLIN R PREFILLED	Human[b]				**Inj**: 100 units/mL
Insulin Lispro			0.25	1 - 1.5	3.5 - 4.5	
	HUMALOG	Human[a]				**Inj**: 100 units/mL **Cartridge**: 1.5 mL **Prefilled Pen**: 3 mL

Isophane Insulin Suspension (NPH)			1 - 2	6 - 12	18 - 26	
	NPH ILETIN II	Purified Pork				**Inj**: 100 units/mL
	HUMULIN N	Human[a]				**Inj**: 100 units/mL
	NOVOLIN N	Human[b]				**Inj**: 100 units/mL
	NOVOLIN N PENFILL	Human[b]				**Inj**: 100 units/mL
	NOVOLIN N PREFILLED	Human[b]				**Inj**: 100 units/mL
Insulin Zinc Suspension (Lente)			1 - 3	6 - 12	18 - 26	
	LENTE ILETIN II	Purified Pork				**Inj**: 100 units/mL
	HUMULIN L	Human[a]				**Inj**: 100 units/mL
	NOVOLIN L	Human[b]				**Inj**: 100 units/mL
Extended Insulin Zinc Suspension (Ultralente)			4 - 8	10 - 18	24 - 36	
	HUMULIN U	Human[a]				**Inj**: 100 units/mL

GENERIC NAME	TRADE NAME	SOURCE OF INSULIN (SPECIES)	ONSET OF ACTION (HOURS)	PEAK ACTIVITY (HOURS)	DURATION OF ACTION (HOURS)	HOW SUPPLIED
70% Isophane Insulin Suspension + 30% Regular Insulin Injection			0.5	2 - 12	up to 24	
	HUMULIN 70/30	Human[a]				**Inj**: 100 units/mL
	NOVOLIN 70/30	Human[b]				**Inj**: 100 units/mL
	NOVOLIN 70/30 PENFILL	Human[b]				**Inj**: 100 units/mL
	NOVOLIN 70/30 PREFILLED	Human[b]				**Inj**: 100 units/mL
50% Isophane Insulin Suspension + 50% Regular Insulin Injection			0.5	2 - 5	up to 24	
	HUMULIN 50/50	Human[a]				**Inj**: 100 units/mL

[a] Produced from proinsulin synthesized by bacteria using recombinant DNA technology.

[b] Produced from baker's yeast using recombinant DNA technology.

ANOREXIANT DRUGS FOR TREATING OBESITY

GENERIC NAME	COMMON TRADE NAMES	MECHANISM OF ACTION	COMMON ADULT DOSAGE	COMMENTS
Amphetamine Sulfate		Norepinephrine releaser	See page 36	High abuse potential
Benzphetamine HCl	DIDREX	Norepinephrine releaser	See page 45	Significant abuse potential
Diethylpropion HCl	TENUATE, TENUATE DOSPAN	Norepinephrine releaser	See page 81	Moderate abuse potential
Mazindol	SANOREX	Norepinephrine reuptake inhibitor	See page 131	Moderate abuse potential
Methamphetamine HCl	DESOXYN	Norepinephrine releaser	See page 135	High abuse potential
Phendimetrazine Tartrate	BONTRIL PDM, PLEGINE, BONTRIL SLOW RELEASE, PRELU-2	Norepinephrine releaser	See page 164	Significant abuse potential
Phentermine HCl	ADIPEX-P	Norepinephrine releaser	See page 164	Moderate abuse potential
Phentermine Resin	IONAMIN	Norepinephrine reuptake inhibitor	See page 165	Moderate abuse potential
Phenylpropanolamine HCl	DEXATRIM	α-Adrenergic receptor agonist & norepinephrine releaser	See page 165	Over-the-counter drug
Sibutramine	MERIDIA	Serotonin and norepinephrine reuptake inhibitor	See page 183	Low abuse potential

COMPARISON OF H_2-RECEPTOR ANTAGONISTS

	Cimetidine (TAGAMET)	Ranitidine HCl (ZANTAC)	Famotidine (PEPCID)	Nizatidine (AXID)
PHARMACOKINETICS				
Oral Bioavailability (%)	60 - 70	50 - 60	40 - 45	90 - 95
Time to Peak Blood Levels (hours)	0.75 - 1.5	1 - 3	1 - 3	0.5 - 3
Plasma Protein Binding (%)	15 - 25	15	15 - 20	35
Liver Biotransformation (%)	30 - 40	10	30 - 35	15 - 20
Major Route of Elimination	Kidney	Kidney	Kidney	Kidney
Elimination Half-life (hours)	2	2.5 - 3	2.5 - 3.5	1 - 2
PHARMACODYNAMICS				
Antisecretory Activity	800 mg hs po inhibited acid output by 85% for 8 hours	150 mg hs po inhibited acid output by 92% for 13 hours	20 mg hs po inhibited acid output by 86% for 10 hours	300 mg hs po inhibited acid output by 90% for 10 hours
Incidence of Adverse Reactions	Low	Low	Low	Low
Inhibition of Microsomal Enzyme Systems (i.e., P-450)	Can be significant	Minimal effect	Minimal effect	Minimal effect
Antiandrogenic Effects	Weak	No effect	No effect	No effect
Elevation of Prolactin Secretion	Transient (after IV use)	Less than with cimetidine	Minimal effect	No effect

PRESCRIPTION WRITING

INTRODUCTION

A **prescription** is an order for a specific medication for a specified patient at a particular time. It is the way in which a physician (or another health care professional) communicates a patient's selected drug therapy to the pharmacist and instructs the patient on how to use the prescribed medication. The prescription order may be given by a physician, dentist, veterinarian, physician assistant, nurse practitioner, or any other legally-recognized medical practitioner; the order may be written and signed or it may be oral, in which case the pharmacist is required to transcribe it into written form and obtain the prescriber's signature, if necessary, at a later time.

The transfer of the therapeutic information from prescriber to pharmacist to patient must be clear. With all of the many drug products available to the prescriber, it is easy to understand how drug strengths, dosage forms, and dosage regimens can be confused. Many drug names may also look alike (especially when written hastily) or may sound alike (when garbled over the telephone). Furthermore, numerous studies have indicated that 25% to 50% of patients do not use their prescription medication properly; the patient often fails to take the drug or uses the medication either in an incorrect dose, at an improper time, or for the wrong condition. Most errors can be traced to the prescription order or the failure of the prescriber to adequately communicate this information to the patient.

In order that these types of errors be avoided and the patient gain the maximum benefit from the prescribed drugs, it is important for the prescriber to understand the basic principles of prescription writing.

COMPOSITION OF THE PRESCRIPTION ORDER

A complete prescription order is composed of eight parts and follows a standardized format which facilitates its interpretation by the pharmacist. The eight major parts of a prescription order include:

1. The date prescribed
2. The name, address, and age of the patient
3. The superscription
4. The inscription
5. The subscription
6. The signa
7. The renewal information
8. The name of the prescriber

Figure 1 illustrates a sample precompounded prescription order with the eight major elements numbered for reference purposes.

1. **The Date Prescribed** - The date on which a prescription was issued is important since a patient may not always have a prescription filled on the day it was written; days, weeks, months, or on occasion, years may pass before a patient presents the prescription to the pharmacist. Medications are intended for a patient at a particular time; the date prescribed may reveal that the presented prescription was not filled when written and now, for example, months later, the patient has "symptoms which are exactly the same as the last time" and is attempting to self-diagnose and self-medicate. Furthermore, drugs controlled by special laws and regulations, e.g., the Controlled Substances Act of 1970, cannot be dispensed or renewed more than six months from the date prescribed. Therefore, the date prescribed provides an accurate record of when a prescription was originally issued to the patient.

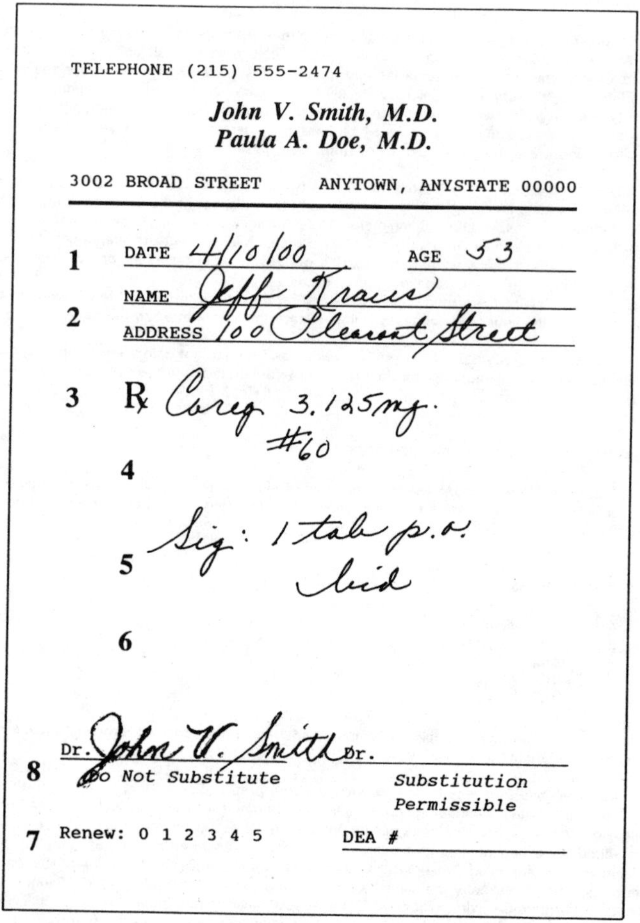

TELEPHONE (215) 555-2474

John V. Smith, M.D.
Paula A. Doe, M.D.

3002 BROAD STREET   ANYTOWN, ANYSTATE 00000

1 DATE 4/10/00   AGE 53

NAME Jeff Kraus
2
ADDRESS 100 Pleasant Street

3 ℞ Coreg 3.125mg.
#60

4

5 Sig: 1 tab p.o.
bid

6

Dr. John V. Smith   Dr.
8 Do Not Substitute   Substitution Permissible

7 Renew: 0 1 2 3 4 5   DEA #

FIGURE 1. A Sample Precompounded Prescription Order

2. **The Name, Address, and Age of the Patient** - This information serves to identify for whom the prescribed medication is intended. The full name of the patient may help to prevent a mixup of drugs within a household when, for example, a parent and child have the same name. If the patient's first name is not known or omitted, the use of the titles Mr., Mrs., Ms. or Miss is appropriate. Information regarding the patient's age should also be indicated, e.g., "adult," "child," or in the case of a young child, the exact age; this allows the pharmacist to monitor the prescribed dosage, especially since the pharmacokinetics of many drugs differ markedly in newborn, pediatric, adult, and geriatric patient populations.

3. **The Superscription** - This portion of the prescription refers to the symbol ℞, a contraction of the Latin verb *recipe*, meaning "take thou." It serves to introduce the drug(s) prescribed and the directions for use.

4. **The Inscription** - The name, strength and quantity of the desired drug is enclosed within this section of the prescription. Although drugs may be prescribed by any known name, i.e., chemical name, trivial name, nonproprietary name (more commonly referred to as the generic name) and manufacturer's proprietary (trade) name, most drugs are prescribed either by the trade name or by the generic name. Chemical and trivial names of drugs are generally not suitable for this purpose and are seldom used. When the trade name is written, the prescription must be filled with product of the specified manufacturer, unless the prescriber and patient approved substitution with another brand. If the generic name is employed, the pharmacist can select from any of the available drug preparations. When two or more drugs are written on the same prescription for compounding purposes, the name and quantity of each should be listed on a separate line directly below the preceding one. To avoid confusion, the salt of a particular medicament should be clearly indicated if more than one is available, e.g., codeine **sulfate** or codeine **phosphate**. The quantities of the ingredients may be written in either the apothecary or metric system. The latter is more popular; it is used exclusively by official pharmaceutical reference texts, and in most cases, in medical schools, hospitals, and other health agencies.

The apothecary system is an older and less popular method of measurement; however, prescriptions are still written in this system and texts may, on occasion, report drug doses in apothecary units. For example, 1 fluid-ounce (apothecary) equals approximately 30 mL (metric) and 1 pint equals 473 mL.

Regardless of which system is employed on the prescription, most patients are more comfortable with household measures, especially with liquid medications. Although the sizes of the household teaspoon and tablespoon vary considerably, the standard household teaspoon should be regarded as containing 5 mL and the tablespoon, 15 mL. Standard disposable plastic teaspoons, tablespoons and graduated two fluid-ounce cups are available in an attempt to reduce liquid dose variability, and the use of these should be encouraged.

5. **The Subscription** - Directions to the pharmacist from the prescriber comprise this section of the prescription; these state the specific dosage form to be dispensed or the desired method of preparation. The subscription is usually a short phrase or sentence such as "Dispense 30 capsules" or "Dispense 90 mL" for a precompounded prescription or "Mix and prepare 10 suppositories" for an extemporaneous preparation.

6. **The Signa** - The directions to the patient are given in this part of the prescription and are usually introduced by the latin *Signa* or *Sig.*, meaning "mark thou". These directions should be as clear and as complete as possible, so that the patient may easily follow the desired dosage schedule and receive the maximum benefit from the medication. Instructions should be provided as to the route of administration, the amount of drug to be taken, and the time and frequency of the dose. Phrases such as "take as directed" and "use as required" are not satisfactory instructions and should be avoided whenever possible.

Latin, often considered to be the language of the medical profession, was used extensively in writing prescription orders until the early part of the 20th century. Although prescription orders in the United States today are almost always written in English, many Latin words and phrases have been retained and are commonly used (as abbreviations) in the Signa. Some of the more commonly-employed Latin terms and abbreviations are given in Table 1. Thus the Signa: "Caps 1 q.i.d. p.c. + H.S. c milk" translates to: "One capsule 4 times daily after meals and at bedtime with milk".

7. **The Renewal Information** - The wishes of the prescriber with regard to refilling the medication should be indicated on every prescription, and if renewals are authorized, the number of times should be designated. Prescription orders for drugs that bear the legend: "Caution: Federal law prohibits dispensing without prescription" may not be renewed without the expressed consent of the prescriber. Prescriptions for drugs covered under Schedule III or IV of the Controlled Substances Act of 1970 may be renewed, if so authorized, not more than five times within six months of date of issue; drugs within Schedule II may not be renewed.

8. **The Name of the Prescriber** - Although in most cases the prescriber's name and address are printed on the prescription blank, the signature of the prescriber affixed to the bottom completes and validates the prescription order. For prescriptions written on hospital prescription blanks, the prescriber must print (or stamp) his/her name on the document, as well as sign it. This is a safe-guard in case a question arises concerning any aspect of the prescription order, the printed name will make it easier to identify and contact the prescriber. On oral prescriptions, the pharmacist adds the prescriber's name to the prescription; however, Federal law requires that prescriptions for Schedule II drugs be validated by the full signature of the prescriber and his/her registered Drug Enforcement Administration (DEA) number. The prescriber's registered DEA number must appear on all prescriptions for drug covered under the Controlled Substances Act (see below).

CLASSES OF PRESCRIPTION ORDERS

Prescription orders may be divided into two general classes based on the availability of the medication. A **precompounded** prescription order requests a drug or a drug mixture prepared and supplied by a pharmaceutical company; prescriptions of this class require no pharmaceutical alteration by the pharmacist. The prescription order shown in Figure 1 is a precompounded prescription. An **extemporaneous** or **compounded** prescription order is one in which the drugs, doses and dosage form, as selected by the prescriber, must be prepared by the pharmacist. Figure 2 shows an example of an extemporaneous prescription order. Most prescriptions written today are of the precompounded type; however extemporaneous prescription orders are not uncommon, especially with liquid, cream and ointment preparations.

CONTROLLED SUBSTANCES ACT

The legal aspects of prescription writing and dispensing are incorporated in various federal, state and local laws, which the medical practitioner must understand and observe; the strictest law regardless of governmental level, always takes precedence unless Federal Law is preemptive. In 1970, the Comprehensive Drug Abuse Prevention and Control Act, commonly called the Controlled Substances Act, was signed into law. This act imposes even more stringent controls on the distribution and use of all stimulant and depressant drugs and substances with the potential for abuse as designated by the Drug Enforcement Administration (DEA), U.S. Department of Justice. This act divides drugs with abuse potential into five categories or schedules as follows:

Schedule I (C-I) — Drugs in this schedule have a high potential for abuse and no currently accepted medical use in the United States. Examples of such drugs include cocaine base ("crack"), heroin, marijuana, peyote, mescaline, some tetrahydrocannabinols, LSD, and various opioid derivatives.

TABLE 1. COMMON LATIN ABBREVIATIONS

WORD OR PHRASE	ABBREVIATION	MEANING
Ad	Ad	Up to
Ana	aa	Of each
Ante cibos	a.c.	Before meals
Aqua	Aq.	Water
Aures utrae	a.u.	Each ear
Aurio dextra	a.d.	Right ear
Aurio laeva	a.l.	Left ear
Bis in die	b.i.d.	Twice a day
Capsula	Caps.	Capsule
Compositus	Comps.	Compounded
Cum	c	With
Et	Et	And
Gutta	Gtt.	A drop, drops
Hora somni	H.S.	At bedtime
Non repetatur	Non rep.	Do not repeat
Oculo utro	O.U.	Each eye
Oculus dexter	O.D.	Right eye
Oculus sinister	O.S.	Left eye
Per os	p.o.	By mouth
Post cibos	p.c.	After meals
Pro re nata	p.r.n.	When necessary
Quaque	q.	Each, every
Quantum satis	Q.S.	As much as is sufficient
Quarter in die	q.i.d.	Four times daily
Semis	ss	A half
Sine	s	Without
Statim	Stat.	Immediately
Tabella	tab	Tablet
Ter in die	t.i.d.	Three times daily
Ut dictum	Ut Dict.	As directed

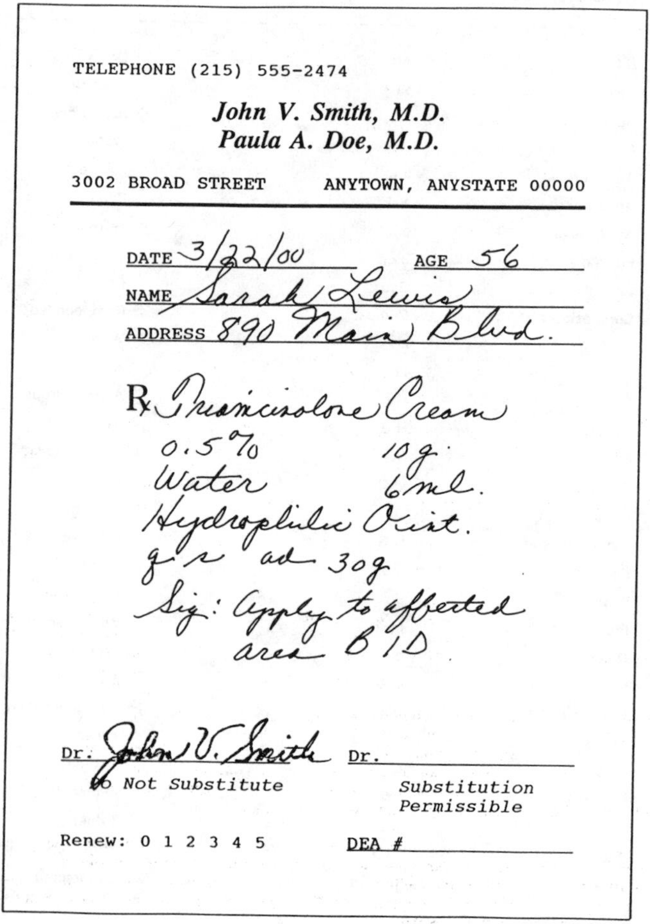

TELEPHONE (215) 555-2474

John V. Smith, M.D.
Paula A. Doe, M.D.

3002 BROAD STREET ANYTOWN, ANYSTATE 00000

DATE 3/22/00 AGE 56

NAME Sarah Lewis

ADDRESS 890 Main Blvd.

℞ Triamcinolone Cream
0.5% 10g.
Water 6ml.
Hydrophilic Oint.
q s ad 30g
Sig: Apply to affected
area BID

Dr. John V. Smith Dr.
Do Not Substitute Substitution Permissible

Renew: 0 1 2 3 4 5 DEA #

FIGURE 2. A Sample Extemporaneous Prescription Order

Substances listed in this schedule are not for prescription use; they may be obtained for chemical analysis, research, or instruction purposes by submitting an application and a protocol of the proposed use to the DEA.

Schedule II (C-II) — The drugs in this schedule have a high abuse potential with severe psychological or physical dependence liability. Schedule II controlled substances consist of certain opioid drugs, preparations containing amphetamines or methamphetamines as the single active ingredient or in combination with each other, and certain sedatives. Examples of opioids included in this schedule are opium, morphine sulfate, codeine sulfate, codeine phosphate, hydromorphone hydrochloride (DILAUDID, DILAUDID-HP), methadone hydrochloride (DOLOPHINE HYDROCHLORIDE), meperidine hydrochloride (DEMEROL), oxycodone hydrochloride (ROXICODONE; and in PERCODAN, PERCOCET, ROXICET, ROXILOX, ROXIPRIN, and TYLOX), oxycodone terephthalate (in PERCODAN, PERCODAN-DEMI), and oxymorphone hydrochloride (NUMORPHAN). Also included are stimulants, e.g., cocaine hydrochloride, dextroamphetamine sulfate (DEXEDRINE), methamphetamine hydrochloride (DESOXYN), methylphenidate hydrochloride (RITALIN, RITALIN SR), and depressants, e.g., pentobarbital sodium (NEMBUTAL SODIUM), and amobarbital sodium and secobarbital sodium (in TUINAL 100 and TUINAL 200).

Schedule III (C-III) — The drugs in this schedule have a potential for abuse that is less than for those drugs in Schedules I and II. The use or abuse of these drugs may lead to low or moderate physical dependence or high psychological dependence. Included in this schedule, for example, are mazindol (SANOREX), and paregoric. Analgesic mixtures containing limited amounts of codeine phosphate (e.g., EMPIRIN W/CODEINE, FIORICET W/CODEINE, FIORINAL W/CODEINE, SOMA COMPOUND W/CODEINE, and TYLENOL W/CODEINE), hydrocodone bitartrate (e.g., ANEXSIA 5/500, ANEXSIA 7.5/650, ANEXSIA 10/660, BANCAP HC, DURATUSS HD, HYDROCET, LORTAB, LORTAB ASA, VICODIN, VICODIN ES, and VICODIN HP), or dihydrocodeine bitartrate (SYNALGOS-DC); or cough mixtures containing hydrocodone bitartrate (e.g., HYCODAN, HYCOMINE, HYCOMINE COMPOUND, HYCOTUSS EXPECTORANT, TRIAMINIC EXPECTORANT DH, TUSSEND, and TUSSEND EXPECTORANT), or hydrocodone polistirex (e.g., TUSSIONEX) are contained within this schedule. Also included in this schedule are certain anabolic steroids (e.g., decanoate and phenpropionate salts of nandrolone (DURABOLIN and DECA-DURABOLIN) and oxandrolone (OXANDRIN)).

Schedule IV (C-IV) — The drugs in this category have the potential for limited physical or psychological dependence and include phenobarbital, phenobarbital sodium, paraldehyde, chloral hydrate, ethchlorvynol (PLACIDYL), meprobamate (EQUANIL, MILTOWN), chlordiazepoxide (LIBRIUM), diazepam (VALIUM), clorazepate dipotassium (TRANXENE-T TAB, TRANXENE-SD), flurazepam hydrochloride (DALMANE), oxazepam (SERAX), clonazepam (KLONOPIN), lorazepam (ATIVAN), quazepam (DORAL), and the salts of propoxyphene (DARVON and DARVON-N). Certain other mixtures are included; for example, the antidiarrheal MOTOFEN and the analgesics DARVON COMPOUND-65, DARVOCET-N 50, DARVOCET-N 100, EQUAGESIC, TALACEN, TALWIN COMPOUND, and WYGESIC.

Schedule V (C-V) — Schedule V drugs have a potential for abuse that is less than those listed in Schedule IV. These consist of preparations containing moderate quantities of certain opioids for use in pain (i.e., buprenorphine hydrochloride (BUPRENEX)) or as antidiarrheals (e.g., diphenoxylate hydrochloride (in LOMOTIL)), or as antitussives (such as codeine-containing cough mixtures, e.g., ROBITUSSIN A-C). Some of the latter may be dispensed without a prescription order, in certain States, provided that specified dispensing criteria are met by the pharmacist.

Every person involved in the manufacture, importing, exporting, distribution or dispensing of any Controlled Drug must obtain an annual registration from the DEA; therefore, a health care practitioner must be registered before he/she can administer or dispense any of the drugs listed in the abuse schedules. Furthermore, the physician's DEA registration number must be indicated on every prescription order for Controlled Substances.

Notes

A

B

C

E

F

G

H

L

M

Q

R

S

U

V

W

X

Y

Z

Notes

ORDERING INFORMATION

If you are paying by credit card, Call Toll Free, Fax, E-Mail or order via the Internet

PHONE	FAX	VIA WEB SITE
1-800-417-3189	1-215-657-1475	MEDICALSURVEILLANCE.COM

E-MAIL	CHECKS OR MONEY ORDERS	MAIL
MEDSURVEILLANCE@AOL.COM	Make check payable to MSI and mail order form	P.O. Box 480 Willow Grove, Pa. 19090

Books	Price	Qty	Sub-Total
Handbook of Commonly Prescribed Drugs, 15th Edition (2000) ISBN # 0-942447-35-2	$ 18.95		
Handbook of Common Orthopaedic Fractures, 4th Edition (2000) ISBN # 0-942447-36-0	$ 18.95		
Travelers Guide to International Drugs, **Western Hemisphere** (2000) ISBN # 942447-30-1	$ 8.95		
Travelers Guide to International Drugs, **European Volume I ** (2000) ISBN # 942447-33-6	$ 8.95		
Travelers Guide to International Drugs, **European Volume II ** (2000) ISBN # 942447-34-4	$ 8.95		
Travelers Guide to International Drugs, **European Volume I & II (2000) **Package** A *savings of $2.00*	$ 15.90		
Travelers Guide to International Drugs, **Middle & Far East** (2000) ISBN # 0-942447-32-8	$ 8.95		
Handbook of Commonly Prescribed Pediatric Drugs, 6th Edition (1999) ISBN # 0-942447-27-1	$ 18.50		
Antimicrobial Therapy in Primary Care Medicine, 1st Edition (1997) ISBN # 0-942447-22-0	$ 17.00		
Drug Charts in Basic Pharmacology, 2nd Edition (1998) ISBN # 0-942447-26-3	$ 18.00		
Warning: Drugs in Sports, 1st Edition (1995) ISBN #0-942447-16-6	$ 14.50		
Textbook			
Basic Pharmacology in Medicine, 4th Edition (1994) ISBN# 0-942447-04-2	$ 49.95		

Shipping and Handling Charges:				
Add $ 6.00 for orders between $10.00 - $49.99	SUB-TOTAL			
Add $ 8.50 for orders between $50.00 - $ 99.99	(*) Shipping & Handling			
Add $ 10.50 for orders between $100.00 - $149.99	PA Residents, Add 6% Sales Tax			
Add $ 12.50 for orders Greater then $ 150.00	TOTAL			

Bookstores subject to standard shipping and handling charges

Name: ____________________

Address: ____________________

City: ____________ **STATE:** ________ **ZIP:** ______

AMT. ENCLOSED ________ **VISA M/C DISCOVER AMERICAN EXPRESS CHECK**

CARD NUMBER: ____________________ **EXP. DATE:** ________

AUTHORIZED SIGNATURE ____________________ **PHONE:** ________

REQUEST FOR INFORMATION

If you wish to be placed on a mailing list for information concerning new publications and updates, please fill out the form below and mail to:

MEDICAL SURVEILLANCE INC.
P.O. Box 480 Willow Grove, PA 19090

(PLEASE PRINT)

Name____

Organization_______________________________________

Street Address______________________________________

City_________________________________State__________

Zip Code_______________

Telephone Number (Optional)___________________________

FOR FURTHER INFORMATION CALL:
800 - 417-3189 or 215 - 784-0976

E-Mail us at **medsurveillance@aol.com**

Visit Us on the **World Wide Web** at
hhtp://www.medicalsurveillance.com